SANFORD GUIDES

熱 病

Thirty – fourth Edi

KU-365-630

THE SANFORD
GUIDE TO
ANTIMICROBI
THERAPY
2004

David N. Gilbert, M.D.
Director of Medical Education & Earl A. Chiles Research Institute
Providence Portland Medical Center
Professor of Medicine
Oregon Health Sciences University
Portland, Oregon

Robert C. Moellering, Jr., M.D.
Physician-in-Chief, Beth Israel Deaconess Medical Center
Herman L. Blumgart Professor of Medicine
Harvard Medical School
Boston, Massachusetts

George M. Eliopoulos, M.D.
Chief, James L. Tullis Firm, Beth Israel Deaconess Hospital
Professor of Medicine
Harvard Medical School
Boston, Massachusetts

Merle A. Sande, M.D.
Clarence M. & Ruth N. Birrer Professor of Medicine
University of Utah School of Medicine
Salt Lake City, Utah

THE SANFORD GUIDE TO ANTIMICROBIAL THERAPY 2004
(34TH EDITION)

Jay P. Sanford, M.D.
1928-1996

EDITORS

David N. Gilbert, M.D.
Robert C. Moellering, Jr., M.D.
George M. Eliopoulos, M.D.
Merle A. Sande, M.D.

The Sanford Guide to Antimicrobial Therapy is published annually by:

ANTIMICROBIAL THERAPY, INC.
P.O. Box 70, 229 Main Street
Hyde Park, VT 05655 USA
Tel 802-888-2855   Fax 802-888-2874
Email: info@sanfordguide.com

www.sanfordguide.com

ISBN 1-930808-14-3
Pocket Edition

PUBLISHER'S PREFACE

To our many readers around the world, we thank you for your continued confidence in the SANFORD GUIDE. For 2004, we are pleased to announce the addition of George M. Eliopoulos, M.D. as our newest editor. Dr. Eliopoulos is Professor of Medicine at Harvard Medical School and Chief of the James L. Tullis Firm at the Beth Israel Deaconess Hospital in Boston. He is also Editor-in-Chief of ANTIMICROBIAL AGENTS AND CHEMOTHERAPY. We welcome him warmly.

Complementing the pocket-sized and larger spiral editions of the SANFORD GUIDE, the electronic edition of the SANFORD GUIDE for Palm ® and Pocket PC ® handheld devices continues to develop a loyal following among a new generation of SANFORD GUIDE users.

Though many readers of the SANFORD GUIDE receive their copy from a pharmaceutical company representative, please be assured that the SANFORD GUIDE has been, and continues to be, independently prepared and published since its inception in 1969. Decisions regarding the content of the SANFORD GUIDE are solely those of the editors and the publisher. We welcome your questions, comments and feedback concerning the Sanford Guide. All of your feedback is reviewed and taken into account in preparing the next edition.

Thanks to the editors for their rigorous review of the relevant literature; to Carolyn Wickwire for preparing the manuscript, and to Gateway Graphics for printing this 34th edition of the SANFORD GUIDE.

Jeb C. Sanford
Publisher

NOTE TO READER

Every effort is made to ensure the accuracy of the content of this guide. However, current full prescribing information available in the package insert of each drug should be consulted before prescribing any product. The editors and publisher are not responsible for errors or omissions or for any consequences from application of the information in this book and make no warranty, express or implied, with respect to the currency, accuracy, or completeness of the contents of the publication. Application of this information in a particular situation remains the professional responsibility of the practitioner.

—TABLE OF CONTENTS —

TABLE 1   Clinical Approach to **Initial Choice** of Antimicrobial Therapy. *Pages 2–45*

TABLE 1B   Prophylaxis and Treatment of Organisms of Potential Use as **Biological Weapons**. *Page 46*

TABLE 1C   Temporal Approach to Differential Diagnosis of Infection After **Organ Transplantation**. *Page 47*

TABLE 2   Recommended Antimicrobial Agents Against **Selected Bacteria**. *Pages 48–50*

TABLE 3   Suggested **Duration** of Antimicrobial Therapy in Immunocompetent Patients. *Page 51*

TABLE 4   Comparison of **Antimicrobial Spectra**. *Pages 52–54*

TABLE 5   Treatment Options for **Highly Resistant Bacteria**. *Pages 55–56*

TABLE 6   Methods for **Penicillin Desensitization** and Sulfonamide Desensitization. *Page 56*

TABLE 7   **Pregnancy Risk Category** of Selected Antimicrobial Agents. *Page 57*

TABLE 8   Antimicrobial Agents Associated With **Photosensitivity**. *Page 57*

TABLE 9   Clinically Useful Selected **Pharmacologic Features** of Antimicrobial Agents. *Pages 58–62*

TABLE 10A   Overview of **Adverse Reactions** of Antibacterial Agents. *Pages 63–65*
10B   **Dosages**, Price, and Selected **Adverse Effects** of Antibacterial Agents. *Pages 66–72*
10C   **Once-Daily Aminoglycoside Therapy**. *Page 73*

TABLE 11A   Recommended **Antifungal, Actinomycotic and Nocardial** Therapy. *Pages 74–82*
11B   **Dosages**, Price, and Selected Adverse Effects of Antifungal Agents. *Pages 82–84*

TABLE 12A   Treatment of Mycobacterial Infections. *Pages 85–90*
12B   **Dosages**, Price, and Selected Adverse Effects of Antimycobacterial Agents. *Pages 91–92*

TABLE 13A   Treatment of **Parasitic Infections**. *Pages 93–100*
13B   **Dosages**, Price, and Selected Adverse Effects of Antiparasitic Agents. *Pages 101–103*

TABLE 14A   Treatment of **Viral Infections**. *Pages 104–112*
14B   **Antiviral Drugs Other Than Retroviral: Dosages**, Price, and Selected Adverse Effects. *Pages 113–115*
14C   **Antiretroviral Therapy in Adults**. *Pages 116–120*
14D   **Antiretroviral Drugs** and Side-Effects. *Pages 120–121*

TABLE 15A   **Antimicrobial Prophylaxis** for Selected Bacterial and Viral Infections. *Pages 122–125*
15B   **Surgical Prophylaxis**. *Pages 125–126*
15C   Prophylaxis for Prevention of **Bacterial Endocarditis**. *Pages 127–128*
15D   Prevention of Opportunistic Infection in **Transplantation**. *Page 128*

TABLE 16   **Pediatric Dosages** of Antimicrobial Agents. *Page 129*

TABLE 17A   Dosages of Antimicrobial Drugs in Adult Patients With **Renal Impairment**. *Pages 130–134*
17B   **No Dosage Adjustment** With Renal Insufficiency. *Page 135*

TABLE 18   Antimicrobials and **Hepatic Disease**. *Page 135*

TABLE 19   Treatment of **CAPD Peritonitis**. *Page 135*

TABLE 20   **Immunizations:**
A. Infants/Children. *Page 136–137*
B. Adults. *Pages 137–139*
C. Urgent Care:
1. **Tetanus**. *Page 139*
2. **Rabies**. *Page 139–140*

TABLE 21   **Directory of Resources**. *Page 140*

TABLE 22A   **Drug/Drug Interactions** of Anti-Infectives. *Pages 141–145*
22B   Drug/Drug Interactions Between **Antiretrovirals**. *Page 146*

TABLE 23   **Generic** and Trade Names. *Pages 147–148*

INDEX   *Page 149*

TABLE 1
CLINICAL APPROACH TO INITIAL CHOICE OF ANTIMICROBIAL THERAPY
Treatment based on presumed site or type of infection. In selected instances, treatment and prophylaxis based on identification of pathogens

ANATOMIC SITE/DIAGNOSIS/ MODIFYING CIRCUMSTANCES	ETIOLOGIES (usual)	SUGGESTED REGIMENS*		ADJUNCT DIAGNOSTIC OR THERAPEUTIC MEASURES AND COMMENTS
		PRIMARY	ALTERNATIVE†	
ABDOMEN: See Peritoneum, page 31; Gallbladder, page 10; and Pelvic Inflammatory Disease, page 16				
BONE: Osteomyelitis General Comment: Regardless of the type of infection, a specific microbiologic diagnosis is essential. It is not possible to predict the microbial etiology based on epidemiology. In chronic osteomyelitis, organism(s) isolated from sinus tract drainage may not accurately reflect organisms present in bone. Ideally, empiric therapy is initiated after collection of blood and infected bone for culture. For review: NEJM 336:999, 1997.				
Hematogenous—Regimens refer to **EMPIRIC THERAPY** in absence of positive culture				
Newborn (<4 mos.)	S. aureus, Gm-neg. bacilli, Group B strep	(**Nafcillin or oxacillin**) + **P Ceph 3** (Dosage in Table 16)	**Vanco + P Ceph 3** (Dosage in Table 16)	Often afebrile. Localizing signs best predictor of osteo. Over 2/3 have positive blood cultures. Risk factors: Preterm and mechanical vent. PIDJ 14:1047, 1995. Treat for minimum of 21 days.
Children (>4 mos.) Often at or adjacent to epiphysis of long bones	S. aureus, Group A strep, coliforms rare	**Nafcillin or oxacillin** Add **P Ceph 3** if Gm-neg. bacteria on Gram stain. Pediatric doses Table 16, adult below	**Vanco or clinda** **Vanco or clinda** on Gram stain. See below	With immunization, H. influenzae almost disappeared. Vanco for nafcillin/oxacillin if pen-allergic or high prevalence of MRSA. IV q8h. If bacterial etiology known, then po or IV rx at home for total of 2-3 wks.
Adult (>21 yrs) More often vertebral than long bones (Review: AJM 101:550, 1996) Vertebral osteo: CID 30:320, 2000; AJM 100:85, 1996	S. aureus most common + variety other aerobic & anaerobic cocci & bacilli; culture before empiric rx unless blood cultures pos.	**Nafcillin or oxacillin** 2.0 gm q4h IV **or cefazolin** 2.0 gm q8h	**Vanco** 1.0 gm q12h IV See Comments	Rx regimens assume empiric rx and either no organism or Gm+ cocci on Gram stain. If high prevalence of MRSA, use vanco. Dx: MRI of spine. **Consider epidural abscess!** If proven MSSA, ceftriaxone another option (CID 30:205, 2000). Linezolid reported effective vs S. aureus osteo (AIM 136:135, 2003).
Adult or child (special circumstances)				
Sickle cell anemia	Salmonella sp.	**FQ** (not in children)	**P Ceph 3**	Sternoclavicular joint and ribs in addition to vertebral and long bones
IV drug abuse, hemodialysis pts	S. aureus, P. aeruginosa	(**Nafcillin or oxacillin**) **+ CIP**	**Vanco + CIP**	
Contiguous Osteomyelitis Without Vascular Insufficiency				
Post-reduction & internal fixation of fracture	Coliforms, S. aureus, P. aeruginosa	**Nafcillin** 2.0 gm q4h IV **+ CIP** 750 mg bid po	**Vanco** 1.0 gm q12h IV **+ P CIP** 750 mg bid po	Usually necessary to remove "hardware" to obtain bone union. Revascularization if needed, e.g., pedicle muscle flaps, myocutaneous flaps.
Post-op sternotomy	S. aureus, S. epidermidis	**Vanco** 1.0 gm q12h IV + **RIF** 600-900 mg qd po	**CIP 3 AP**	Sternal debridement establishes microbial etiology & removes necrotic bone. Use of internal mammary artery (esp. in diabetics) for CABG increases risk of sternal osteo.
Post-prosthetic joint osteo	See Prosthetic Joint, page 21–22			
Post-nail puncture of foot through tennis shoe	P. aeruginosa	**Ceftazidime** 2.0 gm q8h IV or **CFP** 2.0 gm q12h IV	**CIP** 750 mg bid po (not in children)	Osteo evident in only 1–2% plantar puncture wounds; thus, only close observation. No antibiotic unless evidence of infection. P. aeruginosa causes 93%. Debridement necessary to remove foreign body (pieces of sock &/or tennis shoe). See Lung, cystic fibrosis, page 28, for CIP use in children.
Contiguous Osteomyelitis With Vascular Insufficiency				
Pts with neurologic deficit & decubiti; atherosclerotic peripheral vascular disease; diabetic with neuropathy (see Diabetic foot, page 10)	Polymicrobic (Gm+ cocci incl. MRSA & enterococci, Gm-neg. bacilli (aerobic & anaerobic))	**Mild disease—outpatient therapy: AM/CL** 500 mg po tid or **OFX** 400 mg q12h po or (**TC/CL** or **PIP/TZ** or **AM/SB** (**CFP + metro**) or (**aztreonam** + **vanco** + **metro**). (Dosage in footnote*)	**Severe—hospitalized: IMP** or **MER** or **TC/CL** or **PIP/TZ** or **AM/SB** (**CFP + metro**) or (**aztreonam + vanco + metro**). (Dosage in footnote*)	Metal probe to bone correlates with presence of osteomyelitis (JAMA 273:721, 1995). **In extremity, determine extent of atherosclerotic vascular disease and revascularize** if possible. MRI helpful to determine extent of infection. Surgical debridement for culture and removal of necrotic bone. Avoid weight bearing. **Aggressive treatment** (debridement + antibiotics + revascularization) in diabetic decreases need for amputation (CID 23:286, 1995).

---

* Drug dosage: **IMP** 0.5 gm q8h IV, **MER** 1.0 gm q8h IV (not licensed indication but should be effective), **TC/CL** 3.1 gm q6h IV, **PIP/TZ** 3.375 gm q6h or 4.5 gm q8h IV, **CFP** 2.0 gm q12h IV, **metro** 1.0 gm loading dose and then 0.5 gm q6h IV or po or 1.0 gm q12h IV, **aztreonam** 2.0 gm q8h IV, **vanco** 1.0 gm q12h IV. **AM/SB** 3.0 gm IV q6h. (Footnotes and abbreviations on page 45)

† NOTE: All dosage recommendations are for adults (unless otherwise indicated) and assume normal renal function

TABLE 1 (2)

ANATOMIC SITE/DIAGNOSIS/ MODIFYING CIRCUMSTANCES	ETIOLOGIES (usual)	SUGGESTED REGIMENS*		ADJUNCT DIAGNOSTIC OR THERAPEUTIC MEASURES AND COMMENTS
		PRIMARY	ALTERNATIVE†	
BONE (continued)				
Chronic Osteomyelitis (AJM 101:550, 1996) By definition, implies presence of dead bone	S. aureus, Enterobacteriaceae, P. aeruginosa	Empiric rx not indicated. Base systemic rx on results of culture, sensitivity. rx: exacerbation of chronic osteo, rx as acute hematogenous osteo.		Important adjuncts to rx: removal of orthopaedic hardware, surgical debridement, vascularized muscle flaps, distraction osteogenesis (Ilizarov) techniques. Antibiotic-impregnated cement & hyperbaric oxygen adjunctive. NOTE: RIF + (vanco or β-lactam) very effective in animal models + one clinical trial of S. aureus chronic osteo (SMJ 79:947, 1986). Quinolone rx (CID 25:1327, 1997.
BREAST				
Postpartum Mastitis Ref: JAMA 289:1609, 2003	S. aureus, less often S. pyogenes (Gp A or B), E. coli, bacteroides species, & maybe Corynebacterium sp.	**Dicloxacillin** 500 mg q6h po or **cefazolin** 1.0 gm q8h IV. **Nafcillin or oxacillin** 2.0 gm q4h IV or **cefazolin** 1.0 gm q8h IV	**Clinda** 300 mg q6h po	If no abscess, increased frequency of nursing may hasten response: no risk to infant. Corynebacterium sp. assoc. with chronic granulomatous mastitis (CID 35:1434, 2002).
Abscess		**Nafcillin or oxacillin** 2.0 or **cefazolin** 1.0 gm q8h IV (IV as above)	**Vanco** 1.0 gm q12h IV	With abscess, d/c nursing. I&D standard: needle aspiration reported successful (Am J Surg 182:117, 2001). Resume breast feeding from affected breast as soon as pain allows.
Non-puerperal abscess	S. aureus, Bacteroides sp., peptostreptococcus	**Clinda** 300 mg q8h po or IV or (**nafcillin/oxacillin** IV as above) + **metro** 7.5 mg/kg q6h IV	**AM/CL** 875/125 mg q12h po or **AM/SB** 1.5 gm q6h IV or (**vanco** + **metro**)	If subareolar, most likely anaerobes. If not subareolar, staph. Need pretreatment aerobic/anaerobic cultures. Surgical drainage for abscess.
CENTRAL NERVOUS SYSTEM				
Brain abscess Primary rx or contiguous source Ref: CID 25:763, 1997	Streptococci (60–70%), bacteroides (20–40%), Enterobacteriaceae (23–33%), S. aureus (10–15%). Rare: Nocardia (Table 11A, page 81)	**P Ceph 3** (cefotaxime 2.0 gm q4h IV or ceftriaxone 2.0 gm q12h IV) + **metro** 7.5 mg/kg q6h IV (15.0 mg/kg q12h IV). Duration rx or unclear: rx until response by neuroimaging (CT/MRI)	**Pen G** 20–24 MU IV qd + **metro** 7.5 mg/kg q6h or 15 mg/kg q12h IV **P Ceph 3**	If CT scan suggests cerebritis (JNS 59:972, 1983), abscesses <2.5 cm and pt neurologically stable and conscious, start antibiotics and observe. Otherwise, surgical drainage necessary. Neurological deterioration usually mandates surgery. Need culture with Pen G (H-D) + metro without P Ceph 3 or nafcillin/oxacillin has been good. We use P Ceph 3 because of frequency of isolation of Enterobacteriaceae. S. aureus rare without positive blood culture and/or signs of endocarditis. Strep. milleri group esp. prone to produce abscess.
Post-surgical, post-traumatic	S. aureus, Enterobacteriaceae	(**Nafcillin** or **oxacillin**) 2.0 gm q4h IV + **P Ceph 3**	**Vanco** 1.0 gm q12h IV + **P Ceph 3**	If hospital-acquired and MRSA a consideration, substitute vanco for nafcillin or oxacillin. P Ceph 3 dose as for brain abscess, primary.
HIV-1 infected (AIDS)	Toxoplasma gondii	See Table 13, page 97		
Subdural empyema: In adult 60–90% are extension of sinusitis				Rx same as primary brain abscess. Surgical emergency: must drain (CID 20:372, 1995).
Encephalitis/encephalopathy Ref: Ln 359:507, 2002 (See Table 14, page 108, and for rabies, Table 20C, page 139)	Herpes simplex, arboviruses, rabies, West Nile virus. Rarely: Listeria, cat-scratch disease	Start IV **acyclovir** while awaiting results of CSF PCR for H. simplex.		Newly recognized strain of bat rabies. May not require a break in the skin. Eastern equine encephalitis virus focal involvement of basal ganglia and thalamus (NEJM 336:1867, 1997). Cat-scratch ref.: PIDJ 14:866, 1995)
Meningitis, "Aseptic": Pleocytosis of CSF, cells, CSF glucose normal, neg. culture for bacteria (see Table 14, page 104)	Enteroviruses, HSV-2, LCM, HIV, other viruses, drugs (NSAIDs, metronidazole, carbamazepine, TMP/SMX, IVIG), rarely leptospirosis	For all but leptospirosis, IV fluids and analgesics. D/C drugs that may be etiologic. For lepto (**Pen G** 5 mU q6h IV) or (**AMP** 0.5–1.0 gm q6h IV). Repeat LP if suspect partially-treated bacterial meningitis.		If readily available, culture or PCR of CSF for enterovirus. HSV-2 unusual without concomitant genital herpes. Drug-induced aseptic meningitis: AIM 159:1185, 1999. For lepto: positive epidemiologic history and concomitant hepatitis, conjunctivitis, dermatitis, nephritis.

NOTE: All dosage recommendations are for adults (unless otherwise indicated) and assume normal renal function

(Footnotes and abbreviations on page 45)

TABLE 1 (3)

ANATOMIC SITE/DIAGNOSIS/ MODIFYING CIRCUMSTANCES	ETIOLOGIES (usual)	SUGGESTED REGIMENS*		ADJUNCT DIAGNOSTIC OR THERAPEUTIC MEASURES AND COMMENTS
		PRIMARY	ALTERNATIVE[1]	
CENTRAL NERVOUS SYSTEM (continued)				
Meningitis, Bacterial, Acute: Goal is empiric therapy, then CSF cultures to turn neg. in 2 hrs with meningococci & partial response in 4 hrs (Peds 108:1169, 2001)				
Empiric Therapy—CSF Gram stain is negative—immunocompetent				If focal neurologic deficit, give empiric rx, then do CT, then do LP. (NEJM 345:1727, 2001 & 346:1248, 2002). NOTE: In children, treatment caused Gm-neg. bacilli.
Age: Preterm to <1 month	Group B strep 49%, E. coli 18%, listeria 7%, misc. Gm-neg. 10%, misc. 10%.	**AMP + cefotaxime** **AMP + gentamicin**		Primary & alternative regimens active vs Group B strep, most coliforms, & listeria. If premature infant with long maternal stay, i.e., exposure, enterococci, and resistant coliforms potential pathogens. Optional empiric regimens: [nafcillin (cefotaxime or ceftazidime)]. If high risk of MRSA, use vanco + cefotaxime.
		AMP + cefotaxime not recommended. Repeat CSF exam/culture 24–36 hrs after start of rx		Alter regimen after culture/sensitivity data available
		For dosage, see Table 16		
Age: 1 mon.–50 yrs 1999–2000 respiratory disease season, 34.1% of S. pneumo in U.S. were either intermediate in susceptibility to or resistant to concentrations of Pen G (JAMA 286:1857, 2001) (CDC 34 (Suppl.), S4, 2002). See footnote[3] for empiric treatment rationale.	S. pneumo, meningococci, H. influenzae now very rare, listeria unlikely if young & immunocompetent	Adult dose: ((Cefotaxime 2 gm IV q4–6h OR ceftriaxone 2 gm IV q12h) + (**dexamethasone**) + **vanco** (see footnote[3]) Peds: see footnote[3] **Dexamethasone** 0.4 mg/kg q12h IV x2 d. or 0.15 mg/kg IV q6h x4 d. Give with or just before 1st dose of antibiotic to block TNF production (see Comment). See footnote regarding drug-resistant S. pneumo[3] See footnote[3] for rest of ped. dosage	**[(MER** 2.0 gm q8h IV)** (Peds: 40 mg/kg IV q8h)] + **vanco** (see footnote[3] Peds: see footnote[3] **MER** 2.0 gm q8h IV + **vanco** + **dexamethasone** For severe pen. Allergy, see Comment	**Pts with severe pen. allergy:** Chloro 50 mg/kg/d IV div q6h (max. 4 gm/d.) (if for meningococci). OR q8-8h (for listeria if immunocompromised) + vanco. Rare. More frequent in immunocompetent.) + vanco. Rare. More frequent if was chloro. However, high failure rate in pts with DRSP (Ln 339: 405, 1992; Ln 342:240, 1993). The standard alternative for pts with severe pen. allergy was chloro. However, high failure rate in pts with DRSP (Ln 339: 405, 1992; Ln 342:240, 1993). **Value of dexamethasone** documented in children with H. influenzae & now confirmed in adults with S. pneumo & N. meningitidis (NEJM 347:1549 & 1613, 2002). Give 1st dose 15–20 min. Prior to or concomitant with 1st dose of antibiotic. Dose: Either (0.4 mg/kg q12h IV x2 d.) OR (0.15 mg/kg IV q6h x4 **For meningococcal immunization, see Table 20, pages 137–138.**
Age: >50 yrs or alcoholism & other debilitating associated diseases or impaired cellular immunity	S. pneumo, listeria, Gm-neg. bacilli. Note absence of meningococcus	(AMP 2.0 gm IV q4h) + cefotaxime 2.0 gm q12h OR ceftriaxone 2.0 gm q12h IV + **vanco** + **dexamethasone** For vanco dose, see footnote[3] Dosage begin with 1st dose of antibiotic.	MER 2.0 gm IV q8h + **vanco** + **dexamethasone** For severe pen. Allergy, see Comment **MER should work.** 1.0 gm q8h IV, but not an FDA-approved indication	**Severe penicillin allergy:** Vanco 500–750 mg IV + TMP/SMX [≈ TMP/SMX 20 mg/kg/d div q6-8h pending culture results. Chloro has failed vs DRSP (JAC 36(Suppl. A):1, 1995). CSF levels appear adequate (JAC 34:175, 1994) but no clinical data (PIDJ 18:581, 1999). MER active vs listeria in vitro (JAC 26(Suppl. A):1, 1995) **Dexamethasone**: 0.4 mg/kg q12h IV x2 d. 1st dose before or concomitant with 1st dose of antibiotic.
Post-neurosurgery, post-head trauma, or post-cochlear implant (NEJM 349:435, 2003)	S. pneumoniae most common, esp. CSF leak. Other: S. aureus, coliforms, P. aeruginosa	**Vanco** (until known not MRSA) 1.0 gm q8-12h IV + **ceftazidime** 2.0 gm q8h IV (see Comment)	**Vanco** (until known not MRSA) 1.0 gm q8-12h IV + (either cefotaxime 2.0 gm q6h IV) + (either ceftriaxone 2.0 gm q12h IV)	**Vanco** alone to cover suscept. S. pneumo. If/when suscept. S. pneumo. Identified, quickly switch to ceftriaxone or cefotaxime. If culture-proven coliform or pseudomonas meningitis, some add intrathecal gentamicin (4 mg/d) (0.125 mg/kg into lateral ventricles). MER does not have adequate potential of IMP.
Ventriculitis/meningitis due to infected (atrial) shunt	S. epidermidis, S. aureus, coliforms, diphtheroids (rare), P. acnes	**Child** (Vanco 15 mg/kg q6h IV) + (either cefotaxime 50 mg/kg q6h IV) + (either ceftriaxone 50 mg/kg q12h IV)	**Adult** Vanco 1.0 gm q8-12h IV + RIF 600 mg po	Early shunt removal usually necessary for cure. Refs: Adv PID 11:29, 1996; IDCP 4:277, 1995. For adults, can use P Ceph 3 alone if positive Gram stain for Gm-neg. bacilli.

Footnotes:

[1] **Rationale:** Hard to get adequate CSF concentrations of anti-infectives, hence MIC criteria for in vitro susceptibility are lower for CSF isolates (AIM 161:2538, 2001). Cefotaxime/ceftriaxone selected for activity vs meningococci, Hemophilus sp., & pen-sens S. pneumo. For pen-resistant S. pneumo, total of intermediate susceptibility + resistance to cefotaxime/ceftriaxone 88.1% (CID 34(Suppl):S4, 2002). Hence, add vanco until in vitro susceptibility of etiologic organism known.

[2] Low and erratic penetration of **vanco** into the CSF (PIDJ 16:895, 1997). Recommended **dosage in children** is 15 mg/kg q6h IV. **In adults**, a maximum dose of 2–3 gm/day is suggested. 500–750 mg IV (double the standard adult dose).

[3] **Dosages of drugs used to rx children ≥1 mo. of age:** Cefotaxime 200 mg/kg IV div q6h; ceftriaxone 100 mg/kg IV div q12h; vanco 15 mg/kg IV q6h. NOTE: All dosage recommendations are for adults (unless otherwise indicated) and assume normal renal function (Footnotes and abbreviations on page 45)

TABLE 1 (4)

ANATOMIC SITE/DIAGNOSIS/ MODIFYING CIRCUMSTANCES	ETIOLOGIES (usual)	SUGGESTED REGIMENS* PRIMARY	ALTERNATIVE†	ADJUNCT DIAGNOSTIC OR THERAPEUTIC MEASURES AND COMMENTS
CENTRAL NERVOUS SYSTEM *(continued)* **Meningitis, Bacterial, Acute** *(continued)* **Empiric Therapy—Positive CSF Gram stain** Gram-positive diplococci	S. pneumoniae	Either **(ceftriaxone** 2.0 gm IV q12h or **cefotaxime** 2.0 gm IV q4-6h) + **vanco** 15 mg/kg IV q6-12h + **dexamethasone** 0.4 mg/kg q12h IV x2 d.		**For severe penicillin allergy: vanco + RIF 600 mg qd (po or IV).** **Dexamethasone** (1 dose) not reduce penetration of vanco into CSF of **children**, so ceftriaxone + vanco OK; (2) in **adults**, efficacy shown: *NEJM* 347:1549 & 1613, 2002.
Gram-negative diplococci	N. meningitidis	**Pen G** 4 million units IV q4h x5-7 d (if pen. allergic, **chloro** 50 mg/kg (up to 1.0 gm) IV q6h) + **dexamethasone** (dose above)		Listeria ref.: *CID* 24:1, 1997. **If pen.-allergic, use TMP/SMX 15-20 mg/kg/d. div. q6-8h.**
Gram-positive bacilli or coccobacilli	Listeria monocytogenes	**AMP** 2.0 gm IV q4h + **gentamicin** 2 mg/kg loading dose then 1.7 mg/kg q8h		Other possible drugs: aztreonam, CIP, MER. CIP rx success: *CID* 25:936, 1997. Ref. *CID* 37:159, 2003.
Gram-negative bacilli	H. influenzae, coliforms, P. aeruginosa	**Ceftazidime** 2.0 gm IV q8h + **gentamicin** 2 mg/kg 1* dose then 1.7 mg/kg q8h		
Specific Therapy—Positive culture of CSF with in vitro susceptibility results available H. influenzae		**Ceftriaxone** (peds) 100 mg/kg/d, IV q12h		**Pen. allergic: Chloro** 50 mg/kg/d, IV q6h (max. 4 gm/d.)
Listeria monocytogenes		**AMP** 2.0 gm IV q4h + **gentamicin** 2 mg/kg loading dose, then 1.7 mg/kg q8h		**Pen. allergic: TMP/SMX** 15-20 mg/kg/d, div. q6-8h. One report of greater efficacy of AMP + TMP/SMX as compared to AMP + gentamicin (*JID* 33:79, 1996).
N. meningitidis		**Pen G** 50 mg/kg div q6-8h. Adj. pen G 4 mill. units IV q4h x10-14 d.		Rare isolates chloro-resistant (*NEJM* 339:868 & 917, 1998). As few as 3 days of penicillin may suffice in selected pts (*CID* 37:658 & 663, 2003).
S. pneumoniae NOTE: A 2nd CSF exam after 24-48 hrs is suggested both because of difficulty treating resistant S. pneumo & because dexamethasone (if used) may impair clinical assessment	Pen G MIC < 0.1 µg/ml	**Pen G** 4 mill. units IV q4h x5-7 d. (see Comment). If pen. allergic, **chloro** 50 mg/kg div q6h	Treat for 10-14 days	For severe pen. allergy: (**Vanco** IV + **RIF** 600 mg qd po or IV) or **chloro** 50 mg/kg (up to 1.0 gm) IV q6h.
	Pen G MIC > 0.1 µg/ml and/or ceftriaxone MIC > 0.5 µg/ml	**Children:** [(**Ceftriaxone** 50 mg/kg IV q12h to max. of 4 gm/d, or **cefotaxime** 50-75 mg/kg IV q6h) + **vanco** 15 mg/kg IV q6h] + **dexamethasone** 0.4 mg/kg q12h IV x2 d. **Adults:** (**Ceftriaxone** 2.0 gm IV q12h) + (**vanco** 15 mg/kg q6-12h)		For severe pen. allergy: **Vanco** IV + **RIF** 600 mg q6h. In experimental meningitis, vanco + ceftriaxone synergistic even with high ceftriaxone MIC (*AAC* 37:630, 1993). In children, dexamethasone does not ↓ vanco penetration of CSF (*AAC* 39:1988, 1995). MER may work but little clinical experience. **Rx if severe penicillin allergy: Vanco IV + RIF 600 mg qd (po or IV).**
Prophylaxis for H. influenzae and N. meningitidis **Hemophilus Influenzae** Hemophilus influenzae type b Household and/or day care contact: residing with index case or 24 hrs. Day care contact: same day care as index case for 5-7 days before onset		**RIF** 20 mg/kg po (not to exceed 600 mg) qd x4 doses		**Household:** If there is one unvaccinated contact ≤4 yrs in the household, RIF recommended for all household contacts except pregnant women. **Child Care Facilities:** With 1 case, if attended by unvaccinated children ≤2 yrs, consider prophylaxis + vaccinate susceptibles. If ≥2 cases in 60 days & unvaccinated children attend, prophylaxis recommended for children & personnel (*Am J Acad Red Book 1997, page 222*).

(Footnotes and abbreviations on page 45)

NOTE: All dosage recommendations are for adults (unless otherwise indicated) and assume normal renal function

TABLE 1 (5)

ANATOMIC SITE/DIAGNOSIS/ MODIFYING CIRCUMSTANCES	ETIOLOGIES (usual)	SUGGESTED REGIMENS* PRIMARY	ALTERNATIVE†	ADJUNCT DIAGNOSTIC OR THERAPEUTIC MEASURES AND COMMENTS
CENTRAL NERVOUS SYSTEM/Meningitis, Bacterial/Prophylaxis (continued)				
Neisseria meningitidis exposure (close contact) [MMWR 46(RR-5):1, 1997] CDC recommends informing college freshmen living in dormitories & residence halls of available vaccine [MMWR 46(RR-7):1, 2000 & 50:23-487, 2001]		RIF 600 mg po q12h x4 doses. (Children >1 mo. age 10 mg/kg po q12h x4 doses, <1 mo. age 5 mg/kg q12h x4 doses)] or CIP (adults) 500 mg po single dose) or Ceftriaxone 250 mg IM x1 dose (child <15 yrs 125 mg IM x1)]. Spiramycin 500 mg po q6h x5 d. Children 10 mg/kg po q6h x5 d		N. meningitidis spread by respiratory droplets, not aerosols, hence close contact required. ↑ risk if close contact for at least 4 hrs during week before illness onset (e.g., housemates, day care contacts, cellmates) or exposure to pt's naso-pharyngeal secretions (e.g., via kissing, mouth-to-mouth resuscitation, intubation, nasotracheal suctioning). Azithro 500 mg x 1 as effective as RIF 600 mg bid x2 d. [PIDJ 17:816, 1998]. Ceftriaxone equivalent to RIF [JAC 45:909, 2000]. Primary prophylactic regimen in many European countries.
Meningitis, chronic Defined as symptoms + CSF pleocytosis for ≥4 wks	M. tbc 40%, cryptococcus 7%, neoplastic 8%, Lyme, syphilis, Whipple's disease	Treatment depends on etiology. No agent need for empiric therapy.		Long list of possibilities: bacteria, fungi, viruses, neoplasms, vasculitis, and other miscellaneous etiologies—see chapter on chronic meningitis in latest edition of Harrison's Textbook of Internal Medicine.
Meningitis, eosinophilic AJM 114:217, 2003 [See Table 13A, page 97]	Angiostrongyliasis, gnatho-stomiasis, rarely others	Corticosteroids	Not sure antihelminthic rx works	1/3 lack peripheral eosinophilia. Need serology to confirm dx. Steroid ref.: CID 31:660, 2001. Recent outbreak: NEJM 346:668, 2002.
Meningitis, HIV-1 infected (AIDS)	As in adults, >50 yrs: also consider cryptococcus, M. tuberculosis, syphilis, HIV aseptic meningitis, Listeria monocytogenes	If etiology not identified: rx as adult >50 yrs + obtain CSF/serum antigen (see Comments)	For crypto rx, see Table 11A, page 79	C. neoformans most common etiology in AIDS pt. H. influenzae, pneumococci, Tbc, syphilis, viral, histoplasma & coccidioides also need to be considered. Obtain blood cultures. L. monocytogenes risk >60x ↑. ¾ present as meningitis [CID 17:224, 1993].
EAR				
External otitis "Swimmer's ear" PIDJ 22:299, 2003	Pseudomonas sp., Entero-bacteriaceae, Proteus sp. (Fungi rare). Acute infection usually 2° S. aureus	Eardrops: ofloxacin 0.3% soln bid or [(polymyxin B + neomycin + hydrocortisone) qid] or (CIP + hydrocortisone bid) For acute disease: Dicloxacillin 500 mg 4x/d.		Rx should include gentle cleaning. Recurrences prevented (or decreased) by drying ear canal with a hair dryer (1/3 while swimming) after swimming, then antibiotic drops or 2% acetic acid solution. Ointments should not be used in ear. Do not use neomycin if tympanic membrane punctured.
Chronic	Usually 2° to seborrhea	Eardrops: [(polymyxin B + neomycin + hydrocorti-sone qid) + selenium sulfide]		Control seborrhea with dandruff shampoo containing selenium sulfide (Selsun) or [(ketoconazole shampoo) + (medium potency steroid solution, triamcinolone 0.1%)]
Diabetes mellitus, acute "malignant otitis externa"	Pseudomonas sp.	IMP 0.5 gm q6h IV, or MER 1.0 gm q8h IV, or CIP 400 mg q12h IV (or 750 mg q12h po) or ceftaz 2.0 gm q8h IV (or CFP 2 gm q12h) or (PIP 4–6 gm q4-6h IV + tobra) or TC 3.0 gm q4h IV + tobra		CIP especially useful for outpatient rx with early disease. Surgical debridement usually required, but not radical excision. R/O osteomyelitis. CT or MRI scan more sensitive than x-ray. If bone involved, rx for 4-6 wks.

NOTE: All dosage recommendations are for adults (unless otherwise indicated) and assume normal renal function

(Footnotes and abbreviations on page 45)

TABLE 1 (6)

ANATOMIC SITE/DIAGNOSIS/ MODIFYING CIRCUMSTANCES	ETIOLOGIES (usual)	SUGGESTED REGIMENS* PRIMARY	ALTERNATIVE†	ADJUNCT DIAGNOSTIC OR THERAPEUTIC MEASURES AND COMMENTS
EAR (continued) **Otitis media—infants, children, adults** Acute otitis media (NEJM 347:1169, 2002). NOTE: Pending new data, rx children <2 yrs old. If >2 yrs old, afebrile, no ear pain, may be questionable exam—consider symptomatic treatment without antimicrobials	For correlation of bacterial eradication from middle ear & clinical outcome, see *In D* 2:593, 2003. For initial detection in middle ear fluid: No pathogen 25% Virus 5–46% Bact. + virus 48% Bacteria only 55% Role of viruses: *Clin Micro Rev* 16:230, 2003	**If NO antibiotics in prior month:** Amox HD or UD¹ or HD¹ For all doses, see footnotes¹ and ² **All doses are pediatric** Duration of rx: <2 yrs old X10 d; ≥2 yrs old X5–7 d. Appropriate duration unclear. 5 d. may be inadequate for severe disease (NEJM 347:1169, 2002)	**If allergic to β-lactam drugs ?** If history unclear or rash, oral ceph OK; avoid ceph if IgE-mediated (NEJM 347:1169, 2002). High failure rate with TMP/SMX? If etiology is DRSP or H. influenzae (PIDJ 20:260, 2001); azithro x5 d. or clarithro x10 d. (both have ↓ activity vs DRSP; JICAAC Abst. 2324, 2003). **Received antibiotics in prior month:** Amox HD¹ or AM/CL HD¹ or cefdinir or cefpodoxime or cefuroxime axetil For dosage, see footnotes¹ and ² **All doses are pediatric**	**If allergic to β-lactam drugs ?** If history unclear or rash, oral ceph OK; avoid ceph if IgE-mediated (NEJM 347:1169, 2002). High failure rate with TMP/SMX? If etiology is DRSP or H. influenzae (PIDJ 20:260, 2001); azithro x5 d. or clarithro x10 d. (both have ↓ activity vs DRSP; JICAAC Abst. 2324, 2003). **Spontaneous resolution:** 90% pts infected with M. catarrhalis, 50% with H. influenzae, and 10% with S. pneumoniae. DRSP risk ↑ with age <2 yrs, antibiotics last 3 mos., and/or daycare attendance. Selection of drug based on (1) effectiveness against β-lactamase producing H. influenzae & M. catarrhalis and (2) effectiveness against S. pneumo, including DRSP. **Cefaclor, loracarbef, & ceftibuten less active vs DRSP** than other agents listed. Variable acceptance of drug taste/smell by children 4–8 y.o. (PIDJ 19 (Supp 2):S174, 2000). **Clindamycin** not active vs H. influenzae ?S. pneumo resistant to macrolides are usually also resistant to clinda. Definition of failure: no change in ear pain, fever, bulging TM or otorrhea after 3 days of rx. **Pneumococcus** resistant to penicillin: **Vanco is active vs DRSP** **Levo & Gati active vs DRSP, but not approved for use in children.** Ceftriaxone IM x3 d. superior to 1 d. treatment vs DRSP (PIDJ 19:1040, 2000). AM/CL HD reported successful for pen-resistant S. pneumo AOM (PIDJ 20:829, 2001).
Treatment for clinical failure after 3 days rx	Drug-resistant S. pneumoniae main concern	**NO antibiotics in month prior to last 3 days:** AM/CL HD¹ or cefdinir or cefpodoxime or ceftriaxone IM x3 d. For dosage, see footnotes¹ and ² **All doses are pediatric**	**Antibiotics in month prior to last 3 days:** (IM ceftriaxone) or clindamycin and/or (tympanocentesis) *See clindamycin Comments*	
After >48 hrs of nasotracheal intubation	Pseudomonas sp., klebsiella, enterobacter, Pneumococcus, H. influenzae, M. catarrhalis, Staph. aureus, Group A strep (see **Comments**)	Ceftazidime or CFP or IMP or MER or TC/CL or CIP (For dosages, see Ear, malignant otitis externa)		With nasotracheal intubation >48 hrs, about ¼ pts will have otitis media with effusion **Otitis media is a major contributor to emergence of antibiotic-resistant S. pneumoniae**
Prophylaxis: acute otitis media (NEJM 344:403, 2001; PIDJ 22:10, 2003		Sulfisoxazole 50 mg/kg po qd at bedtime or amoxicillin 20 mg/kg po qd	Pneumococcal protein conjugate vaccine decreases freq. AOM in general & due to vaccine serotypes Adenoidectomy at time of tympanostomy tubes ↓ need for future hospitalization for AOM (NEJM 344:1188, 2001).	

---

¹ **Amoxicillin UD or HD** = amoxicillin usual dose or high dose. **AM/CL HD** = amoxicillin/clavulanate high dose. **Dosages in footnote 2**. Data supporting amoxicillin HD: PIDJ 22:405, 2003

² **Drugs and doses suitable for once-daily dosing for acute otitis media: Amoxicillin UD** = 40 mg/kg/d div q12h or q8h. **Amoxicillin HD** = 90 mg/kg/d div q12h or q8h. **AM/CL HD** = 90 mg/kg/d amox component. **Extra-strength AM/CL oral suspension** (Augmentin ES-600) available with 600 mg AM & 42.9 mg CL per 5 ml—dose: 90/6.4 mg/kg/d div q12h. **Ceftriaxone** 50 mg/kg IM x3 d. **Clindamycin** 20–30 mg/kg/d div q8h (may be effective vs DRSP but no activity vs H. influenzae)
Other drugs suitable for this age group (e.g., penicillin)-sensitive S. pneumo: TMP/SMX 8 mg/kg/d of TMP div q12h. **Erythro-sulfisoxazole** 50 mg/kg/d of erythro div q6–8h. **Clarithro** 15 mg/kg/d div q12h; **azithro** 10 mg/kg/d x1 and then 5 mg/kg qd on days 2–5. Other FDA-approved regimens: 10 mg/kg/d x1; 30 mg/kg/d x1. **cefpodoxime proxetil** 10 mg/kg/d as single dose, **cefaclor** 40 mg/kg/d div q8h; **loracarbef** 30 mg/kg/d div q24h; **cefuroxime** 30 mg/kg/d div q12h; **cefprozil** 30 mg/kg/d div q12h; **cefdinir** 14 mg/kg/d div q12h or q24h; **cefixime** 8 mg/kg/d div q12h or q24h; **cefditoren** not approved for <12 yrs old. NOTE: All dosage recommendations are for adults (unless otherwise indicated) and assume normal renal function

(Footnotes and abbreviations on page 45)

TABLE 1 (7)

ANATOMIC SITE/DIAGNOSIS/ MODIFYING CIRCUMSTANCES	ETIOLOGIES (usual)	SUGGESTED REGIMENS* PRIMARY	SUGGESTED REGIMENS* ALTERNATIVE	ADJUNCT DIAGNOSTIC OR THERAPEUTIC MEASURES AND COMMENTS
EAR *(continued)*				
Mastoiditis				
Acute				
Outpatient	Strep. pneumoniae 22%, S. pyogenes 16%, Staph. aureus 7%, H. influenzae 4%, P. aeruginosa 4%, others <1%	Empirically same as Acute otitis media, above: need **nafcillin/oxacillin** if Staph. aureus (decisions on severity) + (**cefotaxime** 1-2 gm IV q4-6h (decisions on severity) or **ceftriaxone** 1-2 gm q24h IV < age 60; 1 gm q24h IV > age 60)		Has become a rare entity, presumably as a result of the aggressive rx of acute otitis media. Small increase in incidence in Netherlands where use of antibiotics limited to children with complicated course or high risk. *(PIDJ 20:140, 2001)*
Hospitalized	Often polymicrobic: anaerobes, S. aureus, Enterobacteriaceae, P. aeruginosa	Treatment for acute exacerbations or perioperatively: ideally, no treatment until surgical cultures obtained. Examples of empiric regimens: **IMP** 0.5 gm q6h IV, **TC/CL** 3.1 gm q6h IV, **PIP/TZ** 3.375 gm q4-6h IV or 4.5 gm q8h IV.		May or may not be associated with chronic otitis media with drainage via ruptured tympanic membrane. Antimicrobials given in association with surgery. Mastoidectomy indications: chronic drainage and evidence of osteomyelitis; chronic draining and evidence of spread to CNS (epidural abscess, suppurative phlebitis, brain abscess).
Chronic				
EYE—General Reviews: *CID 21:479, 1995; IDCP 7:447, 1998*				
Eyelid				
Blepharitis	Etiol. unclear. Factors include Staph. aureus & Staph. epidermidis, seborrhea, rosacea, & dry eye	Lid margin care with baby shampoo & warm compresses q.d. Artificial tears if assoc. dry eye (see *Comment*)		Usually topical ointments of no benefit. If associated rosacea, add doxy 100 mg po bid x2 wks and then qd.
Hordeolum (Stye)				
External (gland of Zeis)	Staph. aureus	Hot packs only. Will drain spontaneously.		Infection of superficial sebaceous gland.
Internal (Meibomian glands)	Staph. aureus	Hot packs & incision & drainage + hot packs		Also called acute meibomianitis. Rarely drain spontaneously.
Conjunctiva: Non-gonococcal (ophthalmia neonatorum): by day of onset post-delivery—all doses pediatric				
Onset 1 day	Chemical due to AgNO₃ prophylaxis	None		Usual prophylaxis is erythro ointment; hence, AgNO₃ irritation rare.
Onset 2-4 days	N. gonorrhoeae	**Ceftriaxone** 25-50 mg/kg IV/IM x1 dose (see *Comment*)		Treat mother and her sexual partners. Hyperpurulent. Topical rx inadequate. **Treat neonate for concomitant Chlamydia trachomatis.**
Onset 3-10 days	Chlamydia trachomatis	**Erythro syrup** 50 mg/kg/d (po in 4 div. doses x14 d.)		Diagnosis by antigen detection. Azithro susp 20 mg/kg po q.d x3 d. reported efficacious *[PIDJ 17:1049, 1998]*. Treat mother & sexual partner.
Onset 2-16 days	Herpes simplex types 1, 2	See keratitis, below.		Consider IV acyclovir if concomitant systemic disease.
Ophthalmia neonatorum prophylaxis: **Silver nitrate** (types 3 & 7 in children), 8, 11 & 19 in adults)				
Pink eye (viral conjunctivitis) Usually unilateral	Adenovirus (types 3 & 7 in children, 8, 11 & 19 in adults)	No treatment. If symptomatic, cold artificial tears may help.		Highly contagious. Onset of ocular pain and photophobia in an adult suggests associated keratitis—rare.
Conjunctivitis:				
Inclusion conjunctivitis (adult) Usually unilateral	Chlamydia trachomatis	**Doxy** 100 mg bid po x1-3 weeks	**Erythro** 250 mg qid po x1-3 weeks	Oculoglandular disease. Diagnosis by culture or PCR—availability varies by region and institution. Treat sexual partner.
Trachoma	Chlamydia trachomatis	**Azithro** 20 mg/kg po single dose—78% effective	**Doxy** 100 mg bid po x14 d. or **tetracycline** 250 mg po x14 d	Starts in childhood and can persist for years with subsequent damage to cornea. Topical therapy of marginal benefit. Avoid doxy/tetracycline in young children. *Ref: CID 24:363, 1997.*
Suppurative conjunctivitis: non-chlamydial	Staph. aureus, S. pneumoniae, H. influenzae, M. catarrhalis. Outbreak due to atypical S. pneumo. *NEJM 348:1112, 2003*	Ophthalmic **bacitracin-polymyxin B** or **TMP** or **tobra** (see *Comment*)	Ophthalmic **gentamicin** or **tobra**	Often self-limited. Eye drops preferred for adults and ointments for young children. Topical gent, tobra, or chloro; neomycin may cause punctate staining of cornea. In children 2 mos – 6 yrs old, topical rx more effective than cefixime *[AJO (PIDJ 20:1039, 2001).*
Gonococcal	N. gonorrhoeae	**Ceftriaxone** 125 mg IM or IV (single dose). See *Genital, page 15*		

(Footnotes and abbreviations on page 45) NOTE: All dosage recommendations are for adults (unless otherwise indicated) and assume normal renal function

TABLE 1 (8)

ANATOMIC SITE/DIAGNOSIS/ MODIFYING CIRCUMSTANCES	ETIOLOGIES (usual)	SUGGESTED REGIMENS* PRIMARY	ALTERNATIVE	ADJUNCT DIAGNOSTIC OR THERAPEUTIC MEASURES AND COMMENTS
EYE *(continued)*				
Cornea (keratitis): Usually serious and often sight-threatening. Prompt ophthalmologic consultation essential. Herpes simplex most common etiology in developed countries; bacterial and fungal infections more common in underdeveloped countries.				
Viral				
H. simplex	H. simplex, types 1 & 2	Trifluridine one drop qh, 9v/d, for up to 21 days	Vidarabine ointment— useful in children. Use 5v/d for up to 21 days.	Fluorescein staining shows topical dendritic figures. 30–50% rate of recurrence within 2 years. 400 mg acyclovir po bid ÷ 4 recurrences, p 0.005 (NEJM 339:300, 1998). If child fails vidarabine, try trifluridine.
Varicella-zoster ophthalmicus	Varicella-zoster virus	Famciclovir 500 mg po or valacyclovir 1.0 gm tid po x10 days	Acyclovir 800 mg po 5x/day x10 days	Clinical diagnosis most common: dendritic figures with fluorescein staining in patient with varicella-zoster staining of ophthalmic branch of trigeminal nerve.
Bacterial		All as listed for bacterial, fungal, & protozoan is topical		
Contact lens users	P. aeruginosa	Tobra or gentamicin (14 mg/ml) + piperacillin or ticarcillin eye drops (6–12 mg/ml) q15–60 min. around clock x24–72 hrs, then slow reduction	CIP or ofloxn 0.3% drops q15–60 min. around clock x24–72 hrs	Pain, photophobia, impaired vision. Recommend alginate swab for culture and sensitivity testing.
Dry cornea, diabetes, immunosuppression	Staph. aureus, S. epidermidis, S. pneumoniae, S. pyogenes, Enterobacteriaceae, listeria	Cefazolin (50 mg/ml) + gentamicin or tobra (14 mg/ml) q15–60 min. around clock x24–72 hrs, then slow reduction	Vanco (50 mg/ml) + ceftazidime (50 mg/ml) q15–60 min. around clock x24–72 hrs, then slow reduction. See Comment	Specific therapy guided by results of alginate swab culture and sensitivity. CIP 0.3% found clinically equivalent to cefazolin + tobra; only concern was efficacy of vs S. pneumoniae (Ophthalmology 163:1864, 1996).
Fungal	Aspergillus, fusarium, candida. No empiric therapy—see Comment	Natamycin (5%) drops q3–5 hrs with subsequent slow reduction	Ampho B (0.05–0.15%) q4-q3 hrs with subsequent slow reduction	No empiric therapy. Wait for results of Gram stain or culture in Sabouraud's medium.
Protozoan Soft contact lens users (overnight use) risk 10–15 fold)	Acanthamoeba, hartmannella	Propamidine 0.1% + neomycin/gramicidin/ polymyxin Eyedrops q waking hour x1 week and then slow taper	Polyhexamethylene biguanide 0.02% or chlorhexidine 0.02%.	Uncommon. Trauma and soft contact lenses are risk factors. Corneal scrapings stained with calcofluor white show characteristic cysts with fluorescent microscopy. Ref. CID 35:434, 2002
Lacrimal apparatus				
Canaliculitis	Actinomyces most common. Rarely, Arachnia, fusobacterium, nocardia, candida	Remove granules & irrigate with pen G (100,000 units/ml) approx. 5 μg/ml + 1 gtt tid	If fungi, irrigate with nystatin	Digital pressure produces exudate at punctum; Gram stain confirms diagnosis. Hot packs to punctal area qid.
Dacryocystitis (lacrimal sac)	S. pneumo, S. aureus, H. influenzae, S. pyogenes, P. aeruginosa	Child: AM/CL or O Ceph 2 Adult:	Often consequence of obstruction of lacrimal duct. Empiric rx based on Gram stain of aspirate—see Comment.	Need ophthalmologic consultation. Can be acute or chronic.

Endophthalmitis: For etiologic agents of post-op endophthalmitis, see Am J Ophthal 122:1, 1996

Bacterial: Haziness of vitreous key to diagnosis. Needle aspirate of both vitreous and aqueous humor for culture prior to therapy. Intravitreal administration of antimicrobials essential.				
Postoperative surgery (cataracts) Early, acute onset	S. epidermidis, S. aureus, Pseudomonas sp.			All require immediate ophthalmologic consultation. With S. aureus or P. aeruginosa, eye may be destroyed within 24 hrs. Rx must be aggressive—early and vitreous therapy. Intravitreal (each in 0.1 ml): Amikacin 0.4 mg + vanco 1 mg (decrease amikacin to 0.1 mg if macular infarction (Br J Ophthal 86:359, 2002); could substitute ceftazidime 2 mg (0.1 ml of 20 mg/ml solution) for amikacin.
Low grade, chronic	Propionibacterium acnes, S. epidermidis, S. aureus			May require removal of lens material. Intraocular vanco.

(Footnotes and abbreviations on page 45)   NOTE: All dosage recommendations are for adults (unless otherwise indicated) and assume normal renal function

TABLE 1 (9)

ANATOMIC SITE/DIAGNOSIS/ MODIFYING CIRCUMSTANCES	ETIOLOGIES (usual)	SUGGESTED REGIMENS* PRIMARY	ALTERNATIVE[1]	ADJUNCT DIAGNOSTIC OR THERAPEUTIC MEASURES AND COMMENTS
EYE: Endophthalmitis (Bacterial) (continued)				
Post filtering blebs for glaucoma	Strep. species (viridans & others), H. influenzae	Intravitreal agent. Intravitreal agent and consider systemic **AM/CL**, **AM/SB** or **P Ceph 2**		
Post-penetrating trauma	Bacillus sp., S. epiderm.	Intravitreal agent as above + systemic **clinda** or **vanco**. Use topical antibiotics (tobra & cefazolin drops)		
None, suspect hematogenous	S. pneumoniae, N. mening- itidis, Staph. aureus	**P Ceph 3** (**cefotaxime** 2.0 gm q4h IV) + **ceftriaxone** 1.0 gm q12h IV pending cultures. Intravitreal antibiotics as with early post-operative.		
IV heroin abuse	Bacillus cereus, Candida sp.			
Mycotic (fungal)	Candida sp.	Intravitreal ampho + systemic **clinda** or **vanco**.		With moderate/marked vitritis, options include systemic rx + vitrectomy ± intra-
Associated broad spectrum antibiotics, often corti- costeroids, indwelling venous catheters	Bacillus cereus, Aspergillus sp.	Intravitreal ampho B (approx 10 mcg) in 0.1 ml. Also see Table 11, pages 74, 75 for concomitant systemic therapy. See Comment.		vitreal ampho B (CID 27:1130 & 1134, 1998). Report of failure of ampho B lipid complex (CID 28:1777, 1999).
Retinitis				
Acute retinal necrosis	Varicella zoster, Herpes simplex	IV **acyclovir** 10–12 mg/kg IV q8h x5–7 d, then 800 mg po 5x/d, x6 wks.		Strong association of VZ virus with atypical necrotizing herpetic retinopathy (CID 24:603, 1997).
HIV+ (AIDS)	Cytomegalovirus	See Table 14, page 107		Occurs in 5–10% of AIDS patients
CD4 usually < 100/mm³				
Orbital cellulitis (see page 36 for erysipelas, facial)	S. pneumoniae, H. influen- zae, M. catarrhalis, S. aureus, anaerobes, group A strep, occ. Gm-neg. bacilli with trauma	**P Ceph 2/3** (**cefuroxime** 1.5 gm q8h IV, **cefoxitin** 2.0 gm q8h IV, **cefotetan** 2.0 gm q12h IV, or **cefotaxime** 2.0 gm q8h IV)	**TC/CL** or **PIP/TZ** (see foot- note[1] for dosages) or **cefo- taxime** 2.0 gm q8h IV or **ceftriaxone** 2.0 gm q24h IV **AM/SB** 3.0 gm q6h IV	See mucor/rhizopus, Table 11, page 80. H. influenzae becoming a rare etiology.
FOOT				
"Diabetic." Reviews: NEJM 343:787, 2000; Ln 361:1545, 2003				
Previously untreated, limited in extent, no osteomyelitis	Aerobic Gm+ cocci: S. aureus, enterococci, Gm-neg. bacilli	**MRSA unlikely:** **Cephalexin** or **AM/CL** or **clinda** + **oral CIP/levo**	**Community-acquired MRSA a concern:** po **TMP/SMX-DS** bid (or po **clinda** 300 mg po q12h)	Reduce weight-bearing. Ensure arterial blood supply adequate. Cultures from ulcers unreliable. Prompt surgical intervention to R/O necrotizing fas- ciitis. As ischemia and nec gangrene become critical need for debridement/ampu-
Chronic, recurrent, limb-threatening (See Bone, page 3, for associated osteomyelitis treatment)	Polymicrobic: aerobic Gm+ cocci, aerobic Gm- neg. bacilli (e.g., E. coli) & strict anaerobes (e.g., B. fragilis), MRSA an increasing problem.	**Non-limb/life-threatening:** **AM/SB** or **TC/CL** or **PIP/TZ** or **CIP** or **levo** or **aztreonam**) + **clinda**. Add **linezolid** or **vanco** for MRSA. **Limb/life-threatening:** (**IMP** or **MER** or **erta**) + **vanco**	Dosages in footnote[2]	tation more likely. Ability to insert probe to bone suggests concomitant osteomyelitis (JAMA 273:721, 1995). MRI cannot distinguish marrow edema than osteo (Radio 203:849, 1997). Avoidance of weight-bearing is key (NEJM 331: 854, 1994). MER less active vs P. aeruginosa than IMP or MER. Charcot foot review. Ln 360:1776, 2002.
Osteomyelitis prognosis depends on blood supply; assess for operable arterial insufficiency early				
Onychomycosis (see Table 11, page 79, fungal infections)				
GALLBLADDER				
Cholecystitis, cholangitis, biliary sepsis, common duct obstruc- tion (partial: 2° to tumor, stones, stricture)	Enterobacteriaceae 68%, enterococci 14%, bacteroi- des 10%, Clostridium sp. 7%	**PIP/TZ** or **AM/SB** or **TC/CL** or **erta** or **MER** If life-threatening: **IMP**	**P Ceph 3 + metro** **Aztreonam + metro** OR **CIP + metro**	For severely ill pts, antibiotic rx is complementary to establishment of adequate biliary drainage. 15–30% pts will require decompression: surgical, percutaneous & or ERCP-placed stent. Whether empirical rx should always cover pseudomonas & anaerobes is uncertain (CID 19:279, 1994). Ceftriaxone associated with biliary sludge (by ultrasound 50%, symptomatic 5%, NEJM 322:1821, 1990); clinical relevance still unclear but has led to surgery (MMWR 42:39, 1993).

[1] **Cephalexin** 500 mg po qid, **cefoxitin** 2.0 gm q8h IV, **CIP** 750 mg po bid (or 400 mg IV q12h), **levo** 750 mg po/IV once daily, **clinda** 300 mg qid po or 450–900 mg IV, **clinda** 600 mg IV q8h, **metro** 1.0 gm q8h IV. **IMP** 0.5 gm q6h IV. **MER** 1.0 gm q8h IV. **AM/CL** 875/125 mg po q12h, **TC/CL** 3.1 gm q6h IV, **PIP/TZ** 3.375 gm q6h IV, **IMP** 0.5 gm q6h IV, **AM/SB** 3.0 gm q6h IV, **AMP** 2.0 gm q6h IV, **aztreonam** 2.0 gm q8h IV. **FQ IV** (**CIP** 400 mg q12h, **gati** 400 mg q24h, **oflox** 400 mg q12h). **Vanco** 15 mg/kg q12h IV. **Linezolid** 600 mg q12h.
[2] **AP Pen** (**ticarcillin** 4.0 gm q6h IV, **PIP** 4.0 gm q6h IV, **PIP/TZ** 3.375 gm q6h IV, **TC/CL** 3.1 gm q6h IV), **erta** 1.0 gm IV, **AM/SB** 3.0 gm q6h IV, **AMP** 2.0 gm q6h IV, **IMP** 0.5 gm q6h IV, **MER** 1.0 gm q8h IV, **TC/CL** 3.1 gm q6h IV, **PIP/TZ** 3.375 gm q6h IV, **metro** 1.0 gm q12h IV, **metro** loading dose then 0.5 gm q6h IV or 1.0 gm q12h IV, **erta** 1.0 gm q8h IV, see previous footnote for **clinda** and **aztreonam** dosage, **P Ceph 3** dose in Table 10B, pages 67, 68, **CIP** 400 mg IV q12h, **levo** 750 mg IV qd. **linezolid** 600 mg IV q12h.

AP Pen (**ticarcillin** 3.0 gm or 4.5 gm q6h IV, **metro** 1.0 gm q12h IV, **levo** 1.0 gm IV q24h) *NOTE: All dosage recommendations are for adults (unless otherwise indicated) and assume normal renal function*

Footnotes and abbreviations on page 45

TABLE 1 (10)

ANATOMIC SITE/DIAGNOSIS/ MODIFYING CIRCUMSTANCES	ETIOLOGIES (usual)	SUGGESTED REGIMENS*		ADJUNCT DIAGNOSTIC OR THERAPEUTIC MEASURES AND COMMENTS
		PRIMARY	ALTERNATIVE†	
GASTROINTESTINAL				
Gastroenteritis—Empiric Therapy (laboratory studies not performed or culture, microscopy, toxin results NOT AVAILABLE) (Ref: *CID* 32:331, 2001)				
Premature infant with necrotizing enterocolitis	Associated with intestinal flora.	Treatment and rationale as for diverticulitis/peritonitis, *page 14, See Table 16, page 129 for pediatric dosages.*		Pneumatosis intestinalis on x-ray confirms dx. Bacteremia–peritonitis in 30–50%. If Staph. epidermidis isolated, add vanco (IV).
Mild diarrhea (≤3 unformed stools/day, minimal associated symptomatology)	Bacterial *(see Severe, below)*, viral, parasitic. Viral usually causes mild to moderate disease. (See *AJM* 106:670, 1999)	Fluids only + lactose-free diet, avoid caffeine		**Rehydration: For po fluid replacement, see Cholera, page 12.** **Antimotility:** Loperamide (Imodium) 4 mg po, then 2 mg after each loose stool to max. of 16 mg/day. Bismuth subsalicylate (Pepto-Bismol) 2 tablets (262 mg) po qid. Do not use if suspect hemolytic uremic syndrome.
Moderate diarrhea (≥4 unformed stools/day and/or systemic symptoms)		Antimotility agents *(see Comments)* + fluids		**Hemolytic uremic syndrome (HUS):** Risk in children infected with E. coli 0157:H7 is 8–10%. Early treatment with TMP/SMX or FQs may ↑ risk of HUS (*NEJM* 342:1930 & 1990; *JAMA* 288:996 & 3111, 2002.
Severe diarrhea (≥6 unformed stools/day, and/or temperature ≥101°F, tenesmus, blood, or fecal leukocytes) **NOTE: Severe afebrile bloody diarrhea should ↑ suspicion of E. coli 0157:H7 infection**—causes only 1–3% all cases diarrhea in U.S.—but causes up to 38% cases of bloody diarrhea (*CID* 32:573, 2001)	Shigella, salmonella, C. jejuni, E. coli 0157:H7, toxin-positive C. difficile, E. histolytica. *For typhoid fever, see page 44*	**FQ (CIP** 500 mg bid x3–5 days) (**CIP** 500 mg po bid x3 d. *TMP/SMX-DS* po bid x3 d. See Table 13A.) **Metro** 500 mg tid po x10–14 days	**TMP/SMX-DS** bid po x3-5 days. Resistance to TMP/ SMX common throughout tropics. **Vanco** 125 mg qid po x10-14 days (C. difficile toxin colitis	**Other potential etiologies:** Cryptosporidia—no treatment in immunocompetent host (see *Table 13A & JID* 170:272, 1994). Cyclospora—usually chronic diarrhea, responds to TMP/SMX (see *Table 12A & AM* 123:409, 1995). **Severe diarrhea** treated with CIP 500 mg bid po decreases duration of diarrhea and other symptoms without consuming duration of fecal carriage of campylobacter. Resistant to FQs (*NEJM* 340:1525, 1999).
Gastroenteritis—Specific Therapy (results of culture, microscopy, toxin assay AVAILABLE). Ref: *CID* 32:331, 2001				
Aeromonas/plesiomonas		**CIP** 500 mg po bid x3 d. TMP/SMX-DS po bid x3 d. See Table 13A.		† worldwide resistance to FQs varies by region from 10% (USA) to 84%
Amebiasis (Entamoeba histolytica, cyclospora and isospora)		Metro 500 mg po tid d. or CIP 500 mg po bid *(See Comment)*	Erythro estearate 500 mg qid po x5 d.	(Thailand) (*CID* 37:24, 2001; *EID* 7:24, 2001; *AAC* 47:2358, 2003). Erythro resistance rarely reported (*CID* 37:131, 2003).
Campylobacter jejuni CAUTION: See Comment. Fever in 53–83%, H/O† bloody stools 37%.		Metro 500 mg tid or 250 mg qid po x10–14 d.	**Vancro** 125 mg tid po x10 d or (**bacitracin** 25,000 u qid po)	Risk of Guillain-Barre syndrome is less than 1/1000 infections (*CID* 32:1201, 2001); responsible for 15% of GBS cases in England (*CID* 37:307, 2003).
C. difficile toxin positive antibiotic-associated colitis (Ref: *NEJM* 346:334, 2002) **Remember: enteric isolation indicated**		If too ill for po, metro 500 mg IV q8h. If ileus, add vanco by N/G or naso-small bowel tube. Consider retrograde cecal catheter &/or vanco enemas *(See Comment)*	**Teicoplanin** 400 mg po bid. *(See Comment)*	**DO antibiotic if possible; avoid antimotility agents; hydration; enteric isolation.** **Relapse occurs in 10–20%:** First, re-treat with metro. For refractory disease, vanco po + RIF po reported effective (*ICHE* 16:459, 1995); metro + RIF should work but no published data. **For severe relapses**, metro x10 d., then (cholestyramine 4 gm po tid + lactobacillus 1 gm po) x4 wks **OR** vanco 125 mg po qod x4 wks **OR** vanco taper, all doses 125 mg po, week 1—qid, week 2—bid, week 3—qod, week 4—qod, weeks 5 & 6 q 3 days.
Fever in 28%. Diagnosis: Tissue culture—detects toxin A&B, most sensitive. Takes 48 h. Rapid immunoassays: Less sens., detect toxin A, B, or both. 10–20% false-neg. rate.				**If metro not possible:** use IV metro + vanco, 500 mg/L saline via small bowel tube and/or via pigtail catheter in cecum (in severe syphilitis pts). Perfuse at 1–3 ml/min to daily max. of 2.0 gm; see *NEJM* 329:583, 1993 & *CID* 35:690, 2002. **NOTE: IV vanco not effective.**

* H/O = history of
(Footnotes and abbreviations on page 45)
† NOTE: All dosage recommendations are for adults (unless otherwise indicated) and assume normal renal function

TABLE 1 (11)

ANATOMIC SITE/DIAGNOSIS/ MODIFYING CIRCUMSTANCES	ETIOLOGIES (usual)	SUGGESTED REGIMENS*		ADJUNCT DIAGNOSTIC OR THERAPEUTIC MEASURES AND COMMENTS
		PRIMARY	ALTERNATIVE†	
Gastrointestinal/Gastroenteritis—Specific Therapy (continued)				
	E. coli O157:H7 Fever in 16–45%, H/O* bloody stools 63%	**NO TREATMENT** with antimicrobials, as may enhance toxin release and risk of hemolytic uremic syndrome (HUS) (NEJM 342:1930 & 1990, 2000).		Natural history: 95% resolve. HUS develops, 5% with antibiotic rx (JAMA 288:996, 2002); conclusion challenged—JAMA 288:3111, 2002. Conservative approach to rx is without antibiotic.
	Listeria monocytogenes	AMP 200 mg/kg/d IV div. q6h	TMP/SMX 20 mg/kg/d IV div. q6–8h	Recently recognized cause of food poisoning, manifest as febrile gastroenteritis. Percentage with complicating meningitis/meningitis unknown. Not detected in standard stool culture (NEJM 336:100 & 130, 1997).
	Salmonella, non-typhi— For typhoid fever see page 41 Fever in 71–91%, H/O* bloody stools in 34%	If pt asymptomatic or illness mild, antimicrobial therapy not indicated. (Also see typhoid fever, page 41) CIP 500 mg po bid x5–7 d. Resistance ↑ (Ln 353:1590, 1999)	**Azithro** 1.0 gm po once, then 500 mg q24h x6 d. (AAC 43:1441, 1999)	If immunocompromised, or pt ill enough to require hospitalization, antimicrobial agents indicated. FQ resistance usually active (see footnote, page 16, for dosage); cefotaxime resistance in Taiwan (EID 9:323, 2003) & FQ resistance in Japan (JAC 9:255, 2003). APAG and azithro less effective. Primary treatment of enteritis is fluid and electrolyte replacement. No adverse effects from FQs in children, rx 14 d. If immunocompromised, rx 14 d. **Peds doses:** TMP/SMX 6/25 mg/kg po x3 d. For severe disease, ceftriaxone 50–75 mg/kg/d x2–5 d. CIP suspension 10 mg/kg bid x5 d. (Ln 352:522, 1998). CIP superior to ceftriaxone in children (LnID 3:537, 2003) **Immunocompromised: children & adults: Treat for 7–10 d.**
	Shigella Fever in 58%, H/O* bloody stools 51%	**FQs** e.g. (**CIP** 500 mg) or (**oflox** 300 mg) x3 d. See Comment in Comment	TMP/SMX-DS bid po x3 d.) or (**azithro** 500 mg po x1, then 250 mg q24 x4 d.)	Azithro superior to cefixime[x1] in trial in children (PIDJ 22:374, 2003)
	Vibrio cholerae Treatment decreases duration of disease, vol losses, and duration of excretion CID 37:272, 2003	**CIP** 1.0 gm po x1 + fluids. **Primary rx is hydration** (see Comment)	**Doxy** 300 mg po x1. For children <8 yrs in pregnancy: **TMP/SMX-DS.** bid po x3 d Peds alternative: azithro x1	Primary rx is fluid. **IV** use (per liter): 4 gm NaCl, 1 gm KCl, 5.4 gm Na lactate, 8 gm glucose. **PO** (per liter potable water): 1 level teaspoon table salt + 4 heaping teaspoons sugar (AMJM 23, 1981.) Volume given = fluid loss + ongoing dehydration, give 5% body weight; for moderate, 7% body weight. (Refs. CID 20:1485, 1995; TRSM 89:103, 1995). Peds azithro: 20 mg/kg (1 gm max.) x1 (Ln 360:1722, 2002).
	Vibrio parahaemolyticus Vibrio vulnificus	Antimicrobial rx does not shorten course. Usual presentation is skin lesions & bacteremia—see page 37		Sensitive in vitro to FQ, doxy. Often history of seafood ingestion.
	Yersinia enterocolitica Ref: PIDJ 14:771, 1995 Fever in 68%, bloody stools in 26%	**CIP** as for Shigella. **TMP/SMX** or **doxy** if not severe (CTID 17:405, 1993)	**Ceftriaxone** 2.0 gm and IV. **Aminoglycoside** and **chloro** also effective.	Mesenteric adenitis pain can mimic acute appendicitis. Lab diagnosis difficult: requires "cold enrichment" and/or yersinia selective agar. Desferrioxamine ↑ severity, discontinue if pt on it. Iron overload states predispose to yersinia (CID 21:362 & 367, 1998).
Gastroenteritis—Specific Risk Groups—Empiric Therapy				
Anorecourse/Intercourse Proctitis (distal 15 cm only).	Herpes viruses, gonococci, chlamydia, syphilis. See Genital Tract, page 15			
Proctocolitis or enterocolitis	Shigella, salmonella, campylobacter, E. histolytica (see Table 13A)	**FQ** e.g. **CIP** 500 mg q12h (po) x3 d. See Table 13A		
HIV-Infected (AIDS): >10 days diarrhea Most/Acid-fast organisms.	[G. lamblia Cryptosporidium parvum, Cryptospora cayetanensis		See Table 13A	
Other:	Isospora belli, microsporidia (Septata intestinalis)		See Table 13A	For influence of highly active antiretroviral therapy, see CID 28:701, 1999
Neutropenic enterocolitis or "typhlitis" (CID 27:695 & 700, 1998)	Mucosal invasion by Clostridium septicum. Occasionally caused by C. sordelli or P. aeruginosa	As for perirectal abscess. Ensure empiric regimen includes drug active vs Clostridia species; e.g., pen G. **AMP** or **clinda** (if resistance); empiric regimen should have predictive activity vs P. aeruginosa also.		See right lower quadrant. Surgical resection controversial but may be necessary **NOTE:** Resistance of clostridia to clindamycin reported.

† = history of
(Footnotes and abbreviations on page 45)   NOTE: All dosage recommendations are for adults (unless otherwise indicated) and assume normal renal function

TABLE 1 (12)

ANATOMIC SITE/DIAGNOSIS/MODIFYING CIRCUMSTANCES	ETIOLOGIES (usual)	SUGGESTED REGIMENS†		ADJUNCT DIAGNOSTIC OR THERAPEUTIC MEASURES AND COMMENTS
		PRIMARY	**ALTERNATIVE†**	
Gastrointestinal/Gastroenteritis—Specific Risk Groups—Empiric Therapy (continued)				
Traveler's diarrhea, self-medication. Patient usually afebrile. (NEJM 342:1716, 2000)	**Acute:** 60% due to toxigenic E. coli, shigella, salmonella, campylobacter. C. difficile, amebiasis (see Table 13). **If chronic:** cyclospora, cryptosporidia, giardia, isospora.	**Azithro** 1.0 gm po x1 dose	**Levo** 500 mg po x1 dose. Alternative: **CIP**[1] or **other FQ** bid x3 d. (see footnote*)	Treatment based on randomized trial (JID 37:1165, 2003). Peds & pregnancy: Avoid FQs. Azithro peds dose: 5–10 mg/kg x1 dose.
		Imodium optional: 4 mg x1, then 2 mg after each loose stool to max. 16 mg/d.		No loperamide if fever or blood in stool.
Prevention			Rarely indicated. Current recommendation is to take **FQ** + **Imodium** with 1st loose stool (NEJM 328:1821, 1993).	Alternative during 1st 3 weeks only if activities are essential: Options: **Bismuth subsalicylate** (Pepto-Bismol) 2 tabs (262 mg) po qid. **Bismuth subsalicylate** can cause black tongue and dark stool.
Gastrointestinal infections by Anatomic Site				
Esophagitis	Candida albicans, HSV, CMV	[See SANFORD GUIDE TO HIV/AIDS THERAPY]		
Duodenal/Gastric ulcer; chronic type B antral gastritis (not 2° NSAIDs) (NEJM 347:1175, 2002)	**Helicobacter pylori.** See Comment: Prevalence of pre-treatment resistance increasing.	**Rx po for 14 days:** Omeprazole[2] 20 mg 2x/day + amox 1 gm + clarithro 500 mg bid. Efficacy 80–95%	**Rx po for 14 days:** **Bismuth** (see footnote*) 4x/d + tetracycline 500 mg 4x/d + metro 500 mg 3x/d + omeprazole 20 mg 2x/d. Efficacy 90–99%	**Dx gold standard:** positive urease on biopsy specimen, histology, or ¹⁴C or ¹³C labeled urea breath test (UBT). Can use antigen-based stool assay, esp. in children—compared to UBT, sens. of 94%, spec. of 90% (PIDJ 19:364, 2000; Hepato-Gastro 49:576, 2002). False-pos stool antigen can occur—other Helicobacter species (BMJ 120:1148, 2002). Confirm cure with UBT or stool antigen ≥1 wks after end of treatment. Rx failure usually 2° to resistance to metronidazole (20–30%) or clarithro (10%); can overcome metro resistance with ↑ dose and clarithro/metro. Resistance higher if prior use of clarithro/metro (AnIM 139:463, 2003).
Whipple's disease (CID 32:457, 2001)	Tropheryma whipplei	**Initial 10-14 days** (**Pen G** 6-24 mill. U/IV qd + **streptomycin** 1.0 gm IM/IV qd) or **ceftriaxone** 2.0 gm IV qd **Then, for approx. 1 year** **TMP/SMX-DS** 1 tab po bid	**TMP/SMX-DS** 1 tab po bid	Rx regimen based on empiricism and retrospective analyses. TMP/SMX CNS relapses during TMP/SMX Rx reported.
Inflammatory bowel disease: Ulcerative colitis, Crohn's disease	Unknown			
Mild to moderate		**Sulfasalazine** 1.0 gm po q6h or **mesalamine** (5ASA) 1.0 gm po q6h. Corticosteroid enemas	**Coated mesalamine** (Asacol) 800 mg bid or qid equally effective.	Check stool for E. histolytica. Try aminosalicylates 1° in mild/mod. disease. See review article for more aggressive therapy.
Severe Crohn's Ref: Ln 359:331, 2002	In randomized controlled trial, CIP[1] metro[1] had no benefit.	**Infliximab**	**Etanercept**	Risk of disseminated TBc [See Table 12A] & other serious infections.

---

[1] **FQ** dosage po for self-use for traveler's diarrhea—mild disease. **CIP** 750 mg x1; severe 500 mg bid x3 d. **Oflox** 500 mg x1, severe 500 mg bid x3 d. Once daily: **Levo** 500 mg; **gati** 500 mg; or **moxi.** 400 mg x3 d. probably would work but not FDA-approved indication.

[2] Can substitute another proton pump inhibitor for omeprazole—all bid. esomeprazole 20 mg, lansoprazole 30 mg, pantoprazole 40 mg, rabeprazole 20 mg

[3] bismuth preparations: (1) In U.S., bismuth subsalicylate (Pepto-Bismol) 2 tabs (524 mg) 4x/day. (2) Outside U.S., colloidal bismuth subcitrate (De-Nol) 120 mg; dose is 1 tablet 4x/day. (3) Another treatment option: Ranitidine bismuth citrate 400 mg, give with metro 500 mg and clarithro 500 mg—all bid x 7 d. Worked despite metro/clarithro resistance. (Gastro 114:A323, 1998)
(Footnotes and abbreviations on page 45)

NOTE: All dosage recommendations are for adults (unless otherwise indicated) and assume normal renal function

TABLE 1 (13)

ANATOMIC SITE/DIAGNOSIS/ MODIFYING CIRCUMSTANCES	ETIOLOGIES (usual)	SUGGESTED REGIMENS*		ADJUNCT DIAGNOSTIC OR THERAPEUTIC MEASURES AND COMMENTS
		PRIMARY	ALTERNATIVE†	
GASTROINTESTINAL/Gastrointestinal Infections by anatomic site *(continued)*				
Diverticulitis, peritoneal abscess, peritonitis. Also see *Peritonitis, page 31 CID (in press)*	Enterobacteriaceae, P. aeruginosa, Bacteroides sp., enterococci	**Outpatient rx—mild diverticulitis, drained peritonitis:**		Must "cover" both Gm-neg. aerobic and Gm-neg. anaerobic bacteria. **Drugs active only vs anaerobic Gm-neg. bacilli:** clinda, metro. **Drugs active only vs aerobic Gm-neg. bacilli:** APAG, aztreonam, CIP, levo. **Drugs active vs both aerobic/anaerobic Gm-neg. bacteria:** cefotetan, TC/CL, PIP/TZ, AM/SB, erta, IMP, MER, gati, & more. Increasing resistance of Bacteroides species:
		TMP/SMX-DS (bid) or (**CIP** 750 mg bid) + **metro** 500 mg q8h. All po x7-10 d.	**AM/CL** 500/125 mg bid po x7-10 d.	
		Mild-moderate disease—Inpatient Rx (e.g., local peri-appendiceal peritonitis, peri-diverticular abscess, endomyometritis)		
				% Resistant: Cefoxitin Cefotetan Clindamycin 16-87 4-25 16-87
		PIP/TZ 3.375 gm IV q6h or <1.5 gm IV q8h or **AM/SB** 3 gm IV q6h, or **TC/CL** 3.1 gm IV q6h or **erta** 1.0 gm IV qd.	(**CIP** 400 mg IV q12h) or (**levo** 750 mg IV q24h) + **metro** 500 mg IV q6h or 1.0 gm IV q12h	**Ertapenem** less active vs P. aeruginosa/Acinetobacter sp. than IMP or MER. Concomitant surgical management important, esp. with moderate-severe disease. Role of enterococci remains debatable. Probably pathogenic in infections of biliary tract. Probably active vs enterococci in pts with valvular heart disease.
		Severe life-threatening disease, ICU patient:		
		IMP 500 mg IV q6h or **MER** 1 gm IV q8h	**AMP + metro** + **CIP** 400 mg IV q12h or **levo** 750 mg IV q24h) **OR** (**AMP** 2 gm IV q6h + **metro** 500 mg IV q6h + **APAG** (see Table 10C, page 73) See Comment	**Severe penicillin/cephalosporin allergy:** (aztreonam 2.0 gm IV q8h) + (metro 500 mg IV q6h) or (1.0 gm IV q12h)] OR [(CIP 400 mg IV q12h) or (levo 750 mg IV qd) + metro]. Based on in vitro data, could sub gati/moxi for CIP/levo, but insufficient clinical data.

GENITAL TRACT: Mixture of empiric & specific treatment. Divided by sex of the patient.
See Guidelines for Dx of Sexually Transmitted Diseases, *MMWR 51(RR-6), 2002 or CID 35(Suppl.2):S135, 2002*

Both Women & Men:

Chancroid	H. ducreyi	**Ceftriaxone** 250 mg IM single dose OR **azithro** 1.0 gm po single dose	**Cipro** 500 mg bid po x3 d. OR **erythro base** 500 mg po x7 d.	In HIV+ pts, failures reported with single dose azithro & cipro. *Ref.: CID 28(Suppl. 1):S14, 1999*
Chlamydia, et al. non-gonococcal or post-gonococcal urethritis, cervicitis NOTE: Assume concomitant N. gonorrhoeae, see treatment gonorrhea. For conjunctivitis, see *Conjunctiva, page 8*	Chlamydia 50%, Mycoplasma hominis. Other known etiologies (10-15%): Ureaplasma, trichomonas. Herpes simplex virus, Mycoplasma genitalium	**Doxy** 100 mg bid po x7 d.1 or **azithro** 1.0 gm po as single dose. Evaluate & rx sex partner **In pregnancy: erythro base** 500 mg po qid x7 d. OR **amox** 500 mg po	(**Erythro base** 500 mg qid po x7 d.) or (**ofloxx** 300 mg po bid x7 d.) or (**levo** 500 mg qd x7 d.) **In pregnancy: azithro** 1.0 **Doxy** & **oflox** contra-indicated	**Diagnosis:** Methods to detect C. trachomatis & N. gonorrhoeae summarized by CDC: *MMWR 51 (RR-15):1-39, 2002*. For C. trachomatis, a nucleic acid ampl. test (on urine, urethral swab (men) or endocervical swab (women) suggested. Doxy & oflox contraindicated: either in pregnancy, either metro 2.0 gm po x1 + either erythro base 500 mg qid x7 d. or erythro ethylsuccinate 800 mg po qid x7 d.
Recurrent/persistent urethritis	Occult trichomonas, tetra-resistant U. urealyticus	**Metro** 2.0 gm po x1 + **erythro base** 500 mg po qid x7 d.	**Metro** or **erythro ethylsuccinate** 800 mg po qid x7 d.	In men with NGU, 26% infected with trichomonas. **Evaluate & treat sex partners.**
Gonorrhea [*MMWR 51(RR-6), 2002 or CID 35(Suppl.2):S135, 2002*]	N. gonorrhoeae			
Conjunctivitis (adult)		**Ceftriaxone** 1 gm IM or IV x1 + lavage with saline x1		

(Footnotes and abbreviations on page 45)   NOTE: All dosage recommendations are for adults (unless otherwise indicated) and assume normal renal function

TABLE 1 (14)

ANATOMIC SITE/DIAGNOSIS/MODIFYING CIRCUMSTANCES	ETIOLOGIES (usual)	SUGGESTED REGIMENS* PRIMARY	ALTERNATIVE†	ADJUNCT DIAGNOSTIC OR THERAPEUTIC MEASURES AND COMMENTS
GENITAL TRACT/Both Women & Men/Gonorrhea [MMWR 51 (RR-6), 2002] (continued)				
Disseminated gonococcal infection (DGI, dermatitis-arthritis syndrome)	N. gonorrhoeae	[Ceftriaxone 1.0 gm IM or IV q24h) or (cefotaxime 1.0 gm q8h IV) or (ceftizoxime 1.0 gm q8h IV)]—see Comment	Spectinomycin 2.0 gm q12h IM or CIP 400 mg IV q12h or oflox 400 mg IV q12h or levo 250 mg IV q24h—see Comment	Continue IM or IV regimen for 24 hrs after symptoms ↓; reliable pts may be discharged 24 hrs after sx resolve to complete 7 days rx with cefixime[A,6] 400 mg po bid or CIP 500 mg po bid or oflox 400 mg po bid or levo 500 mg po qd. Rx meningitis/ endocarditis. **Treat presumptively for concomitant C. trachomatis.**
Endocarditis	N. gonorrhoeae	Ceftriaxone 1-2 gm IV q12h		If chlamydia not ruled out: Azithro 1 gm po x1 or doxy 100 mg po bid x7 d.
Pharyngitis	N. gonorrhoeae	Ceftriaxone 125 mg IM x1	CIP 500 mg po x1	**Treat for both GC & C. trachomatis. Screen for syphilis.**
Urethritis, cervicitis, proctitis (uncomplicated) For prostatitis, see pages 17, 18 **Diagnosis:** Nucleic acid amplification test on urine or urethral swab—see MMWR 51 (RR-15), 2002	N. gonorrhoeae (50% of pts with urethritis, cervicitis have concomitant C. trachomatis —**treat for both**).	[(Ceftriaxone 125 mg IM x1) or (cefixime[A,6] 400 mg po x1) or (levo 250 mg po x1) or (gati 400 mg po x1)] **PLUS** [(Azithro 1 gm po x1) or (doxy 100 mg po 2x/d x7 days)]	[Ceftizoxime[A,6] 400 mg po x1 or (cefixime[A,6] 400 mg po x1) or (levo 400 mg po x1)] **PLUS**	Other alternatives for GC: Spectinomycin 2 gm IM x1. Other single-dose cephalosporins: ceftizoxime 500 mg IM, cefotaxime 500 mg IM, cefotetan 2 gm IM + probenecid 1 gm po. Other single-dose oral quinolones: lome 400 mg, gati 400 mg, norflox 800 mg. Azithro 1 gm po x1 effective for chlamydia but need 2 gm po for GC, not recommended for GC due to GI side-effects. Due to ↑ resistance, do not use a quinolone to treat gonorrhea that may have been acquired in Hawaii, Asia, other Pacific areas, or England. Resistance refs.: Ln 361:1867, 2003; MMWR 51:1041, 2002
Granuloma inguinale (Donovanosis)	Calymmatobacterium granulomatis	Doxy 100 mg bid po x3 wks OR TMP/SMX-DS 2x/d. x3 wks	Erythro 500 mg po bid po x3 wks OR CIP 750 mg po x3 wks OR azithro 1.0 gm po q wk x3 wks	Clinical response usually seen in 1 week. Rx until all lesions healed, may take 4 weeks. Treatment failures & recurrence seen with doxy and TMP/SMX. Report of efficacy with FQ and chloro. Ref.: DCP 25:24, 1997.
Herpes simplex virus	See Table 14, pages 108-109			
Lymphogranuloma venereum	Chlamydia trachomatis, serovars L1, L2, L3.	Doxy 100 mg bid po x21 d.	Erythro 0.5 gm po x21 d.	Dx based on serology; biopsy contraindicated because sinus tracts develop. Rectal LGV may require re-treatment.
Phthirus pubis (pubic lice, "crabs") & scabies	Phthirus pubis & Sarcoptes scabiei See Table 13, page 109			
Syphilis [MMWR 51(RR-6), 2002; JAMA 290:1510, 2003] Early: primary, secondary, or latent < 1 year	T. pallidum	Benzathine pen G (Bicillin L-A) 2.4 mU IM x1	(Doxy 100 mg bid po x14 d) or (tetracycline 500 mg qid po x14 d) or (ceftriaxone 1.0 gm IM/IV daily x8-10 d). Follow-up mandatory	Every effort should be made to document penicillin allergy before choosing alternative (good alternative data). Early or congenital syphilis pts need quantitative VDRL at general ref., NEJM 326:1060, 1992). Early or congenital syphilis pts need quantitative VDRL at 3, 6, 12, & 24 months after rx. If pt had 1° or 2° VDRL should ↓ 2 tubes at 6 months, 3 tubes at 24 months. Early latent: 2 tubes at 12 months. With 1°: 50% will be RPR-seronegative at 12 months, 24% neg. 1° latent at 2-3 yrs (AnIM 114:1005, 1991). Re-treat if (1) clinical signs persist or recur, (2) a sustained 4-fold ↑ in titer occurs, (3) an initially high titer fails to decrease to <1:8 at 1 year. Ref. on syphilis serology: IDCP 5:351, 1996
More than 1 yr's duration (latent of indeterminate duration, cardiovascular, late benign)		Benzathine pen G (Bicillin L-A) 2.4 mU IM q week x3 = 7.2 mU total	Doxy 100 mg bid po x28 d or tetracycline 500 mg qid po x28 d.	No published data on efficacy of alternatives. The value of routine lumbar puncture in asymptomatic late syphilis is being questioned in the U.S. (Ln 348:1461, 1995), but many would LP (CDC): **neurologic symptoms, treatment failure, serum non-treponemal antibody titer ≥1:32, other evidence of active syphilis (aortitis, gumma, iritis), non-penicillin rx.** Serologic criteria for response to rx: 4-fold or greater ↓ in VDRL titer or 6-12 mos.
Neurosyphilis—Very difficult to treat. Includes ocular (retrobulbar neuritis) syphilis		Pen G 3-4 mU q4h IV x10-14 d.	(Procaine pen G 2.4 mU IM + probenecid 0.5 gm po) both x10-14 d.—See Comment	Ceftriaxone 2.0 gm IV or IM x14 d. 23% failure rate reported (AJM 93:481, 1992). For penicillin allergy, either desensitize to penicillin or obtain infectious diseases consultation.

NOTE: All dosage recommendations are for adults (unless otherwise indicated) and assume normal renal/renal function

(Footnotes and abbreviations on page 45)

TABLE 1 (15)

ANATOMIC SITE/DIAGNOSIS/ MODIFYING CIRCUMSTANCES	ETIOLOGIES (usual)	SUGGESTED REGIMENS* PRIMARY	ALTERNATIVE†	ADJUNCT DIAGNOSTIC OR THERAPEUTIC MEASURES AND COMMENTS
GENITAL TRACT/Both Women & Men/Syphilis (continued)				
HIV infection (AIDS) (SEE SANFORD GUIDE TO HIV/AIDS THERAPY for details)	T. pallidum	Adding 10 d. of **amox + probene-cid** to **pen G** improves eff.	For neurosyphilis, recommendations vary, doses & longer periods of rx may be required. VDRL titer (RPR) at 3, 6, 12, 24 months. Higher	Clinical presentations, serology & response to rx may be atypical (AJM 99:55, 1995).
Pregnancy and syphilis		Same as for non-pregnant, some recommend 2nd dose (2.4 mU) **benzathine pen G** 1 wk after initial dose, esp. in 3rd trimester or with 2°syphilis	Skin test for penicillin allergy. Desensitize if necessary.	titer w/ pallidum fall is uncommon, M. pallidum not uncommon. Erytho should not be used as an alternative agent. Re-treat if needed (AJM 93:481, 1992). (see Syphilis, early (above) for indications). Monthly quantitative VDRL or equivalent. If 4-fold ↑, retreat. Doxy, tetracycline contra-indicated because of high risk of failure to cure fetus.
Congenital syphilis		**Aqueous crystalline pen G** 50,000 u/kg IV q8–12h x10–14 d.	Another alternative: **Ceftriaxone** ≤30 days old 75 mg/kg IV/IM qd or >30 days old 100 mg/kg IV/IM qd. Treat 10–14 d. If symptomatic, ophthalmologic exam indicated. If more than 1 day of rx missed, restart entire course. **Need serologic follow-up!**	
Warts, anogenital		See Table 14, pages 111–112		
Women:				
Amnionitis, septic abortion	Bacteroides, esp. Prevotella bivius; Group B, A strepto-cocci; Enterobacteriaceae; C. trachomatis	(**Cefoxitin** or **TC/CL** or **IMP** or **MER** or **erta** or **PIP/TZ**) ± **doxy**, OR [**Clinda** + (**APAG** or **P Ceph 3**)] Dosage: see footnote¹		D&C of uterus. **In septic abortion,** Clostridium perfringens may cause fulminant intravascular hemolysis. **In postpartum patients** with enigmatic fever and/or pulmonary emboli, **consider septic pelvic vein thrombophlebitis** (see Vascular, septic pelvic vein thrombophlebitis, page 44). After discharge, doxy or combine clinda. **NOTE:** IV clinda effective for C. trachomatis, no data on C for both (CID 19:720, 1994).
Cervicitis, mucopurulent	N. gonorrhoeae C. trachomatis	Treat for gonorrhea, page 15 Treat for non-gonococcal urethritis, page 14		Criteria for dx: yellow or green dc on cervical swab; >10 WBC/oil field. Gram stain for GC. If negative for GC or for C. trachomatis. If in doubt, send swab or urine for culture, EIA or nucleic acid amplification test and rx for both.
Endometritis/septic pelvic phlebitis	Bacteroides, esp. Prevotella bivius; Group B, A strepto-cocci; Enterobacteriaceae; C. trachomatis	(**Cefoxitin** or **TC/CL** or **erta** or **IMP** or **MER** or **AM/SB** or **PIP/TZ**) ± **doxy**, OR [**Clinda** + (**APAG** or **P Ceph 3**)] Dosage: see footnote¹		See Comments under Amnionitis, septic abortion
Early postpartum (1st 48 hrs) (usually after C-section)				
Late postpartum (48 hrs to 6 wks) (usually after vaginal delivery)	Chlamydia tracho-matis, M. hominis	**Doxy** 100 mg q12h IV or po x14 d		Tetracyclines not recommended in nursing mothers; discontinue nursing. M. hominis sensitive to tetra, clinda, not erytho (CID 17:S200, 1993).
Pelvic inflammatory disease (PID), salpingitis, tubo-ovarian abscess	N. gonorrhoeae, chlamydia, bacteroides, Enterobacteri-aceae, streptococci	**Outpatient rx:** [(**Ofloxacin** 400 mg po bid or **levo** 500 mg po qd) + (**metro** 500 mg po bid)] **OR** [(**ceftriaxone** 250 mg IV, or IV or IV x1) + **doxy** 100 mg po bid x14 d.] + **doxy** 100 mg po bid x14 d])	**Inpatient regimens:** [(**Cefotetan** 2 gm IV q12h or **cefoxitin** 2 gm IV q6h) + **doxy** 100 mg IV/po q12h]. [**Clinda** 900 mg IV q8h) + (**gentamicin** 2 mg/kg loading dose, then 1.5 mg/kg q8h) x14 d, then **doxy** 100 mg po bid x14d].	Outpatient rx: limit to pts with temp <38°C, WBC <11,000/mm³, minimal evidence of peritonitis, active bowel sounds & able to tolerate oral nourishment

¹ **P Ceph 2 (cefotetan** 2.0 gm q6–8h IV, **cefotetan** 2.0 gm q12h IV, **cefuroxime** 750 mg q8h IV). **TC/CL** 3.1 gm q6h IV. **AM/SB** 3.0 gm q6h IV. **PIP/TZ** 3.375 gm q6h IV or 4.5 gm q8h IV. **doxy** 100 mg q12h IV or po. **clinda** 450–900 mg q8h IV. **APAG (gentamicin** (see Table IIC, 770 mg IV q8h or 5–7 mg/kg q24h IV) or **gentamicin** 2.0 mg/kg q8h IV. **ceftriaxone** 2.0 gm q8h IV. **cefotaxime** 2.0 gm q8h IV. **ceftriaxone** 2.0 gm q8h IV. **cefotaxime** 2.0 gm q8h IV, **cefotaxime** 1.0 gm q8h IV. **IMP** 0.5 gm q6h IV. **MER**
1.0 gm q8h IV, **azithro** 500 mg IV/d), **linezolid** 600 mg q12h IV/po. **vanco** 1.0 gm q12h IV. **etapenem** 1.0 gm qd IV. **IMP** 0.5 gm q6h IV. **MER**
NOTE: All dosage recommendations are for adults (unless otherwise indicated) and assume normal renal function.
(Footnotes and abbreviations on page 4)

Alternative parenteral regimens:
1. (**Ofloxacin** 400 mg IV q12h or **levo** 500 mg IV qd) + metro 500 mg IV q8h
2. **AM/SB** 3 gm IV q6h + **doxy** 100 mg IV/po q12h + levo
Remember: Evaluate and treat sex partner.

TABLE 1 (16)

ANATOMIC SITE/DIAGNOSIS/ MODIFYING CIRCUMSTANCES	ETIOLOGIES (usual)	SUGGESTED REGIMENS* PRIMARY	ALTERNATIVE§	ADJUNCT DIAGNOSTIC OR THERAPEUTIC MEASURES AND COMMENTS
GENITAL TRACT, Women (continued)				
Vaginitis—MMWR 51(RR-6), 2002 or CID 35 (Suppl 2):S135, 2002				
Candidiasis Pruritus, thick cheesy discharge, pH <4.5 See Table 10	Candida albicans 80–90%. C. glabrata, C. tropicalis may be increasing—they are less susceptible to azoles	**Oral azoles:** **Fluconazole** 150 mg po x1 or **Itraconazole** 200 mg po bid x1 day	**Intravaginal azoles:** variety of strengths—from 1 dose x14 d. Less effective. Other rx for azole-resistant strains: gentian violet, boric acid. If recurrent vulvo-candidiasis (4 or more episodes/yr): 6 mos. suppression with: fluconazole 150 mg po q week or itraconazole 100 mg po qd or clotrimazole vag. suppositories 500 mg q week.	Nystatin vag. tabs x14 d. less effective. Other rx for azole-resistant strains: gentian violet, boric acid. If recurrent vulvo-candidiasis (4 or more episodes/yr): 6 mos. suppression with: fluconazole 150 mg po q week or itraconazole 100 mg po qd or clotrimazole vag. suppositories 500 mg q week.
Trichomoniasis Copious foamy discharge, pH >4.5 Treat sexual partners—see Comment	Trichomonas vaginalis	**Metro** 2.0 gm as single dose or 500 mg po bid x7 d. In pregnancy, defer rx until after 1st trimester	Oral azoles: 2002	**Treat male sexual partners (2.0 gm metronidazole as single dose).** **For Rx failure:** Re-treat with metro 500 mg po bid x7 d. If 2nd failure: **Tinidazole** 500 mg po bid + intravaginal 500 mg po bid x14 d. Available from Panorama Pharm: 800-247-9767. Ref. CID 33:1341, 2001.
Bacterial vaginosis Malodorous vaginal discharge, pH >4.5	Polymicrobic: associated with Gardnerella vaginalis, bacteroides non-fragilis, mobiluncus, peptococci, Mycoplasma hominis	**Metro** 0.5 gm po bid x7 d. or **metro vaginal gel¹** (1 applicator intravaginally [5 gm]) q 24h x5 d. or **clinda vaginal cream²** 1 gm intravaginally hs x7 d.	**Clinda** 0.3 gm po bid x7 d. or **Clinda vaginal ovules** 100 mg intravaginally hs x3 d.	Rx of male sex partner **not indicated** unless balanitis present. Exclude cicatricial balanitis (Reiter's syndrome). Plasma cell balanitis (non-infectious) responds to hydrocortisone cream. **Metro 2.0 gm po x1 not as effective as 5–7 day course** (JAMA 268:92, 1992). Metro extended-release tabs 750 mg po qd x7 d. available; no published data. **Pregnancy:** Rx same as non-pregnancy, except avoid clindamycin cream (↑ risk premature birth). Treatment of asymptomatic pts with oral clinda → premature birth (Ln 361:983, 2003)
Men:				
Balanitis	Candida 40%, Group B strep, gardnerella	Oral azoles as for vaginitis		Occurs in ¼ of male sex partners of women infected with candida. Exclude cicatricial balanitis (Reiter's syndrome). Plasma cell balanitis (non-infectious) responds to hydrocortisone cream.
Epididymo-orchitis				
Age <35 years	N. gonorrhoeae, Chlamydia trachomatis	**Ceftriaxone** 250 mg IM x1 + **doxy** 100 mg po bid x10 d. or **oflox** 300 mg bid po x10 d.		Also: bedrest, scrotal elevation, and analgesics.
Age >35 years or homosexual partner (insertive partners in anal intercourse)	Enterobacteriaceae (coliforms)	**FQ: CIP-ER** 500 mg po 1x/d. or **CIP** 400 mg IV bid or **levo** 750 mg IV/po 1x/d.) x10–14 d.	**AM/SB, P Ceph 3, TC/CL, PIP/TZ** (Dosage: see footnote page 16)	Midstream pyuria and edema. Also: bedrest, scrotal pain and analgesics.
Prostatitis—Review: AJM 106:327, 1999				
Acute	N. gonorrhoeae, C. trachomatis	**Oflox** 400 mg po x1 then 300 mg po bid x10 d. or **cef-triaxone** 250 mg IM x1 then **doxy** 100 mg bid x10 d.		Ofloxacin effective vs gonococci & C. trachomatis and penetrates prostate. In AIDS pts, prostate may be focus of Cryptococcus neoformans.
<35 years of age	N. gonorrhoeae, C. trachomatis	**FQ** (dosage: see Epididymo-orchitis, >35 yrs., above)		Treat as acute urinary infection. 14 days (not single dose regimen). Some authorities recommend 3–4 week rx (IDCP 4:325, 1995).
≥35 years of age	Enterobacteriaceae (coliforms)	**TMP/SMX** 1 DS tablet (160 mg TMP) po x10–14 d.	**TMP/SMX-DS** 1 tab po bid x1–3 mos.	
Chronic bacterial	Enterobacteriaceae 80%, enterococci 15%, P. aeruginosa	**FQ** (CIP 500 mg po x4 wks, **oflox** 300 mg bid po x6 wks)—see Comment		With rx failures consider infected prostatic calculi. Levo mg FDA-approved but should work: dosage unclear—500–750 mg qd.

---

¹ 1 applicator contains 5.0 gm of gel with 37.5 mg metronidazole

NOTE: All dosage recommendations are for adults (unless otherwise indicated) and assume normal renal function

(Footnotes and abbreviations on page 45)

TABLE 1 (17)

ANATOMIC SITE/DIAGNOSIS/ MODIFYING CIRCUMSTANCES	ETIOLOGIES (usual)	SUGGESTED REGIMENS*		ADJUNCT DIAGNOSTIC OR THERAPEUTIC MEASURES AND COMMENTS
		PRIMARY	ALTERNATIVE†	
GENITAL TRACT, Men/Prostatis (continued)				
Chronic prostatitis syndrome (New NIH classification, JAMA 282:236, 1999)	The most common prostatis syndrome. Etiology is unknown; molecular probe data suggest infectious etiology (Clin Micro Rev 11: 604, 1998)	α-adrenergic blocking agents are controversial (AnIM 133:367, 2000)		Pt has sx of prostatitis but negative cultures and no cells in prostatic secretions. Rev.: IJAC 46:157, 2000.
HAND: (Bites: See Skin)				
Paronychia				
Nail biting, manicuring	Staph. aureus, anaerobes	Clinda 300 mg po	Erythro 500 mg qid po	Onset usually 2-5 days after trauma. No lymphangitis.
Contact with oral mucosa—dentists, anesthesiologists, wrestlers	Herpes simplex (Whitlow)	Acyclovir 400 mg tid po x10 days	Famciclovir or valacyclovir should work, see Comment	Gram stain and routine culture negative. Famciclovir/valacyclovir doses used for primary genital herpes should work, see Table 14, page 108
Dishwasher (prolonged water immersion)	Candida sp.	Clotrimazole (topical)		Avoid immersion of hands in water as much as possible
HEART				
Atherosclerotic coronary artery disease	Chlamydia pneumoniae— under study	New name: Chlamydophila pneumoniae. Ref.: JAMA 290:1459 & 1515, 2003		
Infective endocarditis— Native valve—empiric rx awaiting cultures	NOTE: Diagnostic criteria include evidence of continuous bacteremia (multiple positive blood cultures), new murmur (worsening of old murmur) of valvular insufficiency, definite emboli and echocardiographic (transthoracic or transesophageal) evidence of valvular vegetations. Review: NEJM 345:1318, 2001.			
See Table 15 for prophylaxis	Viridans strep 30-40%, enterococci 5-18%, staphylococci 20-35%	[(Pen G 20 mU od IV, continuous or div. q4h) or (AMP 12 gm od IV continuous or div. q4h) + nafcillin or oxacillin 2.0 gm q4h IV) + gentamicin 1.0 mg/kg q8h IM or IV, not once daily dosing)]	Vanco 15 mg/kg q12h (not to exceed 2 gm od unless serum levels monitored) + gentamicin 1.0 mg/kg q8h IM or IV	If patient not acutely ill and not in heart failure, we prefer to wait for blood culture results. If initial 3 blood cultures neg. after 24-48 hrs, obtain 2-3 more blood cultures before empiric rx started. Nafcillin/oxacillin may not be adequate coverage, relative to addition of penicillin G pending cultures. When blood cultures +, modify regimen from empiric to specific based on organism, in vitro susceptibilities, clinical experience.
Infective endocarditis—Native valve—culture positive (Consensus opinion on rx [see Table 17,				
Viridans strep, S. bovis	Viridans strep, S. bovis with penicillin G MIC ≤0.1 μg/ml	[(Pen G 12-18 mU/d IV continuous or q4h x2 wks) PLUS (gentamicin IV 1 mg/kg q8h IV x2 wks)] OR (Pen G 12-18 mU/d IV continuous or q4h x4 wks) OR (ceftriaxone 2.0 gm od IV x4 wks)	Vanco 30 mg/kg IV in 2 div. doses to max. 2 gm/d unless serum levels measured x4 wks	1995/Review: NEJM 345:1318, 2001]/Combination rx: CID 36:615, 2003) Also effective: (ceftriaxone 2.0 gm qd) + (gentamicin[NS] 4 mg/kg qd) x2 wks (CID 21: 1406, 1995). Target gent levels: peak 3 μg/ml, trough <1 μg/ml. If very obese pt, recommend consultation for dosage adjustment.
	Viridans strep, S. bovis with penicillin G MIC >0.1 to <0.5 μg/ml	Pen G 18 mU/d IV (continuous or q4h) PLUS gentamicin 1 mg/kg q8h IV x2 wks NOTE: Low dose of gentamicin	Vanco 30 mg/kg/d IV in 2 div. doses to max, 2 gm/d unless serum levels documented x4 wks	Can use cefazolin for pen G in pt with allergy that is not IgE-mediated (e.g., anaphylaxis). Alternatively, can use vanco. (See Comment above on gent and vanco)
	Viridans strep, S. bovis nutritionally variant streptococci, tolerant strep†	Pen G 18-30 mU/d IV continuous or q4h PLUS gentamicin 1 mg/kg q8h IV x4 wks	Vanco 30 mg/kg/d IV in 2 div. doses to max. 2 gm/d unless serum levels documented x4 wks	

* Assumes estimated creatinine clearance ≥80 ml/min, see Table 17
† Tolerant streptococcus = MBC 32-fold greater than MIC
(Footnotes and abbreviations on page 45)   NOTE: All dosage recommendations are for adults (unless otherwise indicated) and assume normal renal function

TABLE 1 (18)

ANATOMIC SITE/DIAGNOSIS/ MODIFYING CIRCUMSTANCES	ETIOLOGIES (usual)	SUGGESTED REGIMENS PRIMARY	ALTERNATIVE[*]	ADJUNCT DIAGNOSTIC OR THERAPEUTIC MEASURES AND COMMENTS
HEART/Infective endocarditis—Native valve–culture positive *(continued)*				
For viridans strep or S. bovis with pen G MIC ≤0.1 and enterococcus susceptible. AMP: pen G allergic, consider vanco. NOTE: Int. Dis. consultation suggested	Susceptible enterococci, viridans strep, bovis, nutritionally variant streptococci	(Pen G 18–30 mu/24h continuous or div. q4h x4–6 wks) PLUS (gentamicin 1–1.5 mg/kg q8h IV x4–6 wks) OR (AMP 12 gm/24 IV, continuous or div q4h x4–6 wks + gent as above x4–6 wks)	Vanco 30 mg/kg/d IV in 2 div doses to max. of 2 gm/d unless serum levels measured. Target serum levels: peak 20–50 µg/ml, trough 5–12 µg/ml NOTE: Be careful, not all enterococci causing endocarditis should be tested in vitro for susceptibility to penicillin, β-lactamase	4 wks of rx if symptoms <3 mos; 6 wks of rx if symptoms >3 mos. Vanco for pen-allergic pts; do not use cephalosporins Do not give gent once-daily for enterococcal endocarditis. Once-daily gentamicin rx not efficacious in an animal model of E. faecalis endocarditis (JAC 49:437, 2002).
Enterococci: MIC streptomycin >2000 µg/ml, MIC gentamicin >500–2000 µg/ml; no resistance to penicillin	Enterococci, high-level aminoglycoside resistance	Pen G or AMP IV as above x8–12 wks (approx. 50% cure)	If prolonged pen G/AMP fails, consider surgical removal of infected valve. See Comment	Case report of success with combination of AMP, IMP, and vanco (Scand J Inf Dis 29:628, 1997).
Enterococci: β-lactamase production test is positive and no resistance to penicillin	Enterococci, penicillin resistance	AM/SB 3.0 gm q6h IV x4–6 wks PLUS gentamicin 1–1.5 mg/kg q8h IV x4–6 wks Low dose of gent	AM/SB 3.0 gm IV q6h PLUS vanco 30 mg/kg IV in 2 div. doses (check levels if >2 gm)	β-lactamase not detected in E. faecium. Detection requires testing with the chromogenic cephalosporin nitrocefin. Once-daily gentamicin not efficacious in pt with E. faecalis endocarditis (CID 37:e29, 2003).
Enterococci: β-lactamase test neg., pen G/AMP MIC >16 µg/ml; no gentamicin resistance	Enterococci, intrinsic pen G/AMP resistance	Vanco 30 mg/kg/d IV in 2 div. doses PLUS gent 1–1.5 mg/kg q8h IV x4–6 wks	Teicoplanin 6 mg/kg IV q12h x >4 wks (check levels if >2 gm) + gent Teicoplanin is not available in U.S.	Desired vanco serum levels: peak 20–50 µg/ml, trough 5–12 µg/ml
Enterococci: Pen/AMP resistant + high-level gent/strep resistant (vancomycin sensitive) VRE Consultation suggested	Enterococci, vancomycin-resistant, usually E. faecium	No reliable effective rx. Can try Synercid (quinupristin/dalfopristin) (Synercid—see Comment and Table 5, footnote[*]), or linezolid—see Comment. Consultation suggested.	Catclavin 2.0 gm q8h IV x4–6 wks PLUS (gentamicin 1.0 mg/kg IV in 2 doses). Low dose of gent	Synercid activity limited to E. faecium and is usually bacteriostatic, therefore expect high relapse rate. Dose: 7.5 mg/kg IV q8h. **Linezolid** 600 mg IV or po. q12h. Dose: 600 mg 2x/d IV or po. Linezolid active most enterococci, but bacteriostatic.
Staphylococcal endocarditis Aortic and/or mitral valve infection	Staph. aureus, methicillin-sensitive	Nafcillin (oxacillin) 2 gm q4h IV PLUS gentamicin 1 mg/kg q8h IV x3–5 d NOTE: low dose of gent	OR Vanco 30 mg/kg/d IV in 2 doses (check levels if >2 gm) x4–6 wks	Avoid cephalosporins in pts with immediate allergic reaction to penicillin; cefazolin recognition of penicillin rx. At present, favor q8h dosing 3–5 d. If TEE neg., can need 2 wks of therapy in this series.
Tricuspid valve infection (usually IVDUs); MSSA	Staph. aureus, methicillin-sensitive	Nafcillin (oxacillin) 2 gm q4h IV PLUS gentamicin 1 mg/kg q8h IV x2 wks	If penicillin allergic: Not clear, but failure rate with 2-week regimen higher, consider longer duration of rx or vanco x4–6 wks. RIF (if sensitive)	**2-week regimen not recommended** if metastatic infection (e.g. osteo) or **left-sided endocarditis.** Oxacillin IV without gentamicin 89% successful (AnIM 125:969, 1996). CIP 750 mg bid + RIF 300 mg po bid x28d, 20(?). Can tx in 90% of reports of success with 4-week oral regimen. **Daptomycin:** FDA-approved for soft tissue infection.
Methicillin resistance (MRSA)	Staph. aureus, methicillin-resistant	Vanco 30 mg/kg/d IV in 2 div. doses (check levels if >2 gm) x4–6 wks	Fails/intolerant to vanco, can try daptomycin, quinu/dalfo, or linezolid	For MRSA, no difference in duration of bacteremia or fever between pts with vanco or nafcillin rx (CID 17:674, 1991). Daptomycin, Linezolid 600 mg IV or po q12h. Endocarditis studies in progress.

[*] Three interesting recent reports: (1) Successful rx of vanco-resistant E. faecium prosthetic valve endocarditis with Synercid without change in MIC (CID 25:163, 1997); (2) resistance to Synercid emerged during therapy of E. faecium bacteremia (CID 24:91, 1997); and (3) super-infection with vanco-resistant E. faecalis during rx of Synercid rx of E. faecium (CID 24:91, 1997).
[*] **Daptomycin** 6 mg/kg IV (daptomycin (Synercid) IV PLUS ampicillin, mitral valve endocarditis q8h. **Linezolid** 600 mg IV or po q12h.

(footnotes and abbreviations on page 45)   NOTE: All dosage recommendations are for adults (unless otherwise indicated) and assume normal renal function

TABLE 1 (19)

ANATOMIC SITE/DIAGNOSIS/ MODIFYING CIRCUMSTANCES	ETIOLOGIES (usual)	SUGGESTED REGIMENS*		ADJUNCT DIAGNOSTIC OR THERAPEUTIC MEASURES AND COMMENTS
		PRIMARY	ALTERNATIVE†	
HEART, Infective endocarditis—Native valve–culture positive (continued)				
Slow-growing fastidious Gm-neg. bacilli	**HACEK** (see Comments) (Mayo Clin Proc 72: 532, 1997)	**Ceftriaxone** 2.0 gm qd IV x4 wks	**AMP** 12 gm qd (continuous or div. q4h) IV x4 wks + **gentamicin** 1.0 mg/kg q8h IV or IM x4 wks	**HACEK** (acronym for **H**emophilus paraphrophilus, **H. aphrophilus, Actinobacillus, Cardiobacterium, Eikenella, Kingella**). H. aphrophilus should be susceptible to AM/SB + gentamicin. Penicillinase-positive HACEK organisms should be susceptible to AM/SB + gentamicin. For hemophilus, see CID 24:1087, 1997.
Bartonella species [for bacteremia, see page 40—*Urban trench fever*] Ann Int Med 163: 226, 2003; CID 35:684, 2002	B. henselae, B. quintana	Optimal rx evolving. Retrospective study suggest prospective trials for optimal rx. Suggest **gentamicin** 3 mg/kg IV once daily x minimum of 14 days + **doxy** 200 mg po as single dose x28 days		**Dx:** Immunofluorescent antibody titer ≥1:800; blood cultures only occ. positive, or PCR. **Surgery:** Over ½ pts require valve surgery; relation to cure unclear. B. quintana transmitted by body lice among homeless; asymptomatic colonization of RBCs described (Ln 360:226, 2002).
Infective endocarditis—culture negative				
Fever, valvular disease (see ECHO vegetations ± emboli and below), psittacosis, brucellosis, bartonella (see above), fungi	C. whippelii, Q fever (see below), psittacosis, brucellosis, bartonella (see above), fungi	Emphasis on diagnosis. See specific organism for treatment regimens.		For Q fever, see CID 33:1347, 2001. 4 pts with afebrile culture-neg. endocarditis had T. whippelii identified by PCR on resected heart valves (Ln 131:112 & 144, 1999). Review Whipple's endocarditis: CID 33:1309, 2001.
Infective endocarditis—Prosthetic valve—empiric therapy (cultures pending)				
Early (<2 months post-op)	S. epidermidis, S. aureus. Rarely, Enterobacteriaceae, diphtheroids, fungi	**Vanco** 15 mg/kg IV q12h + **gentamicin** 1.0 mg/kg q8h IV + **RIF** 600 mg po daily		Early surgical consultation advised. Watch for evidence of heart failure.
Late (>2 months post-op)	S. epidermidis, viridans strep, enterococci, S. aureus			
Infective endocarditis—Prosthetic valve–positive blood cultures				
Staphylococcal,	Staph. epidermidis	**(Vanco** 15 mg/kg IV q12h + **RIF** 300 mg q8h po) **x6 wks** + **gentamicin** 1.0 mg/kg q8h IV **x14 d.**	If S. epidermidis is susceptible to nafcillin/(oxacillin in vitro (not common), then substitute nafcillin (or oxacillin) for vanco.	
	Staph. aureus	Methicillin sensitive: (**Nafcillin** 2.0 gm q4h IV + **RIF** 300 mg q8h po) **x6 wks** + **gentamicin** 1.0 mg/kg q8h IV **x14 d.** Methicillin resistant: (**Vanco** 1.0 gm q12h IV + **RIF** 300 mg q8h po) **x6 wks** + **gentamicin** 1.0 mg/kg q8h IV **x14 d.**	Methicillin sensitive: substitute nafcillin (or oxacillin) for vanco.	High mortality. Valve replacement plus antifungal therapy standard therapy but some success with antifungal therapy alone (CID 22:262, 1996).
	Enterobacteriaceae or P. aeruginosa	See infective endocarditis, native valve, culture positive, pages 18, 19		
	Candida, aspergillus	**Ampho B** ± an azole, e.g. fluconazole (Table 11, page 77)	In theory, could substitute CIP for APAG, but no clinical data.	
Infective endocarditis—Q fever LnID 3:709, 2003	Coxiella burnetii	**Doxy** 100 mg po bid + **hydroxychloroquine** 600 mg/d, x1.5–3 yrs		**Dx:** Antibody to phase I antigen. Ref. MMWR 51:924, 2002. Surgical resection of infected heart valve does not ensure cure.
Pericarditis, purulent	Staph. aureus, Strep. pneumoniae, Group A strep, Enterobacteriaceae	**(Nafcillin** or **oxacillin)** + **APAG** (Dosage, see footnote)	**IMP** or **TC/CL** or **PIP/TZ** or **AM/SB** or **MER** or **CFP** (see footnote)	Drainage required if signs of tamponade. If MRSA suspected, use vanco 1.0 gm q12h IV
Rheumatic fever with carditis Ref. CID 33:806, 2001 For acute rheumatic fever, see page 41; reactive arthritis p. 21	Post-infectious sequelae of Group A strep infection (usually pharyngitis)	Diuretics, ASA, and usually prednisone 2 mg/kg/d po		Clinical features: Carditis, polyarthritis, chorea, subcutaneous nodules, erythema marginatum. For Jones criteria: Circulation 87:302, 1993. Prophylaxis: see page 41

*APAG (Table 10C, page 73), **IMP** 0.5 gm q6h IV, **MER** 1.0 gm q8h IV, **nafcillin** or **oxacillin** 2.0 gm q4h IV, **TC/CL** 3.1 gm q4-6h IV, **PIP/TZ** 3.375 gm q6h IV or 4.5 gm q8h IV, **AM/SB** 3.0 gm q6h IV, **P Ceph 1 (cephalothin** 2.0 gm q4h IV), **CFP 750** mg bid po or 400 mg bid IV, **vanco** 1.0 gm q12h IV, **azithromycin** 2.0 gm q8h IV, **CFP** 2.0 gm IV q12h.
NOTE: All dosage recommendations are for adults (unless otherwise indicated) and assume normal renal/renal function.

(Footnotes and abbreviations on page 45)

TABLE 1 (20)

ANATOMIC SITE/DIAGNOSIS/ MODIFYING CIRCUMSTANCES	ETIOLOGIES (usual)	SUGGESTED REGIMENS*		ADJUNCT DIAGNOSTIC OR THERAPEUTIC MEASURES AND COMMENTS
		PRIMARY	ALTERNATIVE†	
JOINT—Also see Lyme Disease, page 39				
Reactive arthritis				
Reiter's syndrome (See Comment for definition)	Occurs wks after infection with C. tra- chomatis, Campylobacter jejuni, Yersinia enterocolitica, Shigella/Salmonella.	Only treatment is non-steroidal anti-inflammatory drugs		Definition: Urethritis, conjunctivitis, arthritis, and sometimes uveitis and rash. Arthritis: asym- metrical oligoarthritis of ankles, knees, feet, sacroiliitis. Rash: palms and soles—keratoderma blennorrhagica, circinate balinitis of glans penis. HLA-B27 positive predisposes to Reiter's.
Poststreptococcal reactive arthritis	Immunologic reaction after strep pharyn- gitis. (1) arthritis onset in <10 days, (2) lasts months, not responsive to ASA	Treat strep pharyngitis (prednisone needed in some pts)		A reactive arthritis after a β-hemolytic strep infection in absence of sufficient Jones criteria for acute rheumatic fever. Ref.: Mayo Clin Proc 75:144, 2000.
Acute Rheumatic Fever, see page 20				
Septic arthritis: Treatment requires both adequate drainage of purulent joint fluid and appropriate antimicrobial therapy.				
of blood and joint fluid but for culture, review Gram stain of joint fluid. For full differential, see JAMA 297:1478, 2007				There is no need to inject antimicrobials into joints. Empiric therapy after collection
Infants <3 months (neonate)	Staph. aureus, Enterobac- teriaceae, Group B strep, N. gonorrhoeae	**(Nafcillin or oxacillin) + P Ceph 3** (Dosage, see Table 16, page 129)	**Nafcillin or oxacillin + APAG** (If MRSA prevalent, use vanco in place of nafcillin/ oxacillin).	Blood cultures frequently positive. Adjacent bone involved in 2/3 pts. Group B strep and gonococci most common community-acquired etiologies.
Children (3 months–14 years)	Staph. aureus 27%, S. pyo- genes & S. pneumo 14%, H. influenzae 3% (was 41% pre- H. influenzae vaccine), Gm-neg. bacilli 6%, other (GC, N. men- ingitidis) 14%, unknown 36%	**(Nafcillin or oxacillin) + P Ceph 3**	**Vanco + P Ceph 3** See Table 16 for dosage Steroids ?—see Comment	Marked ↓ in H. influenzae since use of conjugate vaccine. NOTE: Septic arthritis due to salmonella has no association with sickle cell disease, unlike salmonella osteomyelitis. Duration of treatment varies with specific microbial etiology. Short-course steroid: Benefit reported (PIDJ 22:883, 2003).
Adults (review Gram stain): See page 39 for Lyme Disease				
Acute monoarticular				
At risk for sexually- transmitted disease	N. gonorrhoeae (see page 15), S. aureus, streptococci, rarely aerobic Gm-neg. bacilli	**Gram stain negative:** Ceftriaxone 1.0 gm IV or cefotaxime 1.0 gm q8h IV or **ceftizoxime 1.0** gm q8h IV	If Gram stain shows Gm+ cocci in clusters: **nafcillin** (or oxacillin) 2.0 gm q4h IV	For rx comments, see Disseminated GC, page 15
Not at risk for sexually- transmitted disease	S. aureus, streptococci, Gm-neg. bacilli	**Nafcillin/oxacillin + P Ceph 3** For treatment duration, see Table 3 For dosage see footnote page 23	**Nafcillin/oxacillin – CIP**	Differential includes gout and chondrocalcinosis (pseudogout). Look for crystals in joint fluid. Levo has appropriate in vitro spectra and should work, but no clinical data. NOTE: Substitute vanco for nafcillin/oxacillin if MRSA suspected or proven. For bites, see page 35
Chronic monoarticular	Brucella, nocardia, myco- bacteria, fungi.		See Tables 2, 11, & 12	
Polyarticular, usually acute	**Gonococci.** B. burgdorferi, acute rheumatic fever, disseminated N. gonorrhoeae, B19 virus, hepatitis B, rubella vaccine, parvo B19	Gram stain usually negative for GC. If sexually active, culture urethra, cervix, anal canal, throat, blood, joint fluid, and then: ceftriaxone 1.0 gm IV daily		If GC, usually associated petechiae and/or pustular skin lesions and tenosynovitis. Lyme disease (if exposure areas known to harbor infected ticks. See page 39. Expanded differential includes gout, pseudogout, reactive arthritis (HLA-B27 pos).
Prosthetic joint, postoperative or infection post intra-articular injection (CID 36[Suppl 2]:S94, 2001)	MSSE/MRSE 40%, MSSA/ MRSA 20%, Enterobacteri- aceae, Pseudomonas sp.	**Vanco + CIP** (or aztreo- nam or APAG or CFP) (for dosage, see footnote page 23)	**[CIP 750 mg bid po + RIF 900 mg x1(1 po) or oflox 400 mg po + RIF 900 mg x1.(1 po)]**	For infections after intra-articular injections, arthroscopy or joint washout, and treatment depends on extent of infection. Most infections at bone-prosthesis interface = osteomyelitis. 2 strategies: open debridement, prosthesis retention, 6 wks antibiotics vs 2-stage exchange arthroplasty with 6 wks antibiotics (see CID 32:419–430, 2001; CID 35[Suppl 2]:S94, 2001).
Empiric rx, no culture data		**Culture first isolation/in vitro susceptibility of etiologic organisms essential.**		Management after joint aspiration if acute 4 days. **Prosthetic joint** remains variable.

NOTE: All dosage recommendations are for adults (unless otherwise indicated) and assume normal renal function

(Footnotes and abbreviations on page 45)

TABLE 1 (21)

ANATOMIC SITE/DIAGNOSIS/ MODIFYING CIRCUMSTANCES	ETIOLOGIES (usual)	SUGGESTED REGIMENS*		ADJUNCT DIAGNOSTIC OR THERAPEUTIC MEASURES AND COMMENTS
		PRIMARY	ALTERNATIVE†	
JOINT/Prosthetic joint, postoperative or infection post intra-articular injection (continued)				
Culture results known: NOTE: Salvage of prosthesis unlikely after ~2 wks of symptomatic infection (CID 29:292 & 296, 1999)	[MRSA/MRSE or MSSA] MSSE] **CIP/RIF suscep- tible**	FQ + RIF] in dosage on previous page for Empiric rx (Footnote, page 20), then	Oxacillin 2.0 gm q4h IV + RIF 900 mg x1/d. po	Data on staph species infection of stable implants treated by debridement and prolonged oral antimicrobials: (1) po RIF + oflox x3-9 mos., 74% success (AAC 37:1214, 1993); (2) Initial IV nafcillin/oxacillin or vanco, then CIP + RIF x3 mos. (hip) or 6 mos. (knee). Cure in 100% (knee) & 69% (hip) (JAMA 279:1537 & 1575, 1998). (3) po TMP/SMX (20 mg/kg/d of TMP) successful in 2/3 pts with staph species (AAC 42:3086, 1998). Most S. aureus are sensitive to MSSE/MRSE; most MRSA and roughly ⅙ of MSSE/MRSE are resistant to RIF.
	[MRSA/MRSE or MSSA/ MSSE] **CIP resistant**	Vanco + RIF (no published studies)	Another alternative: Linezolid + RIF (no published studies)	
Rheumatoid arthritis	Treatment with TNF inhibitors (adalimumab, etanercept, infliximab) increases risk of disseminated tuberculosis or invasive fungal infection.			
Septic bursitis	Staph. aureus ~80%, M. tuberculosis (rare), M. marinum (rare)	oxacillin or oxacillin 2 gm IV q4h or dicloxacillin 500 mg qid	Cefazolin 2 gm IV q8h or vanco 1 gm IV q12h or CIP 750 mg q12h po or CIP 300 mg po bid po	Initially aspirate daily and treat for a minimum of 2-3 weeks. If recurrence, surgical excision of bursa may be necessary often if treated for 3 weeks + RIF. Ref.: Semin Arth & Rheum 24:391, 1995.
Other doses, see footnote page 23				
KIDNEY, BLADDER AND PROSTATE [For review, see AJM 113(Suppl 1A):1S, 2002 & NEJM 349:259, 2003]				
Acute uncomplicated urinary tract infection (cystitis-urethritis) [NOTE: Routine urine culture not necessary; self-rx works (AnIM 135:9, 2001)]				
NOTE: **Resistance of E. coli** to TMP/SMX approx. 15–20% (CID 36:183, 2003) & corre- lates with microbiological/ clinical failure (CID 34:1061 & 1165, 2002). **Recent reports of E. coli resistant to CIP & levo**	Enterobacteriaceae (E. coli) Staph. saprophyticus, enterococci	If local E. coli resistant to TMP/SMX <20%, **TMP/SMX-DS** 1 tab po bid x3 d. If resistant >20%, use **FQ x3 d**: **CIP 250** mg bid or **CIP-ER 500** mg qd, **levo 250** mg qd, **ofIox 200** mg bid po. Most: See Comment	**TMP/SMX-DS** 1 tab bid x3 d. Other options: **O Ceph. NF TMP** or **AM/CL** Usual dura- tion of rx is 3 d. for dosage, see footnote d.	7-day rx recommended in pregnancy [discontinue or do not use sulfonamides (TMP/SMX) near term (2 weeks before EDC) because of potential ↑ in kernicterus]. If failure on 3-day course, culture and rx 2 weeks. **Fosfomycin** 3.0 gm po x1 less effective vs E. coli than multi-dose TMP/SMX or FQ (Med Lett 39:66, 1997). **Moxifloxacin & gemifloxacin:** Neither approved for UTIs. Do not use; inadequate urine concentration. c. Phenazopyridine (Pyridium)—non-prescription—may relieve dysuria. 200 mg tid x2 days. d. Hemolysis if G6PD deficient.
Risk factors for STD. Dipstick: positive leucocyte esterase or hemoglobin	C. trachomatis	**Doxy** 100 mg bid x7	**Azithro** 1.0 gm single dose	Pelvic exam for vaginitis & herpes simplex, urine LCR/PCR for GC and C. trachomatis.
Recurrent (3 or more episodes/ year) in young women	Any of the above bacteria	Eradicate infection, then TMP/SMX tab od pro long term	TMP/SMX single-strength tab po qd	A cost-effective alternative to continuous prophylaxis is self-administered single dose rx (TMP/SMX DS, 2 tabs, 320/1600 mg) at symptom onset. Another alternative: 1 DS tablet, TMP/SMX post-coitus.
Child ≤5 yrs and grade 3-4 reflux	Coliforms	**TMP/SMX**		Definition: ≥3 culture + symptomatic UTIs in 1 year or 2 UTIs in 6 months.
Recurrent UTI in postmenopausal women. See CID 30:152, 2000	E. coli & other Enterobac- teriaceae, enterococci, S. saprophyticus	Treat as for uncomplicated UTI. Evaluate for potentially correctable urologic factors—see Comment. NF not effective if creatinine clearance <50; in increasing frequency, but Editors worry about pulmonary fibrosis with long-term NF rx (CID 36:1362, 2003).		Urologic factors: (1) cystocele, (2) incontinence, (3) residual urine volume (≥50 ml).

* **O Ceph** listed in Table 10B, page 68; **nitrofurantoin** 100 mg po qid or sustained release 100 mg po bid; **TMP** 100 mg po bid; **doxy** 100 mg po bid; **AM/CL** 875/125 mg po bid (severe infection) or 500/125 mg po bid (mild infection)   NOTE: All dosage recommendations are for adults (unless otherwise indicated) and assume normal/renal function
* (Footnotes and abbreviations on page 45)

TABLE 1 (22)

ANATOMIC SITE/DIAGNOSIS/ MODIFYING CIRCUMSTANCES	ETIOLOGIES (usual)	SUGGESTED REGIMENS		ADJUNCT DIAGNOSTIC OR THERAPEUTIC MEASURES AND COMMENTS
		PRIMARY	ALTERNATIVE[1]	
KIDNEY, BLADDER AND PROSTATE (continued)				
Acute uncomplicated pyelonephritis (usually women 18–40 yrs. temperature >102°F; definite costovertebral tenderness)				[NOTE: Culture of urine and blood indicated prior to therapy. Report of hemolytic uremic syndrome as result of toxin-producing E. coli UTI (NEJM 335,635, 1996).]
Moderately ill (outpatient)	Enterobacteriaceae (most likely E. coli)	An **FQ** po x 7 d, **CIP** 500 mg bid or **CIP-ER** 1000 mg q24h, **levo** 250 mg qd, **oflox** 400 mg bid	**AM/CL, O Ceph,** or **TMP/SMX-DS.** Treat for 14 days.	In randomized double-blind trial, bacteriologic and clinical success higher for 7 days of oral CIP than for 14 days of TMP/SMX; failures correlated with TMP/SMX in vitro resistance (JAMA 283:1583, 2000).
NOTE: Increasing resistance of E. coli to both TMP/SMX & FQs is a concern	(Gm (–) urinary **unfringed** urine may allow identification of Gm-neg. bacilli vs Gm(+) cocci.)			Since CIP worked with 7-d. rx, suspect other FQs effective with 7 d. of rx. Do not use more due to low concentrations.
Hospitalized	E. coli most common, enterococci 2nd in frequency	**FQ** (IV) or (**AMP** + **gent**-**ate** or **P Ceph 3**) or **TC/CL** or **AP Pen.** Treat for 14 d.	**TC/CL** or **AM/SB** or **PIP/TZ** or **erta.** Treat for 14 d. Dosages in footnote[1]	Treat IV until afebrile 24–48 hrs; then complete 2-wk. course with oral drugs (as above). If no clinical improvement in 3 days, we recommend imaging. On CT if single focal mass-like lesion & moderately ill, response 13 d. (AJM 93:289, 1992). **If pt hypotensive, prompt imaging (Echo or CT) is recommended to ensure absence of obstructive uropathy.**
		Do not use P Ceph 3 for suspect or proven enterococcal infection		**NOTE: P Ceph 3 & ertapenem not active vs enterococci.**
Complicated UTI/catheters	Enterobacteriaceae, P. aeruginosa, enterococci	(**AMP** + **gent**) or **PIP/TZ** or **TC/CL** or **IMP** or **MER** x2–3 wks	[IV **FQ: CIP, gati, levo,** x2–3 Dosages in footnote[1] For dosages, see footnote[1]	Rule out obstruction. Watch out for enterococci and P. aeruginosa—not all listed drugs have predictable activity. **CIP-ER dose: 1000 mg qd**
Obstruction, reflux, azotemia, transplant, Foley catheter-related		Switch to **FQ** or **TMP/SMX** when possible	Switch to **FQ** or **TMP/SMX** when possible	
Asymptomatic bacteriuria Preschool children		Base regimen on C&S, not empirical		Diagnosis requires ≥10⁵ CFU/ml urine of same bacterial species in 2 specimens obtained 3–7 days apart.
Pregnancy	Aerobic Gm-neg. bacilli & Staph. hemolyticus	Screen 1st trimester. If positive, rx 3 d. with **amox, NF O Ceph, TMP/SMX,** or **TMP** alone		Screen monthly for recurrence. Some authorities treat continuously until delivery (stop TMP/SMX 2 wks before EDC). ↑ resistance of E. coli to TMP/SMX.
Before and after invasive urologic intervention, e.g.,	Aerobic Gm-neg. bacilli	Obtain urine culture and then rx 3 d. with TMP/SMX/DS bid		In one study, single dose of TMP/SMX DS 80% effective (AnIM 114:713, 1991). Use of silver-alloy Foley catheter may ↓ risk of clinically significant bacteriuria (AJM 105:236, 1998; AIM 160:3294, 2000).
Neurogenic bladder	No rx if asymptomatic	No rx if asymptomatic; intermittent catheterization if possible		Ref.: AJM 113(1A):67S, 2002
Symptomatic, advanced age, male or female	No rx indicated unless in conjunction with surgery to correct obstructive uropathy; measure residual urine vol. in females; prostate exam/PSA in males.			
Malacoplakia	E. coli	**Bethanechol chloride** + **CIP** or **TMP/SMX**	**Vanco**	Chronic pyelo; often with abnormal inflammatory response. See CID 29:444, 1999
Perinephric abscess				
Associated with staphylococcal bacteremia	Staph. aureus	**Nafcillin/oxacillin** or **P Ceph 1** (Dosage, see footnote[1])	**Vanco**	Drainage, surgical or image-guided aspiration
Associated with pyelonephritis	Enterobacteriaceae	See pyelonephritis, complicated UTI, above		Drainage, surgical or image-guided aspiration
Prostatitis		See prostatitis, pages 17–18		

---

[1] **AM/CL** IV 875/125 mg q12h or 500/125 mg tid po, **aztreonam** 2.0 gm IV q6h, **FQ (IV): CIP** 400 mg bid, **gati** 400 mg IV, **levo** (250 mg qd for mild uncomplicated disease, 500 mg qd for hospital **Ceph 3 cefotaxime** 1.0 gm IV q8h or **ceftriaxone** 1.0 gm IV q24h) (for life-threatening infections, **ceftriaxone** 2.0 gm IV q24h) (use 2.0 gm under age 65). **AP Pen** (**PIP** 3.0 gm q4h IV, **AM/SB** 3.0 gm q6h IV, **PIP/TZ** 3.375 gm q6h or 4.5 gm q8h IV, **gentamicin** (see Table 9C, page 71), **TMP/SMX** 2.0 mg/kg (TMP) q6h IV, **P Ceph 3 AP ceftazidime** 2.0 gm q8h IV, **CFP** 2.0 gm q12h IV), **erta** 1.0 gm qd IV, **Nafcillin** or **oxacillin** 2.0 gm q4h IV. For oral cephalosporin dosages, see Table 9B, page 66. **Dicloxacillin** 500 mg po qid. **Metronidazole** 500 mg po qid. **MER** 1.0 gm IV q12h, **linezolid** 600 mg IV/po q12h. **Vanco** 1.0 gm IV q12h. (unless otherwise indicated) and assume normal renal function

(Footnotes and abbreviations on page 45)

TABLE 1 (23)

ANATOMIC SITE/DIAGNOSIS/ MODIFYING CIRCUMSTANCES	ETIOLOGIES (usual)	SUGGESTED REGIMENS*		ADJUNCT DIAGNOSTIC OR THERAPEUTIC MEASURES AND COMMENTS
		PRIMARY	ALTERNATIVE¹	
LIVER (for spontaneous bacterial peritonitis, see page 31)				
Cholangitis		See Gallbladder, page 31		
Hepatic abscess	Enterobacteriaceae, bacteroides, enterococci, Entamoeba histolytica, Yersinia enterocolitica (rare) For echinococcus, see Table 13, page 99. For calcio-scratch disease (CSD), see pages 30 & 38.	Metro + (P Ceph 3 or cefoxitin or PIP/TZ or AM/SB or TC/CL or IMP/CIL Metro + APAG + metro traditional & effective but AMP-resistant Gm-neg. bacilli increasing.	Metro (for amoeba) + either IMP or MER (Dosage, see footnote page 23)	**Serological tests for amebiasis should be done on all patients;** if neg, surgical drainage or percutaneous aspiration. In pyogenic abscess, ½ have identifiable GI source. If amoeba serology positive, treat with metro alone without surgery. Metro included for both E. histolytica & bacteroides. **Hemochromatosis** associated with Yersinia enterocolitica liver abscess (CID 18:938, 1994); regimens listed are effective for yersinia.
Leptospirosis, see page 40	Leptospirosis, see page 40			
Peliosis hepatis in AIDS pts	Bartonella henselae and B. quintana	See page 38		
Viral hepatitis	Hepatitis A, B, C, D, E, G	See Table 14		
LUNG/Bronchi				
Bronchiolitis/wheezy bronchitis (expiratory wheezing) Infants/children (≤ age 5)	**Respiratory syncytial virus** (RSV) 50%, parainfluenza 25%, other viruses 20%	Antibiotics not useful, mainstay of rx is oxygen. Ribavirin of no benefit (AJRCCM 160:829, 1999). 2 products available for prevention: **RSV-immune globulin** and a humanized mouse monoclonal antibody, **palivizumab**. See Table 14, page 112		RSV most important. Rapid dx with antigen detection methods. Ribavirin: No data on IV ribavirin but little enthusiasm. Emphasis now on vaccine development and preventive modulation with immunoglobulins. Reviews: PIDJ 19:773, 2000; Red Book of Peds 2002, 26ʰ Ed.
Bronchitis Infants/children (≤ age 6)	≤ Age 2: Adenovirus, age 2–5: Respiratory syncytial virus, parainfluenza 3 virus.	Antibiotics indicated only with associated sinusitis or heavy growth on throat culture for S. pneumo, Group A strep, H. influenzae, or no improvement in 1 week. Otherwise rx is symptomatic.		
Adolescents and adults with acute tracheobronchitis (Acute bronchitis) Ref., AJM 162:256, 2002; AnIM 134:521, 2001	Usually viral. No pneumonia 5%; C. pneumoniae 5%. See Persistent cough, below	Antibiotics not indicated. Antitussives ± inhaled bronchodilators		Purulent sputum alone not an indication for antibiotic rx. Azithro was no better than low-dose vitamin C in a controlled trial (Ln 359:1648, 2002). Expect cough to last 2 weeks. If fever/rigors, get chest x-ray. M. pneumoniae & C. pneumoniae ref.: Ln ID 1:334, 2001. Rare pt with true C. pneumo infection may require 6 wks of clarithro to clear organism (J Med Micro 52:265, 2003).
Persistent cough (>14 d.), afebrile during community outbreak: Pertussis (whooping cough) 10–20% adults with cough >14 d. (AnIM 128:1691, 2001). Rev.: Ln ID 2:744, 2002	Bordetella pertussis: occ. Bordetella parapertussis. Also consider asthma, gastroesophageal reflux, post-nasal drip	Peds doses: Azithro OR clarithro OR erythro estolate po 40 mg/kg/d div q6-12h x14 d. OR TMP/SMX 8 mg/kg/d div. q6h x14 d	Adult doses: Erythro estolate 500 mg qid x14 d. OR TMP/SMX-DS 1 tab bid x14 d. OR (clarithro 500 mg po bid or 1.0 gm ER qd x7 d.)	**3 stages of illness:** catarrhal (1–2 wks), paroxysmal coughing (2–4 wks), and convalescence (1–2 wks). Pts most contagious during catarrhal stage: erythro does not shorten paroxysmal stage if started during paroxysmal stage, but may ↓ pharyngeal secretions of C. pertussis–toxin (antitox). **Rx aimed at decreasing spread by eradicating nasopharyngeal carriage.** Hypertrophic pyloric stenosis reported in infants under 6 wks of age given erythro (MMWR 48:1117, 1999).
Prophylaxis of household contacts		**Erythromycin—Children:** clarithro 7.5 mg/kg po bid x14 d. **Alternative: clarithro** 7.5 mg/kg po bid x14 d. **See footnote**		Recommended by Am. Acad. Ped. Red Book 2003 for all household or close contacts, community-wide prophylaxis not recommended.

¹ Peds doses: azithro 10 mg/kg/d day 1, then 5 mg/kg 1x/d. x4 d. (PIDJ 22:847, 2003) or clarithro 7.5 mg/kg po bid x5–7 d.
² Compliance with erythro poor due to nausea/vomiting; clarithro costs more but compliance should be better.
(Footnotes and abbreviations on page 45)   NOTE: All dosage recommendations are for adults (unless otherwise indicated) and assume normal renal function

TABLE 1 (24)

ANATOMIC SITE/DIAGNOSIS/ MODIFYING CIRCUMSTANCES	ETIOLOGIES (usual)	SUGGESTED REGIMENS*		ADJUNCT DIAGNOSTIC OR THERAPEUTIC MEASURES AND COMMENTS
		PRIMARY	**ALTERNATIVE†**	
LUNG/Bronchi/Bronchitis (continued) **Acute bacterial exacerbation of chronic bronchitis (AECB), adults** (almost always when with COPD) Refs.: AnM 134:595 & 600, 2001; NEJM 346:988, 2002; AnM 1:62:256, 2002	Viruses 20–50%, C. pneumoniae <1%, S. pneumo, H. influenzae & M. catarrhalis controversial. Tobacco use, air pollution contribute.	**Severe AECB** = ↑ dyspnea, ↑ sputum volume, ↑ sputum viscosity/purulence. For severe AECB: (1) consider chest x-ray, esp. if febrile &/or low O₂ sat, (2) inhaled anticholinergic bronchodilator vs non-invasive positive pressure ventilation. Role of antimicrobial rx debated even for severe disease, no antimicrobial treatment or maybe amox, doxy, TMP/SMX, or O Ceph. For severe disease, AM/CL, azithro, clarithro, or O Ceph with enhanced activity vs drug-resistant S. pneumo: see Comment. Drug & doses in footnote¹. Duration varies with drug; range 3–10 d.		For severe ABECB: (1) consider chest x-ray, esp. if febrile (2) oral corticosteroid, taper over 2 wks.; (4) D/C tobacco use; (5) non-invasive positive pressure ventilation.
Pneumonia				Role of antimicrobial treatment or maybe no antimicrobial treatment or maybe
Neonatal: Birth to 1 month	CMV, rubella, H. simplex Bacteria: Group B strep, listeria, coliforms, S. aureus, P. aeruginosa Other: Chlamydia trachomatis, syphilis	**AMP + gentamicin** ‡ **cefotaxime** If MRSA a concern. For chlamydia rx, **erythro** 12.5 mg/kg po or IV qid x14 d.	**vanco** (add)	Blood cultures indicated. Consider C. trachomatis if afebrile pneumonia, staccato cough, IgM > 1:8; rx with erythro or sulfisoxazole. If MRSA documented, **vanco**. **TMP/SMX**, & **linezolid** alternatives. **Linezolid** dosage birth to age 11 yrs is **10 mg/kg q8h**. Ref.: PIDJ 22(Suppl.)S158, 2003.

CONSIDER TUBERCULOSIS IN ALL PATIENTS; ISOLATE ALL SUSPECT PATIENTS

Age 1–3 months Pneumonitis syndrome. Usually afebrile.	C. trachomatis, RSV, parainfluenza virus 3, Bordetella, S. pneumoniae, S. aureus (rare)	**Outpatient: po erythro** 10 mg/kg q6h or po **azithro** 10 mg/kg x1, then 5 mg/kg x4 d.	**Inpatient: If afebrile erythro** 10 mg/kg IV q6h or **azithro** 2.5 mg/kg IV q12h **If febrile,** add **cefotaxime** 200 mg/kg/d div q8h	Pneumonitis syndrome: cough, tachypnea, dyspnea, diffuse infiltrates, afebrile. Usually requires hospital care. Reports of hypertrophic pyloric stenosis after erythro under age 6 wks: not sure about azithro. If lobar pneumonia, give AMP 200–300 mg/kg/d div q6h. No azithro/ coverage for S. aureus, as it is rare etiology.
Age 4 months–5 years For RSV, see bronchiolitis, page 24, & Table 14, page 24, NEJM 346:429, 2002	RSV, other resp. viruses, S. pneumo, H. flu, myco- plasma, S. aureus (rare), M. tbc	For RSV, see bronchiolitis. **Outpatient: Amox** 100 mg/kg/d po q8h. **Inpatient (not ICU):** No antibiotic if viral. If bacterial, AMP 200 mg/kg/d div q6h	**Inpatient (ICU): Cefotaxime** 200 mg/kg/d IV div q8h or **ceftriaxone** 50–75 mg/kg/d IV 1x/d.	Common 'other' viruses: rhinovirus, influenza, parainfluenza, adenovirus (PIDJ 19: 293, 2000). Often of mild to moderate severity. S. pneumo, non-type B H. flu in 4–21%: test x10–14 d. NOTE: High frequency of resistance of DRSP to ceftriaxome. See footnote†, footnote 1 page 24, footnote¹ page 26, and Table 5, page 55, for rx of drug-resistant S. pneumo.
Age 5 years–15 years, Non-hospitalized, immunocompetent NEJM 346:429, 2002; PIDJ 21:592, 2002	Mycoplasma, Chlamydo- phila pneumoniae, S. pneumo, Mycobac- terium tuberculosis	**(Amox** 100 mg/kg/d) + **(Clarithro** 500 mg po bid or 1 gm ER qd). Peds dose: 7.5 mg/kg q12h **OR (azithro** 10 gm po x1 (max 500 mg), then 5 mg/kg/d (max. 250 mg)	**(Doxy** 100 mg/kg/d) in pts >8 yrs old) or **erythro** 500 mg po q6h]	If otherwise healthy and if not concomitant with post-influenza. S. pneumoniae uncommon in this subset; suspect S. pneumo if sudden onset and large amount of purulent sputum, macrolide-resistant S. pneumo in pts <5 yrs old (JAMA 286:1857, 2001). Mycoplasma PCR/viral culture usually not done for outpatients. Mycoplasma requires 2–3 wks of rx. C. pneumoniae up to 6 wks. (Ln ID 1:334, 2001; J Med Micro 52:265, 2003).

| | See Comment regarding macrolide resistance | | | |

---

¹ **TMP/SMX**, 1 double-strength tab (160 mg TMP) bid po. **doxy** 100 mg bid po. **amox** 500 mg tid po. adult dose of **O Ceph** [**cefaclor** 500 mg q8h or 500 mg CD (extended release) q12h po. **cefdinir** 300 mg bid, or 600 mg qd po. **cefixime** 400 mg qd po. **cefpodoxime** 200 mg q12h po. **loracarbef** 400 mg q12h po. **cefprozil** 250–500 mg q12h po. **cefuroxime axetil** 250 or 500 mg q12h po. **ceftibuten** 400 mg qd po]. **AM/CL** 875/125 mg bid or 500/125 mg tid po. **AM/CL-ER** two 1000/62.5 mg tabs q12h po. **levo** 500 mg qd po x7 d. **dirithromycin** 500 mg qd x7 d. **clarithro** ER 1000 mg qd x7 d; or regular dose then 250 mg x4 d. **clarithro** 500 mg q12h po x14 d. **clarithro** 500 mg bid po. **gati** 400 mg qd po. **gemi** 320 mg qd po. **levo** 500 mg qd po. **moxi** 400 mg qd po.

Ketolide: Telithromycin 800 mg po x5 d.

NOTE: CIP and cefibuten have relatively poor activity vs S. pneumo.

* All dosage recommendations are for adults (unless otherwise indicated) and assume normal renal function
NOTE: All dosage recommendations are for adults (unless otherwise indicated) and assume normal renal function
(Footnotes and abbreviations on page 45)

TABLE 1 (25)

ANATOMIC SITE/DIAGNOSIS/ MODIFYING CIRCUMSTANCES	ETIOLOGIES (usual)	SUGGESTED REGIMENS*		ADJUNCT DIAGNOSTIC OR THERAPEUTIC MEASURES AND COMMENTS
		PRIMARY	ALTERNATIVE†	
LUNG/Pneumonia (continued) Hospitalized, Immunocompetent	S. pneumoniae, viruses, S. pneumoniae, S. aureus if abscesses or necrotizing	**Cephalosporins** 50 mg/kg/d IV (to max. 2 gm/d) or Vanco 40 mg/kg/d IV q6h to 500 mg + IV div q12h, Add anti-staph drug if evidence of lung necrosis	**Alternatives are a problem in children:** No doxy under age 8, no FQs under age 18. For S. pneumo, MIC ≥2 μg/ml, see Table 5, page 55 for options; e.g., Vanco. Linezolid reported efficacious in children (PIDJ 22:677, 2003). Cefotaxime failures vs DRSP (CID 29:482, 1999).	
Adults (over age 18)—See IDSA Guidelines (CID 37:1405, 2003) Community-acquired, not hospitalized Empiric therapy	Varies with clinical setting. Atypicals—M. pneumoniae, et al., S. pneumo, viral Alcoholism: S. pneumo, anaerobes, coliforms Bronchiectasis: see Cystic fibrosis COPD: H. influenzae, M. catarrhalis, S. pneumo MDU: Hematogenous S. aureus Post-CVA aspiration: Oral flora, anaerobes Post-obstruction of bronchi: S. pneumo, anaerobes Post-viral: e.g., influenza	**No co-morbidity:** **Azithro** 0.5 gm po x1, then 0.25 gm/d OR **clarithro** 500 mg po bid or clarithro-ER 1 gm po qd OR **doxy** 100 mg po bid **OR** if antibiotic within 3 months: **azithro** or **clarithro** + **H** OR **clarithro**[3] 1.0 gm po bid	**Co-morbidity present:** **Respiratory FQ** (see footnote[2]) **azithro** + (high dose) OR **clarithro** + (high dose AM/CL) **cefdinir, cefpodoxime, or cefprozil** + **azithro** or **clarithro** OR **H** New drug (10/03): **Telithromycin** Doses in footnote[4]	**Azithro/clarithro:** Pro: appropriate spectrum of action, more in vitro resistance than clinical failure [CID 34(Suppl 1):S27, 2002]; qd dosing. Breakthrough infections reported (NEJM 346:630, 2002; CID 34(Suppl.1):S4, 2002). Con: S. pneumo resistance ↑ in vitro 20–30% (CID 34(Suppl 1):S27, 2002) **Amoxicillin:** Pro: Active 90–95% S. pneumo at 3–4 gm/d Con: No activity atypicals or β-lactamase + bacteria. Need 3–4 gm/day **AM/CL:** Pro: spectrum includes β-lactamase + H. influenzae, M. catarrhalis, MSSA & Bacteroides sp. Con: No activity atypicals **Cephalosporins**—po: Ceftdiren, cefpodoxime, cefprozil, cefuroxime & others—see footnote[3] Pro: Active 75–85% S. pneumo & H. influenzae. Cefuroxime least active & higher mortality rate when S. pneumo resistant (CID 37:230, 2003). **Doxycycline:** Pro: Active vs S. pneumo but resistance may be increasing, Active vs H. influenzae, atypicals, & bioterrorism agents (anthrax, plague, tularemia) Con: Resistance of S. pneumo 15–20% (CID 35:633, 2002). Sparse clinical data (AnIM 159:266, 1999). QD dosing. **FQs—Respiratory FQs:** Pro: In vitro & clinically effective vs pen-sensitive & pen-resistant S. pneumo. Gemi only available po. Con: Reports of emerging resistance with clinical failure (NEJM 346:747, 2002). Drug-drug interactions (see Table 22A, page 142)
		Duration of rx: —Bacteremic: 10-14 days C. pneumoniae—Unclear. Some reports suggest 21 days. Some bronchitis pts required 5–6 wks of rx (J Med Micro 43:265, 2003) Legionella—10–21 days[2] Nonbacteremic pneumonia 2° to coliforms, S. aureus, anaerobes: ≥2 weeks		
Community-acquired, hospitalized—NOT in the ICU Empiric therapy	Etiology by co-morbidity & risk factors as above	**P Ceph 3[3]** + **azithro** 500 mg IV or IV qd	**Gati** 400 mg IV qd or **levo** 750 mg IV qd or **moxi** 400 mg IV qd	**Ceftriaxone/cefotaxime:** Pro: Drugs of choice for pen-sens. S. pneumo, active H. influenzae, M. catarrhalis, & MSSA Con: Inactive atypicals or pharyngeal anaerobes. Add macrolide for atypicals. **Dx:** Sputum Gram stain + culture. Blood ± pleural fluid culture. Pneumococcal urine antigen (S 32:824, 2000) sensitivity & simple. May augment other diagnostic tests. Positive in healthy asymptomatic children (CID 32:824, 2000).

---

[1] Atypical pathogens: Chlamydophila pneumoniae, Legionella sp., M. pneumoniae, C. psittaci, C. burnetii (Q fever). LnID 3:709, 2003
[2] Respiratory FQs with enhanced activity vs S. pneumo with HLR to penicillin: **gati** 400 mg IV/po qd, **gemi** 320 mg po qd, **levo** 750 mg IV/po qd, **moxi** 400 mg IV/po qd. Also active: **telithro** 800 mg po qd.
[3] O Ceph dosage: **Cefdinir** 300 mg po q12h; **cefditoren pivoxil** 200 mg, 2 tabs po bid, **cefpodoxime proxetil** 200 mg po q12h, **cefprozil** 500 mg po q12h, **cefuroxime axetil** 250–500 mg po q12h; high dose amox 1.0 gm po bid. **high dose AM/CL**—use **AM/CL-ER** 1000/62.5 mg, 2 tabs po bid
[4] Cephalosporin, penicillin & carbapenem dosages. **P Ceph 3: cefotaxime** dose ranges from 2.0 gm q6h IV for severe infection to 2.0 gm q4h IV for life-threatening infection, **ceftriaxone** 1.0 gm IV qd standard. However, unpublished data suggest possible underdosing in younger pts, hence would consider 2 gm IV < age 65; 1 gm IV > age 65.) **Other cephalosporins: Ceftazidime** 2.0 gm q8h IV; **cefepime** 2.0 gm q12h IV. **If P. aeruginosa**, ceftazidime 2.0 gm q8h or 4.5 gm q8h IV. Aztreonam 2.0 gm q8h IV. **tobra** 5 mg/kg IV once daily, or (PIP/TZ 3.375 gm q4h + tobra 5 mg/kg once daily). **If no P. aeruginosa, PIP/TZ** can be 3.375 gm q6h or 4.5 gm q8h IV. **Carbapenems: IMP** 0.5 gm IV q6h, **MER** 1.0 gm IV q8h

TABLE 1 (26)

ANATOMIC SITE/DIAGNOSIS/ MODIFYING CIRCUMSTANCES	ETIOLOGIES (usual)	SUGGESTED REGIMENS† PRIMARY	ALTERNATIVE†	ADJUNCT DIAGNOSTIC OR THERAPEUTIC MEASURES AND COMMENTS
LUNG/Pneumonia/Adults *(continued)* **Community-acquired, hospitalized—IN ICU** Empiric therapy P. aeruginosa **unlikely** etiology: P. aeruginosa possible etiology + other pathogens above, esp. S. pneumo & legionella		*Same as above: Community-acquired, not in the ICU* **[PIP/TZ]** + (**tobra** or **CIP**) + **azithro** or (**IMP** or **cefepime** or **ceftazidime**) + **azithro**	**Aztreonam** + (**levo** or **tobra**) or (**IMP** or **cefepime** or **ceftazidime**) + **FQ†** (**gati, levo** or **moxi**)	**Prognosis:** Retrospective analyses of S. pneumo pneumonia show better outcomes when macrolide is part of combination rx (AJM 161:1837, 2001; CID 36:389, 2003). P. aeruginosa uncommon etiology: usually with risk factors: bronchiectasis, cystic fibrosis, mechanical ventilation. Empiric therapy options should have predictive activity vs S. pneumo, legionella, & P. aeruginosa. Urine for legionella urine antigen for all ICU pts. If suspect legionella, rx with gati, levo, or azithro.
Hospital-acquired ± mechanical ventilation, NOT neutropenic *For rx of specific bacteria, see below & Table 2, page 48*	**By clinical setting: Post-OA aspiration:** S. pneumo, anaerobes. **Water:** Legionella. **Organ failure:** Coliforms. P. aeruginosa, S. aureus, Stenotrophomonas. **Airway obstruction:** Anaerobes. **Steroids:** yeast, PCP (see AIDS)	*Dosages in footnote 4 page 26* (**IMP** 0.5 gm IV q6h or **MER** 1.0 gm IV q8h) plus **tobra.** Add **resp. FQ** if suspect legionella or bioterrorism. *Dosages: See footnotes pages 16, 23, 25, & 26*	**Cefepime** OR **PIP/TZ†** ± **tobra.** Add **resp. FQ** if suspect legionella or bioterrorism, **respiratory FQ** (**gati, levo** or **moxi**) *See Comment regarding diagnosis*	**Dx of ventilator-associated pneumonia:** Fever & lung infiltrates often **not** pneumonia (Chest 106:221, 1994). Quantitative cultures helpful: bronchoalveolar lavage (>10⁴/ml pos.) or protected brush (>10³/ml pos.) Ref.: AJRCCM 165:867, 2002. **Microbial etiology:** No empiric regimen covers all possibilities. Regimens listed active vs majority of S. pneumo, legionella, & most coliforms. Regimens not active vs MRSA, Stenotrophomonas & others; see below: *Specific rx when culture results known.* **Ventilator-associated pneumonia—Prevention:** If possible, keep head of bed elevated 30° or more. Remove N-G, endotracheal tubes as soon as possible. If available, continuous subglottic suctioning. Limit stress ulcer prophylaxis. Ref.: NEJM 340:627, 1999.
Hospital- or community-acquired, neutropenic pt (<500 neutrophils/mm³)	Any of organisms listed under community- & hospital-acquired + fungi (aspergillus, Candida sp.)	*See Hospital-acquired, immediately above.* Vanco not included in initial rx unless high suspicion of infected IV access or drug-resistant S. pneumo. Ampho not used unless still febrile after 3 days or high clinical likelihood. See Comment		See consensus document on management of febrile neutropenic pt: CID 34:730, 2002.
Adults—Selected specific rx when culture results (sputum, blood, pleural fluid, etc.) available. Also see Table 2, page 48				
	Gram-negative			
Burkholderia (Pseudomonas) pseudomallei (etiology of melioidosis) Ref.: Ln 361:1715, 2003		**Initial parenteral rx: Ceftazidime** 40 mg/kg IV q8h or **IMP** 20 mg/kg IV q6h. Rx minimum 10 days & improving, then po therapy →	**Post-parenteral rx:** For **Adults** (see Comment for **children**) **Chloro** 10 mg/kg q6h, **Doxy** 2–2.2 mg/kg bid x20 wks. **TMP/SMX** (TMP component) bid x20 wks	For oral regimen, use **AM/CL-ER** 1000/62.5, 2 tabs po bid. **Children ≤8 yrs old & pregnancy:** 2 tabs bid po. Even with compliance, relapse rate is 10%.
Haemophilus influenzae	β-lactamase negative	**AMP** IV, **amox** po, **TMP/SMX**, **azithro/clarithro**, **doxy**		25–35% strains β-lactamase positive. * resistance to both TMP/SMX See Table 2, page 66 for dosages.
	β-lactamase positive	**AM/CL**, **O Ceph 2/3**, **O Ceph 2/3**, **azithro/clarithro**, **doxy**		
Legionella species	Hospitalized/immunocom promised	**Azithro** IV or **levo** IV or **gati** or **moxi.** See Table 108,	**Erythro** ± **rifampin**, **clarithro**, **telithro**	**FQ, TMP/SMX**. Best legionella levofloxacin only option. **Dx:** Urine antigen and culture. See Table 108, page 108 for dosages.
Moraxella catarrhalis	90% β-lactamase positive	**AM/CL**, **O Ceph 2/3**, **O Ceph 2/3**, **macrolide**,² **telithro**, **FQ**, **TMP/SMX**. **Doxy** another option. See Table 108, page 108 for dosages.		

---

1 **Telithro** = telithromycin 800 mg po qd
2 **Macrolide** = azithromycin, clarithromycin, dirithromycin, and erythromycin. Dirithromycin serum levels inadequate for bacteremic S. pneumo.
(Footnotes and abbreviations on page 45) NOTE: *All dosage recommendations are for adults (unless otherwise indicated) and assume normal renal function*

TABLE 1 (27)

ANATOMIC SITE/DIAGNOSIS/ MODIFYING CIRCUMSTANCES	ETIOLOGIES (usual)	SUGGESTED REGIMENS*		ADJUNCT DIAGNOSTIC OR THERAPEUTIC MEASURES AND COMMENTS
		PRIMARY	ALTERNATIVE†	
LUNG/Pneumonia/Adults, when culture results available (continued)				
Staphylococcus aureus	MSSA/MRSA	**MSSA:** Oxacillin/nafcillin; **MRSA:** vanco, linezolid	**MSSA:** TMP/SMX, linezolid	In retrospective analysis of MRSA nosocomial pneumonia, linezolid superior to vanco, p <0.01 (Chest 124:1789, 2003).
Stenotrophomonas maltophilia [a]		TMP/SMX	TC/CL± aztreonam	In vitro synergy (AAC 39:2220, 1995; CMR 11:57, 1998.
Streptococcus pneumoniae	Penicillin-susceptible	AMP 2.0 gm IV q6h; amox 1.0 gm po q8h, penicillin, cephalosporins, macrolide (see footnote 4 page 27), doxy	**P Ceph 2,3, (telithro** 800 mg po qd
	Penicillin-resistant, high level	FQs with enhanced activity (gati, gemi, levo, moxi) IV, (vanco IV ± RIF)—see Table 5, page 55 for more data. If allergic, all options not possible (e.g., allergy), linezolid alone		
LUNG—Other				
Anthrax	Bacillus anthracis			1. Clinda may block toxin production
Inhalation (applies to oro-pharyngeal & gastrointestinal forms): Treatment (Cutaneous: See page 34)	**To report possible bioterrorism event: 770-488-7100**	**Adults (including pregnancy):** CIP 400 mg IV q12h) or (doxy 100 mg IV q12h) plus (clindamycin 900 mg IV q8h) and/or RIF 300 mg IV q12h) Switch to po when able & lower CIP to 500 mg po bid, or clinda to 450, and/or RIF 300 mg po q12h. Treat x60 days.	**Children:** CIP 10-15 mg/kg IV q12h; or (Doxy: >8 y/o & <45 kg: 100 mg IV q12h; ≤8 y/o: 2.2 mg/kg IV q12h) plus clindamycin 7.5 mg/kg IV q8h and/or RIF 20 mg/kg (max. 600 mg) IV q12h. Treat x60 d. See Table 16, page 129 for oral doses.	2. Rifampin penetrates CSF & intracellular sites. 3. If isolate shown penicillin-susceptible: a. **Adults: Pen G** 4 mU IV q4h b. **Children: Pen G** <12 y/o: 50,000 U/kg IV q6h; >12 y/o: 4 mU IV q4h c. Constitutive & inducible β-lactamases—do not use pen or amp alone. 4. Do not use cephalosporins or TMP/SMX. 5. Erytho, azithro activity borderline; clarithro active. 6. No person-to-person spread.
	Refs: JAMA 287:2236, 2002 & MMWR 50:909, 2001. For distinguishing clinical features, see AnIM 139: 337, 2003			
Post-exposure prophylaxis	Info: www.bt.cdc.gov	**Adults (including pregnancy):** CIP 500 mg po bid x60 d. **Children:** CIP 20-30 mg/kg/d div q12h x60 d.	**Adults (including pregnancy): Doxy** 100 mg po bid x60 d. **Children:** Doxy: >8 y/o & >45 kg: 100 mg po bid; >8 y/o & <45 kg: 2.2 mg/kg po bid; ≤8 y/o: 2.2 mg/kg po bid. All for 60 days.	Once organism shows suscept. to amoxicillin 80 mg/kg/d div. q8h (max. dose 500 mg tid) in children 80 mg/kg; pregnant (if fails to amoxicillin 500 mg tid). Do not use cephalosporins or TMP/SMX. Other FQs (gati, levo, moxi) & clarithro should work but no clinical experience.
Aspiration pneumonia & lung abscess (CJM 88:409, 1995)	Bacteroides sp. (~15% B. fragilis), peptostreptococci, Fusobacterium sp., S. milleri group, nocardia (pts taking steroids)	**Clinda** 450-900 mg q8h IV for nocardia, see Table 11, page 61	**Cefoxtin** 2.0 gm q8h IV, or **TC/CL** 3.1 gm q6h IV, or 4.5 gm q6h IV, or AM/SB 3.0 gm q6h IV. Initially when IV po q8h (PIP or ticar-cillin) can also be effective.	Bronchoscopy to R/O neoplasm if fails to clear or recurs. Metro not as effective in putrid lung abscess as clinda. Occasionally Type 3 pneumococci, Staph. aureus, Klebsiella pneumoniae are etiologic. A recent review questioned the etiologic role of anaerobic bacteria; the editors respectfully disagree (NEJM 344:665, 2001).
Chronic pneumonia with fever, night sweats and weight loss	M. tuberculosis, coccidioidomycosis, histoplasmosis	See Tables 11, 12		HIV+, foreign-born, alcoholism, contact with TB, travel into developing countries
Cystic fibrosis	S. aureus or H. influenzae early in disease; P. aerug-nosa later in disease	**For P. aeruginosa:** Tobra 3.3 mg/kg q8h or 10 mg/kg q24h IV + (ticar or tobra with [PIP or ticar-cillin 100 mg/kg q8h] or with ceftaz 50 mg/kg q8h) IV. Also see footnote² & Comment	**For S. aureus: (1) MSSA-oxacillin/nafcillin** 2.0 gm IV q4h; (2) **MRSA** vanco 1.0 gm q12h & check serum levels. See Comment	Additional therapy: Claritho synergistic with tobra vs P. aeruginosa (AAC 46:1105, 2002); + anti-inflammatory agents (Pharmacotherapy 22:227, 2002) Azithro 250 mg/day improved FEV, pts chronically infected with P. aeruginosa (JAMA 290: 1749, 2003). For pharmacodynamics of aminoglycosides in CF, see JAC 50:553, 2002. For chronic suppression of P. aeruginosa, inhaled phenol-free tobra 300 mg bid x28 d, then no x28 d, then repeat cycle (AJRCCM 167:841, 2003; NEJM 340:23, 1999; Chest 120:107S, 2001).
Acute exacerbation of pulmonary symptoms Refs: LnID 3:87, 661, 2003; AJRCCM 168:918, 2003				

---

1 **IV Pen G dosage:** Blood cultures neg., 1 mU IV q4h; blood cultures pos. & no meningitis, 2 mU IV q4h. Another option is continuous infusion (CI) 3 mU loading dose & then CI of 10–12 mU over 12 hrs (Chest 122:1471, 2007). CIP IV/po + (clinda or metro), e.g., CIP IV/po + clinda IV (LnID 3:537, 2003).

2 Other options: (Tobra 1x: aztreonam 50 mg/kg q8h IV; (TMP 15–25 mg/kg q8h IV + tobra). **CIP commonly used in children**, 20 mg/kg q12h IV, but not approved for adults (unless otherwise indicated) and assume normal renal function.

(Footnotes and abbreviations on page 45)

TABLE 1 (28)

ANATOMIC SITE/DIAGNOSIS/ MODIFYING CIRCUMSTANCES	ETIOLOGIES (usual)	SUGGESTED REGIMENS*		ADJUNCT DIAGNOSTIC OR THERAPEUTIC MEASURES AND COMMENTS
		PRIMARY	ALTERNATIVE†	
LUNG/Other (continued) Cystic fibrosis (continued)	Burkholderia (Pseudomonas) cepacia	**TMP/SMX** 5.0 mg/kg (TMP) q6h IV	**Chloro** 15–20 mg/kg IV or q6h po *For other alternatives, see Table 2*	B. cepacia has become a major pathogen. Patients develop progressive respiratory failure. Patients develop progressive respiratory failure, 62% mortality at 1 year. **Fail to respond to APAG,** piperacillin, & ceftazidime. Patients with B. cepacia should be isolated from other CF patients. **NOTE:** 3- & 4-drug combinations under study in refractory pts (AAC 43:213, 1999)
Empyema. Refs: CID 22:747, 1996. Pleural effusion review: NEJM 346:1971, 2002				
Neonatal	Staph. aureus, Strep. pneumoniae	See Pneumonia, neonatal, page 25		Drainage indicated.
Infants/children (1 month–5 yrs)	Staph. aureus, Strep. pneumoniae, H. influenzae	See Pneumonia, age 1 month–5 years, page 25		Drainage indicated.
Child >5 yrs to ADULT—Diagnostic thoracentesis, chest tube for empyemas Acute, usually parapneumonic	Strep. pneumoniae, Group A strep	**Cefotaxime or ceftriaxone** (Dosage, see footnote 4, page 26)	**Vanco**	Randomized trial showed benefit of intrapleural streptokinase (250,000 units in 20 ml saline via 24hr dwell x3 days) if organisms. R/O tuberculosis or tumor (AJRCCM 159:37, 1997). Urokinase 100,000 IU/d, x3 d, effective in double-blind study (AJRCCM 159:37, 1997).
Subacute/chronic	Staph. aureus	**Nafcillin or oxacillin** + **P Ceph 3**	**Vanco**	Gram(+), cocci in clusters
	Anaerobic strep, Strep. milleri, Enterobacteriaceae, M. tuberculosis	**Clinda** 450–600 mg q8h IV or q6h po **+ P Ceph 3**	**TMP/SMX or AM/SB Cefoxitin or IMP or TC/CL or PIP/TZ or AM/SB** (Dosage, see footnote 4 page 26)	Pleomorphic, Gm-neg, bacilli. ↑ resistance to TMP/SMX. If organisms not seen, treat as subacute. Drainage. R/O tuberculosis or tumor (CID 22:747, 1996) Pleura biopsy with culture and histology if TBc suspected (CID 22:747, 1996)
Human immunodeficiency virus infection (HIV+)				
CD4 T-lymphocytes <200/ mm3 or clinical AIDS	Pneumocystis (carinii) most likely, also M. tbc, fungi, Kaposi's sarcoma, & others. NOTE: AIDS pts may develop pneumonia due to PCP or other pathogens—see next box below	**Rx** listed here is for **severe** pneumonias; see Table 13, page 98 for mild-moderate & alternatives. **Prednisone 1st (see Comment), then : Prednisone 40 mg bid po x5 d, then 40 mg qd po x5 d then 20 mg qd po x11 d.** Initiation of anti-PCP rx: **initiate steroid x15–30 min prior to 1st dose anti-PCP rx.**	**Pentamidine 30 mg/kg qd po) or pentamidine isethionate 4 mg/kg/IV)] d** See Comment	Diagnostic procedure of choice is sputum induction; if negative, bronchoscopy. Pts with PCP (pO2 <200, CD4 cells/mm3 should be on anti-PCP prophylaxis for life. If PCP (pO2 <70 mmHg), should be given at initiation of anti-PCP rx, don't wait until pt's condition deteriorates (Table 13, page 98). If PCP studies negative, consider bacterial pneumonia, TBc, cocci, histo, crypto, Kaposi's sarcoma or lymphoma. **Pentamidine not active vs bacterial pathogens.**
Prednisone first if suspect pneumocystis (see Comment)				
CD4 T-lymphocytes normal Acute onset, purulent sputum ± pulmonary infiltrates ± pleuritic pain. **Isolate pt until tbc ruled out.**	Strep. pneumoniae; H. influenzae, aerobic Gm-neg. bacilli (including P. aeruginosa); Legionella rare; M. tbc.	**P Ceph 3** (Dosages in footnotes on pages 16 & 23) ± **azithro.** Could use **gati, levo,** or **moxi** (see Comment)	**If Staph. aureus resistant to TMP/SMX, albeit rare, does exist.** If Gram stain of sputum shows Gm-neg. bacilli, options include P Ceph 3 AP, TC/CL, PIP/TZ, IMP, MER FQs: Levo 500 mg po/IV qd; gati 400 mg IV/po qd; moxi 400 mg po/IV qd	
As above: Children	Same as adult + lymphoid interstitial pneumonia (LIP)	As for HIV+ adults with pneumonia. If diagnosis is LIP, rx with steroids.	**rx**	In children with AIDS, LIP responsible for 1/3 of pulmonary complications, usually >1 yr of age vs PCP, which is seen at <1 yr of age. Alveolar-interstitial, hepatosplenomegaly, salivary glands enlarged but no fever (differs from PCP).
Viral (interstitial) pneumonia suspected (See Table 14, page 104)	Consider adenovirus, hantavirus, influenza, metapneumovirus, parainfluenza virus, respiratory syncytial virus	**For influenza A: rimantadine** 100 mg po x2/d or **amantadine** 100 mg po	**For influenza A: rimantadine** 75 mg po bid x5 d or **zanamivir** 10 mg inhaled bid x5 d. Start within 48 hrs of symptom onset	No known efficacious drugs for adenovirus, coronavirus (SARS), hantavirus, metapneumovirus, parainfluenza or RSV. Need travel (SARS) & exposure (Hanta) history.
LYMPH NODES (approaches below apply to lymphadenitis without an obvious primary source)				
Lymphadenitis, acute Generalized	Etiologies: EBV, early HIV infection, syphilis, toxoplasma, tularemia, Lyme disease, sarcoid, lymphoma, systemic lupus erythematosus, and Kikuchi-Fujimoto disease. Complete history and physical examination followed by appropriate serological tests. Treat specific agent(s).			

Footnotes and abbreviations on page 45

NOTE: All dosage recommendations are for adults (unless otherwise indicated) and assume normal renal function

TABLE 1 (29)

ANATOMIC SITE/DIAGNOSIS/ MODIFYING CIRCUMSTANCES	ETIOLOGIES (usual)	SUGGESTED REGIMENS* PRIMARY	ALTERNATIVE†	ADJUNCT DIAGNOSTIC OR THERAPEUTIC MEASURES AND COMMENTS
LYMPH NODES/Lymphadenitis, acute *(continued)*				
Regional				
Cervical—see cat-scratch disease (CSD), below	CSD (B. henselae), Grp A strep, Staph. aureus, anaerobes, M. TBc (scrofula), M. avium, M. scrofulaceum, M. malmoense, toxo, tularemia.			History & physical exam directs evaluation. If nodes fluctuant, aspirate and base rx on Gram & acid-fast stains. Review of *mycobacterial etiology: CID 20:954, 1995.* Kikuchi-Fujimoto disease causes fever and benign self-limited adenopathy: the etiology is unknown (AJM 171:401, 1996).
Inguinal				
Sexually transmitted	HSV, chancroid, syphilis, LGV			
Not sexually transmitted	GAS, SA, tularemia, CSD.			
Axillary	GAS, SA, CSD, tularemia, Y. pestis, sporotrichosis	Treatment varies with specific etiology.		
Extremity, with associated nodular lymphangitis	Sporotrichosis, leishmania, Nocardia brasiliensis, Mycobacterium marinum, Mycobacterium chelonae, tularemia			A distinctive form of lymphangitis characterized by subcutaneous swellings along inflamed lymphatic channels. Primary site of skin invasion usually present; regional adenopathy variable.
Cat-scratch disease— **immunocompetent patient** Axillary/epitrochlear nodes 46%, neck 26%, inguinal 17%	Bartonella henselae Review: *IDC No. Amer. 12:* 137, 1998	**Azithro dosage—Adults** (>45.5 kg): 500 mg po x1, then 250 mg/d x4 d. **Children** (<45.5 kg): liquid azithro 10 mg/kg x1, then 5 mg/kg/d x4 d. Rx is controversial—see Comment	No rx: resolves in 2–6 mos. Needle aspiration relieves pain in suppurative nodes. Avoid I&D.	**Clinical:** Approx. 10% nodes suppurate. Atypical presentation in <5% pts., i.e., lung nodules, liver/spleen lesions, Parinaud's oculoglandular syndrome, CNS manifestations in 2% of pts (encephalitis, peripheral neuropathy, retinitis). **Dx:** Cat exposure. Positive IFA serology. Rarely need biopsy. **Rx:** Only 1 prospective randomized blinded study, used azithro with ↑ rapidity of resolution of enlarged lymph nodes (PIDJ 17:447, 1998).
MOUTH				
Odontogenic infection, including Ludwig's angina Can result in more serious parapharyngeal space infection (see page 33)	Oral microflora: infection polymicrobial	**Clinda** 300–450 mg q6h po or 600 mg IV q6–8h		Surgical drainage and removal of necrotic tissue essential. β-lactamase producing organisms are ↑ in frequency. Ref: *Canad Dental Assn J 64:508, 1998* Other parenteral alternatives: AM/SB, PIP/TZ, or TC/CL.
Buccal cellulitis Children <5 yrs	H. influenzae	**Cefuroxime** or **P Ceph 3**	**AM/CL** or **TMP/SMX** *Dosage: see Table 14, page 129*	With Hib immunization, invasive H. influenzae infections have ↓ by 95%. Now occurring in infants prior to immunization.
Herpetic stomatitis	Herpes simplex virus 1 & 2			
Aphthous stomatitis, recurrent, HIV-neg.	Etiology unknown	Topical steroids (Kenalog in Orabase) may ↓ pain and swelling; if AIDS, see SANFORD GUIDE TO HIV/AIDS THERAPY.		
MUSCLE				
"Gas gangrene" Contaminated traumatic wound. Spontaneous without trauma (CID 28:159, 1999)	Cl. perfringens, other histotoxic Clostridium sp.	**(Clinda** 900 mg q8h IV) + **(pen G** 24 mU/d div. q4–6h IV)	**Ceftriaxone** 2.0 gm q12h IV or **erythro** 1.0 gm q6h IV (not by bolus)	Surgical debridement primary rx. Hyperbaric oxygen adjunctive: efficacy debated, consider if debridement not complete or possible (NEJM 334:1642, 1996). Clinda ↓ toxin production.
Pyomyositis	Staph. aureus, Group A strep, (rarely Gm-neg. bacilli), rarely anaerobic organisms	**(Nafcillin** or **oxacillin** 2.0 gm q4h IV) or **(P Ceph 1** [cefazolin 2.0 gm q8h IV])	**Vanco** 1.0 gm q12h IV	Has been common in tropics, rare but cases in temperate zones (IDCP 7:265, 1998). Follows exercise or muscle injury, see Necrotizing fasciitis. Now seen in HIV/AIDS (Variety of anaerobic organisms Add clinda or metro if anaerobes suspected/proven (IDCP 8:252, 1999)
PANCREAS: Review—NEJM 340:1412, 1999; Ln 361:1447, 2003 Acute alcoholic, viral (mumps) (idiopathic) pancreatitis	Not bacterial	None		1–9% become infected (source of bacteria unclear) (Surgery 119:519, 1996). Observe for pancreatic abscesses or necrosis which require rx.
Pancreatic abscess, infected pseudocyst, infected necrosis	Enterobacteriaceae, enterococci, S. aureus, S. epidermidis, anaerobes, candida	**(IMP** or **MER)** Start IMP or MER early (within 48h) for necrotizing pancreatitis; prevents infection of necrotic tissue (Ann Surg 232:619, 2000)		For necrotizing pancreatitis (>30% necrosis: contrast-enhanced CT. Accuracy >90% if >30% gland necrosis); if infected, debride: prophylactic antimicrobials (Ln 346:652, 1995). Role of prophylactic antibiotics uncertain (pending FDA-approved study) CID 37:208, 2003 (sens. 90%, spec. 99%). Candida (CID 37:208, 2003

(Footnotes and abbreviations on page 45) NOTE: All dosage recommendations are for adults (unless otherwise indicated) and assume normal renal/renal function

TABLE 1 (30)

ANATOMIC SITE/DIAGNOSIS/ MODIFYING CIRCUMSTANCES	ETIOLOGIES (usual)	SUGGESTED REGIMENS*		ADJUNCT DIAGNOSTIC OR THERAPEUTIC MEASURES AND COMMENTS
		PRIMARY	ALTERNATIVE†	
PAROTID GLAND "Hot" non-tender parotid swelling	S. aureus, oral flora, & aerobic Gm-neg. bacilli (rare), influenza	**Nafcillin** or **oxacillin** 2.0 gm IV q4h.		Predisposing factors: stone(s) in Stensen's duct, dehydration. Rx depends on ID of specific etiologic agent.
"Cold" non-tender parotid swelling	Granulomatous disease (e.g., mycobacteria, fungi, sarcoidosis, Sjögren syndrome), drugs (iodides, et al.), diabetes, tumors			History/lab results may narrow differential; may need biopsy for dx
PERITONEUM/PERITONITIS: Reference—*CID 31:997, 2003*				
Primary (spontaneous) bacterial peritonitis, SBP) Ref: *CID 26:1035, 1998* ESBL ref: *CID 26:683, 1999* Microbiology: *CID 31:513, 2001*	Enterobacteriaceae 63%, S. pneumo. 15%, enterococci 6–10%, anaerobes <1%.	**Cefotaxime** 2.0 gm q8h IV or **TC/CL** 3.1 gm IV q6h **OR** [**AM/SB**] OR [**ceftriaxone** 2.0 gm q24h IV] or **erta** 1.0 gm IV qd If resistant E. coli/klebsiella problem (ESBL+?): **IMP** or **MER** or **erta** (Dosage in footnote)	**TMP/SMX** ↓ peritonitis or spontaneous bacteremia from 27% to 3% (*AJM 122:595, 1995*). Ref. for CIP. or **CIP** 750 mg IV q12h Ref.: *Hepatol 32:171, 1995* then: **CIP/FQ: CIP, levo, gati, moxi)**	One-way path of SBP in pts with ascites and cirrhosis as high as 29% (*Gastro 104:1133, 1993*). 30–40% of pts have neg. cultures of blood and ascitic fluid. % pos. cultures ↑ if 10 ml of pt's ascitic fluid added to blood culture bottles. Duration of rx unclear. Suggest 5 wks if blood cultures pos. One report suggests repeat paracentesis after 48 hrs of cefotaxime. If PMNs <250/mm³ and ascitic fluid sterile, success with 5 days of rx (*AJM 37:69, 1994; Hepatol 5:457, 1985*). IV albumin (1.5 gm/kg at dx then 1 gm/kg on day 3) may ↓ frequency of renal impairment (p 0.002) & ↓ hospital mortality (p 0.01) (*NEJM 341:403, 1999*).
Prevention of SBP Cirrhosis & ascites		**TMP/SMX-DS** 1 tab po 5 d/ wk or **CIP** 750 mg po q wk		
Cirrhosis & UGI bleeding		**CIP** 500 mg po q12h		
Secondary (bowel perforation, ruptured appendix, ruptured diverticulum) Refs.: *NEJM 338:1521, 1998 & CID 31:997, 2003*	Enterobacteriaceae, Bacteroides sp., enterococci, P. aeruginosa (3–15%)	**Mild–moderate disease—Inpatient—parenteral rx:** (e.g., focal periappendiceal peritonitis, periverticular abscess, endometriitis) **PIP/TZ** 3.375 gm q6h IV q12h OR or 4.5 gm IV q8h, **OR AM/SB** 3.0 gm IV q6h OR **TC/CL** 3.1 gm IV q6h OR **erta** 1 gm IV qd **Severe life-threatening disease—ICU patient:** **IMP** 500 mg q6h or **MER** 1 gm IV q8h	**CIP** 400 mg IV q12h or **levo** 750 mg IV q24h] + (**CIP** 400 mg IV q12h or **levo** 750 mg IV q24h)] OR [**AMP** 2 gm IV q6h + **metro** (see Comment) **APAG** (see Table 10C, page 73) See Comment [**AMP** + **metro** + (**CIP** 400 mg IV q12h or **levo** 750 mg IV q24h)] OR [**AMP** 2 gm IV q6h + **metro** 1 gm IV q8h + **APAG** (see Table 10C, page 73)]	Must "cover" both Gm-neg. aerobic & Gm-neg. anaerobic bacteria. **Drugs active only vs aerobic Gm-neg. bacilli:** APAG, P Ceph 2/3/4, aztreonam, AP Pen, CIP, levo. **Drugs active vs both aerobic and anaerobic Gm-neg. bacteria:** cefotetan, cefoxitin, PIP/TZ, AM/SB, IMP, MER, gati, moxi. Cefoxitin Cefotetan Clindamycin Cefotaxime % R 16–44 5–10 Essentially no resistance: metro, PIP/TZ (*CID 35:S126, 2000*) **Ertapenem** less active vs P. aeruginosa/Acinetobacter species than IMP or MER. Based on in vitro activity, could sub **gati/levo** for CIP/levo, but insufficient clinical data. It absence of ongoing fecal contamination, aerobic/anaerobic culture of peritoneal exudate, abscess often not helpful in guiding specific therapy. Less need for aminoglycosides. **With severe pen allergy:** can "cover" Gm-neg. aerobes with CIP or aztreonam, **Concomitant surgical management important.**
		Concomitant surgical management important.		
Associated with chronic ambulatory peritoneal dialysis (defined as > 100 WBC/μL, > 50% PMNs)	Staph. aureus (most common), Staph. epidermidis, P. aeruginosa 7%, Gm-neg. bacilli 11%, sterile 20%, M. fortuitum (rare)	If of moderate severity, can rx by adding drugs to dialysis fluid—see **Table 17** for dosage. Reasonable empiric combinations: **vanco** + **P Ceph 3 AP** or **vanco** + **APAG**. If severely ill, add **systemic** rx. If not last dose for renal function, **Table 17B** via addition to dialysis fluid. Excellent ref.: *Perit Dialysis Int 13:14, 1993*	For diagnosis: concentrate several hundred ml of removed dialysis fluid by centrifugation. Gram stain concentrate and then inject into aerobic/anaerobic blood culture bottles. A positive Gram stain is unusual. If culture neg. after 3–4 days, look for fungi, mycobacteria. For "saving" dialysis catheter: if multiple Gm-neg. bacilli cultured, consider bowel perforation and catheter removal.

† Parenteral IV therapy for peritonitis: **TC/CL** 3.1 gm q6h, **PIP/TZ** 3.375 gm q6h or 4.5 gm q8h, **AM/SB** 3.0 gm q6h, **IMP** 0.5 gm q6h, **MER** 1.0 gm q8h, **FQ** (**CIP** 400 mg q12h, **oflox** 400 mg q12h, **levo** 500 mg qd, **gati** 400 mg qd, **moxi** 400 mg po q4–6h), **AMP** 2.0 gm q4–6h, **ceftizoxime** 1–2 gm qd, **ceftriaxone** 2.0 gm q24h, **cefotaxime** 2.0 gm q8h, **cefepime** 2.0 gm q12h, **cefoperazone** (see Table 10C, page 73), **P Ceph 3 AP** (**ceftazidime** 2.0 gm q8h, **cefepime** 2.0 gm q12h, **aztreonam** 2.0 gm q8h), **P Ceph 4** (**ticarcillin** 4.0 gm q4–6h), **PIP** 4.0 gm q4–6h, **AP Pen** (**ticarcillin** 2.0 gm q6h), **cefotaxime** 2.0 gm q8h. NOTE: All dosage recommendations are for adults (unless otherwise indicated) and assume normal renal function.

(Footnotes and abbreviations on page 45)

TABLE 1 (31)

ANATOMIC SITE/DIAGNOSIS/ MODIFYING CIRCUMSTANCES	ETIOLOGIES (usual)	SUGGESTED REGIMENS*		ADJUNCT DIAGNOSTIC OR THERAPEUTIC MEASURES AND COMMENTS
		PRIMARY	ALTERNATIVE†	
PHARYNX **Pharyngitis**—Reviews: *NEJM 344:205, 2001; AnIM 134:506 & 509, 2001.* **"viral,"** (Group A,C,G strep, "viral," *C. pneumoniae*, mononucleosis (*NEJM 329:156, 1993*), C. diphtheriae, A. haemolyticum, Mycoplasma pneumoniae*) *For relationship to acute rheumatic fever, see footnote[1]* Rheumatic fever ref.: *Ln 349:935, 1997*	In children & adults: Group A,C,G strep, "viral," *C. pneumoniae*, mononucleosis (*NEJM 329:156, 1993*), C. diphtheriae, A. haemolyticum, Mycoplasma pneumoniae* In children & adults pharyngitis due to Group A strep	**Pen V** po x10 d, or if compliance a problem, **benzathine pen** IM x1	**Erytho V** po x10 d, or **O Ceph 2** or **Ceph 3** x5–10 d, or **clarithro** x10 d, or **azithro** x5–d, or **dirithro** x10 d.	**Dx:** In children & adults—Rapid strep test or culture. In adults, culture most cost-effective (*AnIM 139:113, 2003*). **Pen Allergy/Resistance:** No penicillin or cephalosporin-resistant S. pyogenes, but now macrolide-resist. S. pyogenes. Need culture & in vitro susceptibility testing. Clinical failure w/ empiric azithro/clarithro. **S. pyogenes Groups C & G cause pharyngitis but not a risk for post-strep rheumatic fever.** To prevent rheumatic fever, eradicate Group A strep. Requires 10 d. of pen V po; 4–6 d of po O Ceph 2; 5 d. of po azithro; 10 d. of clarithro. In controlled trial, 4–6 d of po O Ceph 2 had better eradication rate with 10 d. azithro (91%) than 5 d. azithro (82%)*CID 32:1798,2001*. Acetaminophen effective for pain relief (*Br J Gen Pract 50:817, 2000*). *See footnote[2] for adult and pediatric dosages.*
	Gonococci	**Ceftriaxone** 125 mg IM x1 (+ **azithro** or **doxy**) *(see Comment)*	(**CIP** 500 mg po x1) or **gati** 400 mg po x1 or (**ofox** 400 mg po x1) + (**azithro** or **doxy**) *(see Comment)*	Because of risk of concomitant genital *C. trachomatis*, add either **azithro** 1.0 gm po x1) or (doxy 100 mg po 2x/d x7 d). See pages 15 for more options
Asymptomatic post-rx carrier	**Group A strep**	No rx required		Routine post-rx throat culture not advised
Multiple repeated culture-positive episodes (*CID 25:574, 1997*)	**Group A strep**	**Clinda** or **AM/CL** po	Parenteral **benzathine pen** (± **RIF** Dosages in footnote[3]	Small % fail to have recurrent culture-pos. "Group A strep w/ symptomatic pharyngitis. Hard to tell if true Group A strep infection or active viral infection in chronic Group A strep carrier. One regimen that may help: 20 mg/kg/d x4 d. to max. of 300 mg bid x10 d (*J Ped 106:481 & 876, 1985*).
Whitish plaques, HIV+, (thrush) **Vesicular, ulcerative**	Candida albicans (see *Table 11, page 77*) Coxsackie A9, B1-5, ECHO (multiple types), Enterovirus 71, Herpes simplex 1,2		**acyclovir** 400 mg tid po x10 d.	Antibacterial agents not indicated, but for HSV–
Membranous—Diphtheria or Vincent's angina	**C. diphtheriae**	**Antitoxin** + **erythro** 20–25 mg/kg q12h IV x7–14 d. or (**benzyl pen** [**benzyl pen G** 50,000 U/kg/d div q12h x5 d.)		Diphtheria occurs in immunized individuals. Antibiotics ↓ toxin production, ↓ spread of organisms. Erythro superior to pen G in randomized trial (*CID 27:845, 1998*)
	Vincent's angina (anaerobes/spirochetes)	**Pen G** 4 mU q4h IV	**Clinda** 600 mg IV	May be complicated by F. necrophorum bacteremia, see jugular vein phlebitis (Lemierre's), page 53.
Epiglottitis (*IDCP 6:500, 1997*) Children	H. influenzae (rare), S. pyogenes, S. pneumoniae, S. aureus	**Peds dosage:** Cefotaxime 50 mg/kg q8h IV or **ceftriaxone** 50 mg/kg q24h IV	**Peds dosage: AM/SB** 100-200 mg/kg/d div q6h or **TMP/ SMX** 8–12 mg TMP comp./kg/d. div q12h	Have tracheostomy set * at bedside. * Chloro is effective, but potentially less toxic alternative agents available. Review (adults): *JAMA 272:358, 1994)*

---

[1] Primary rationale for treatment is eradication of Group A (GAS) strep. This was associated with clearance of GAS on pharyngeal cultures (*CID 19:1110, 1994*). Subsequent studies have been based on cultures, not actual prevention of ARF. Treatment, ↓ duration of symptoms.

[2] **DOSAGE—Group A strep:** **All po unless otherwise indicated. PEDIATRIC DOSAGE: Benzathine penicillin** 25,000 U/kg IM to max. 1.2 mU; **Pen V** 25–50 mg/kg/d div. q6h x10 d; **AM/CL** 45 mg/kg div. q12h x10 d.; **erythro estolate** 20 mg/kg div. bid or **succinate** 40 mg/kg/d div. bid x10 d.; **cefadroxil** 30 mg/kg q24h x10 d.; **cefprozil** 15 mg/kg bid x10 d.; **cefpodoxime proxetil** 10 mg/kg bid x10 d.; **cefdinir** 7 mg/kg q12h x5–10 d. or 14 mg/kg q24h x10 d; **azithro** 12 mg/kg q24h x5 d (max. 500 mg). **ADULT DOSAGE: Benzathine penicillin** 1.2 mU IM x1; **Pen V** 500 mg bid or 250 mg qid x10 d.; **erythro**. dosage varies—w/ erythro base 500 mg qid x10 d.; **cefadroxil** 500 mg bid x10 d.; **cefuroxime axetil** 250 mg bid x4 d.; **cefpodoxime proxetil** 100 mg bid x4 d.; **cefdinir** 300 mg q12h x5–10 or 600 mg q24h x10 d.; **cefprozil** 500 mg bid x10 d.; **clarithro** 250 mg bid x10 d or 500 mg XL q24h x10 d.; **dirithromycin** 500 mg q24h x10 d. **NOTE:** All dosage recommendations are for adults (unless otherwise indicated) and assume normal renal function
(Footnotes and abbreviations on page 45)

TABLE 1 (32)

ANATOMIC SITE/DIAGNOSIS/ MODIFYING CIRCUMSTANCES	ETIOLOGIES (usual)	SUGGESTED REGIMENS*		ADJUNCT DIAGNOSTIC OR THERAPEUTIC MEASURES AND COMMENTS
		PRIMARY	ALTERNATIVE†	
PHARYNX/Epiglottitis *(continued)*				
Adults	Group A strep, H. influenzae (rare)	**Adult dosage: See footnote¹ for epiglottitis**		
Parapharyngeal space infection Poor dental hygiene, dental extractions, foreign bodies (e.g., toothpicks, fish bones)	submandibular, submaxillary (Ludwig's = angina, used loosely for these), lateral pharyngeal, retropharyngeal, pretracheal Polymicrobic: Strep sp., anaerobes, Eikenella corrodens	**[Clinda** (600–900 mg IV q8h) or **pen G²** 24 mU q4h IV q6h] or **pen G² 24** mU by cont. infusion or div. q4–6h IV + **metro** 1.0 gm load and then 0.5 gm q6h IV]	**Clinda** 600–900 mg q8h IV	Usual rx includes external drainage of lateral pharyngeal space. Emboli, pulmonary and systemic common. Erosion into carotid artery can occur.
Jugular vein septic phlebitis (Lemierre's) (see footnote 2 [PID 22:921, 2003])	Fusobacterium necrophorum in vast majority	**Pen G²** 24 mU q4 IV by cont. infusion or div. q4–6h	**Clinda** 600–900 mg q8h IV	
Laryngitis (hoarseness)/tracheitis	Viral (90%)	Not indicated		
SINUSES, PARANASAL				
Sinusitis, acute; current terminology: acute rhinosinusitis. Obstruction of sinus ostia, viral infection, allergens	Strep. pneumoniae 31%, H. influenzae 21%, M. catarrhalis 2%, Group A strep 2%, anaerobes 6%, viruses 15%, Staph. aureus 4% **By CT scans, sinus mucosa inflamed in 87% of viral URIs; only 2% develop bacterial rhinosinusitis**	**Reserve antibiotic rx for pts given decongestants/facial analgesics for 7 d, who have (1) maxillary/facial pain & (2) purulent nasal discharge; if severe illness (pain, fever), treat sooner—usually requires hospitalization.** For mild/mod. disease: Antibiotics in prior season and/or DRSP prevalence >30%²²	For pts with pen/cephalosporin allergy, esp. severe IgE-mediated allergy, e.g., hives, anaphylaxis, **treatment options: clarithro, azithro, telithro, TMP/SMX, doxy or FQs. Avoid FQs if under age 18. Dosages in** *footnote 2 page 32.* If allergy just skin rash, can use cephalosporin OK. **YES:** FQ (adults). For pen. allergy, see Comments. **Severe Disease:** Gati, levo, moxi	**Rx goals: (1)** Resolve infection, (2) prevent complications of bacterial disease, e.g., bacteremia, meningitis, brain abscess, (3) avoid chronic sinus disease, (4) avoid unnecessary antibiotic rx. High rate of spontaneous resolution. For pts with pen/cephalosporin allergy, see above. Avoid FQs if under age 18. Dosages in footnote 2 page 32. Watch for pts with fever & fascial cellulitis: 1 risk of S. aureus infection, requires IV **nafcillin/oxacillin** (antistaphylococcal penicillin, penicillinase-resistant). In areas with prevalence of DRSP >30% and recent prior antibiotic use, consider increasing amoxicillin dose to 3–3.5 gm/d; use extra amox, do not increase AM/CL beyond standard dosage.
		For mild/mod. disease: AM/CL-ER (adults) or cefdinir or cefpodoxime or cefprozil or telithro Amox or AM/CL-ER (adults) or cefdinir or cefpodoxime or cefprozil or telithro Treat x10 days. Adult and pediatric doses in footnote 2 page 32 & footnote 2 page 7 (Otitis)		Usual 10 days. In 1 study, results of 3 & 10 d. of TMP/SMX the same (JAMA 273:1015, 1995). Pts aged 1–18 yrs with clinical diagnosis of sinusitis randomized to placebo, amox, or AM/CL for 14 d. **No difference** in multiple measures of efficacy (Pediatrics 107:619, 2001). Similar study in adults (AtM 163:1793, 2003).
Clinical failure after 3 days	As above; consider diagnostic tap/aspirate	**Mild/Mod. Disease:** AM/CL-ER OR (cefpodoxime, cefprozil, or cefdinir) See Table 11, page 80. Ref: NEJM 357:254, 1997		
Diabetes mellitus with acute ketoacidosis, neutropenia, deferoxamine rx	Rhizopus sp. (mucor), aspergillus			

---

¹ **Ceftriaxone** 2.0 gm IV qd: **cefotaxime** 2.0 gm IV q4–8h IV; **AM/SB** 3.0 gm IV q6h.

² **Penicillin** may be given in divided doses q4–6h or by continuous infusion.

³ **Pediatric doses for sinusitis (all oral): Amoxicillin** high dose 90 mg/kg/d div. q8h or q12h; **AM/CL-ES** (cefuroxime axetil) div q6h, q8h, or q12h; then 3.75 mg/kg, **clarithro** 15 mg/kg/d div. q12h; **cefpodoxime** 10 mg/kg/d div. daily or div. q12–24h, **cefdinir** 14 mg/kg/d once daily or divided bid.
TMP/SMX 8–12 mg TMP/40–60 mg SMX/kg/d div. q12h.

Amox/clav doses: **amox** 2000/125 mg **amox** 1.0 gm IV, **clarithro** 500 mg qid or **clarithro ext. release** 1.0 gm; **amox**, **doxy** 100 mg bid, FQs (**gati** 400 mg qd)
gemi 320 mg qd *(not FDA indication for sinusitis)* **levo** 750 mg qid, **moxi** 400 mg qd), **Oceph** (**cefdinir** 300 mg q12h or 600 mg qd), **cefpodoxime** 200 mg bid, **cefprozil** 250–500 mg bid.
cefuroxime 250 mg bid, **TMP/SMX** 1 double-strength (TMP 160 mg) bid, **telithro** 800 mg qd *(not FDA approved 10/03)*.
(Footnotes and abbreviations on page 45) NOTE: All dosage recommendations are for adults (unless otherwise indicated) and assume normal renal function

TABLE 1 (33)

ANATOMIC SITE/DIAGNOSIS/ MODIFYING CIRCUMSTANCES	ETIOLOGIES (usual)	SUGGESTED REGIMENS*		ADJUNCT DIAGNOSTIC OR THERAPEUTIC MEASURES AND COMMENTS
		PRIMARY	ALTERNATIVE†	
SINUSES, PARANASAL/Sinusitis, Acute				
Hospitalized + nasotracheal or nasogastric intubation	Gm-neg. bacilli 47% (pseudomonas, acinetobacter, E. coli common), Gm+ (S. aureus) 35%, yeasts 18%. Polymicrobial in 80%.	Remove nasotracheal tube and if fever persists, recommend sinus aspiration for C/S prior to empiric rx	**IMP** 0.5 gm q6h or **vanco†** (or **CFP** 2.0 gm IV q12h IV)	After 7 d. of nasotracheal or gastric tubes, bacterial sinusitis (fluid in sinuses), but on transnasal puncture only 38% culture + (AJRCCM 150:776, 1994). With nasotracheal mechanical ventilation for ≥1 wk, bacterial sinusitis occurs in 10%. (CID 27:851, 1998). May need fluconazole if yeast on Gram stain of aspirate. Review: CID 25:1441, 1997. Epidemiology study: CID 27:463, 1998.
Sinusitis, chronic **Adults**	Prevotella, anaerobic strep. & fusobacteria—common anaerobes. Strep sp. hemophilus, P. aeruginosa, S. aureus, & moraxella—aerobes. (CID 35:428, 2002)	Antibiotics usually not effective	Otolaryngology consultation, if sinusitis exacerbation, rx as acute	Pathogenesis unclear and may be polyfactorial: damage to ostiomeatal complex during acute bacterial sinusitis, allergy ± polyps, occult immunodeficiency, and/or odontogenic disease (periodontitis in maxillary teeth).
SKIN				
Acne vulgaris (NEJM 336:1156, 1997; Ln 351:1871, 1998; Med Lett 44:52, 2002)				
Comedonal acne. "blackheads," "whiteheads," earliest form, no inflammation	Excessive sebum production & gland obstruction. No Propionibacterium acnes	Once-daily: Topical **tretinoin** (cream 0.025 or 0.05%) or (gel 0.01 or 0.025%)	All once-daily: Topical **adapalene** 0.1% gel OR **azelaic acid** 20% cream bid	Goal is prevention. ↓ number of new comedones and create an environment unfavorable to P. acnes. Adapalene causes less irritation than tretinoin. Azelaic acid less potent but less irritating than retinoids.
Mild inflammatory acne: small papules or pustules	Proliferation of P. acnes + abnormal desquamation of follicular cells	Topical **erythro** 3% + **benzoyl peroxide** 5%, bid	Can substitute **clinda** 1% gel for erythro	Topical metro has anti-inflammatory activity but P. acnes not susceptible.
Inflammatory acne: comedones, papules & pustules. Less common: deep nodules (cysts)	Progression of above events	Topical **erythro** 3% + **benzoyl peroxide** 5%, bid) ± oral antibiotic	Oral drugs: (**doxy** 100 mg bid) or (**minocycline** 50 mg bid) + topical benzoyl peroxide. Other oral antibiotics: **erythro, TMP/SMX, clinda**	Systemic **isotretinoin** reserved for pts with severe widespread nodular (cystic) lesions that fail oral antibiotic rx; 4–5 mo. course of 0.1–1.0 mg/kg/day. Aggressive/violent behavior reported. Tetracyclines stain developing teeth. Doxy can cause photosensitivity. Minocycline side-effects: urticaria, vertigo, pigment deposition in skin or oral mucosa.
Acne rosacea	? skin mite Demodex folliculorum	**Azelaic acid gel** bid, topical	Metro topical cream bid	More pt satisfaction with azelaic acid (J Am Acad Derm 40(6, Pt 1):961, 1999).
Anthrax, cutaneous, inhalation (pulmonary, mediastinal) **To report bioterrorism event:** 770-488-7100; **For info: www.bt.cdc.gov** Refs.: JAMA 281:1735, 1999, & MMWR 50:909, 2001	**B. anthracis.** See Lung, page 28, and Table 1B, page 46	**Adults (including pregnancy):** CIP 500 mg po bid OR **Doxy** 100 mg po bid. **Children:** CIP 20–30 mg/kg/d div q12h (to max 1 gm/d.) x60 d.	**Adults (including pregnancy): Doxy** 100 mg (po bid) x60 d. **Children: Doxy** >8 y/o & >45 kg: 100 mg po bid; ≤8 y/o & ≤45 kg: 2.2 mg/kg po bid; >8 y/o & ≤45 kg: 2.2 mg/kg po bid x60 d.	1. If penicillin susceptible, then: **Adults: Amox** 500 mg po q8h x60 d. **Children: Amox** 80 mg/kg/d div. q8h (max. 500 mg q8h) 2. Treatment of cutaneous anthrax is 7–10 d.; 60 d. in setting of bioterrorism with presumed aerosol exposure 3. Other **FQs** (gati, levo, moxi) should work based on in vitro susceptibility data
Bacillary angiomatosis: For other Bartonella infections, see Cat-scratch disease lymphadenitis, page 30, and Bartonella, page 38	Bartonella henselae and quintana	**Clarithro** 500 mg bid po or **azithro** 250 mg qd po or **CIP** 500–750 mg bid po (see Comment)	**Erythro** 500 mg qid po or **Doxy** 100 mg bid po	In immunocompetent pts with severe disease, doxy 100 mg po/IV bid + RIF 300 mg po bid reported effective (IDC Nor Amer 12:37, 1998; Adv PID 11:1, 1996).
In immunocompromised (HIV-1, bone marrow transplant) patients *Also see SANFORD GUIDE TO HIV/AIDS THERAPY*				In immunocompromised pts with severe disease

NOTE: All dosage recommendations are for adults (unless otherwise indicated) and assume normal renal function

(Footnotes and abbreviations on page 45)

NOTE: All dosage recommendations are for adults (unless otherwise indicated) and assume normal renal function

TABLE 1 (34)

ANATOMIC SITE/DIAGNOSIS/ MODIFYING CIRCUMSTANCES	ETIOLOGIES (usual)	SUGGESTED REGIMENS*		ADJUNCT DIAGNOSTIC OR THERAPEUTIC MEASURES AND COMMENTS
		PRIMARY	**ALTERNATIVE†**	
SKIN (continued)				
Bite: Prophylaxis within 12 hrs of bite or empirical rx of established infection. Ref.: CID 14:633, 1992; remember tetanus prophylaxis—see Table 20C. See Table 20C for rabies prophylaxis				
Bat, raccoon, skunk	?	AM/CL 875/125 mg bid or 500/125 mg tid po	Doxy 100 mg bid po	In Americas, antirabies rx indicated, antirabies immune globulin + vaccine. (See Table 20C, page 155)
Cat (Ref., NEJM 340:85 & 138, 1999)	Pasteurella multocida, Staph. aureus	AM/CL 875/125 mg bid or 500/125 mg tid po	Cefuroxime axetil 0.5 gm q12h po or doxy 100 mg bid po. Do not use cephalexin	80% cat bites become infected. P. multocida resistant to dicloxacillin, cephalexin, clinda; many strains resistant to erythro (most sensitive to azithro but no clinical data). P. multocida infection develops within 24 hrs. Observe for osteomyelitis. If culture + for only P. multocida, can switch to pen VK po.
Catfish sting	Toxins	See Comments		Presents as immediate pain, erythema and edema. Resembles strep cellulitis. May become secondarily infected. PCG is reasonable choice for prophylaxis.
Dog (Ref. NEJM 340:85 & 138, 1999)	P. multocida, S. aureus, Bacteroides sp., Fusobacterium sp., EF-4, Capnocytophaga	AM/CL 875/125 mg bid or 500/125 mg tid po	Clinda 300 mg qid po + FQ (adults) or clinda + TMP/SMX (children)	Only 5% dog bites become infected. Prophylaxis may be worthwhile (AcEM 23:535, 1994). Consider antirabies rx, rabies immune globulin + vaccine (Table 20C). May transmit blastomycosis. Capnocytophaga in splenectomized pts may cause local eschar, sepsis with DIC. P. multocida resistant to dicloxacillin, cephalexin, clinda and erythro, sensitive to FQs in vitro (AAC 43:1475, 1999). For in vitro susceptibility vs macrolides see JAC 41:391, 1998.
Human	Viridans strep 100%, Staph epidermidis 53%, coryne-bacterium 41%, Staph. aureus 29%, eikenella 15%, bacteroides 82%, peptostrep 26%.	Early (not yet infected): AM/CL 875/125 mg po x5 d. Later: Signs of infection (usually in 3–24 hrs) + cefoxitin 2.0 gm q8h IV or TC/CL 3.1 gm q6h IV or PIP/TZ 3.375 gm q6h or 4.5 gm q8h IV]	Pen allergy: Clinda + (either CIP or TMP/SMX) P Ceph 3 or TC/CL or IMP	Eikenella resistant to clinda, nafcillin/oxacillin, metro, P Ceph 1, and erythro; susceptible to FQs and TMP/SMX.
Pig (swine)	Polymicrobic: Gm+ cocci, Gm-neg. bacilli, anaerobes, Pasteurella sp.	AM/CL 875/125 mg bid po	P Ceph 3 or TC/CL or IMP	Information limited but infection is common and serious (Ln 348:886, 1996).
Primate, non-human	Herpesvirus simiae	Acyclovir: See Table 14B, page 113		CID 20:421, 1995
Rat	Spirillum minus & Streptobacillus moniliformis	AM/CL 875/125 mg bid po	Doxy	Antibacks rx is not indicated.
Snake: pit viper (Ref. NEJM 347:347, 2002)	Pseudomonas sp., Enterobacteriaceae, Staph. epidermidis, Clostridium sp.	AM/CL 875/125 mg bid po		Primary therapy is antivenom. Penicillin generally used but would not be effective vs organisms isolated. Ceftriaxone should be more effective than AM/CL.
Spider Widow (Latrodectus)	Not infectious	None		May be confused with "acute abdomen." Diazepam or calcium gluconate helpful to control pain, muscle spasm. Tetanus prophylaxis.
Brown recluse (Loxoscoeles) (not west of Nebraska)	Not infectious (Ref: JID 35:426, 2001	Dapsone 50 mg q4 po (see Comments)		Systemic antibiotics do not shorten clinical course: theoretically lower risk of bacteremia
Boils—Furunculosis—Subcutaneous abscesses in drug addicts ("skin poppers")				
	Staph. aureus, both MSSA & MRSA	Guided by in vitro susceptibilities, Staph, epidermidis, Staph. MRSA	Hot packs, incision, & drainage	Epidemic of community-acquired MRSA, often susceptible to TMP/SMX, clinda, minocycline, & linezolid. If erythro-resistant, probably clinda-resistant. Seems reasonable in pts with large abscesses and/or fever to rx: (1) I&D culture & sens, & (2) empiric TMP/SMX-DS, 1 bid
To lessen number of recurrences	MSSA & MRSA	Dapsone 50 mg qd po		Plus: Nasal & under fingernail treatment with either bacitracin ointment or mupirocin ointment bid
		Dicliox 500 mg po qid or TMP/SMX-DS 1 tab po bid) + RIF 600 mg po qd, all x10 d		Plus: Shower with Hibiclens daily x3 d, then 3x/week. Others have tried 5% povidone-iodine cream intranasal 4x/d, x5 d. Reports of S. aureus resistant to bacitracin & mupirocin.

(Footnotes and abbreviations on page 45)   NOTE: All dosage recommendations are for adults (unless otherwise indicated) and assume normal renal function

TABLE 1 (35)

ANATOMIC SITE/DIAGNOSIS/ MODIFYING CIRCUMSTANCES	ETIOLOGIES (usual)	SUGGESTED REGIMENS*		ADJUNCT DIAGNOSTIC OR THERAPEUTIC MEASURES AND COMMENTS
		PRIMARY	ALTERNATIVE†	
SKIN/Boils—Furunculosis (continued)				
Hidradenitis suppurativa	Lesions secondarily infected: S. aureus, Enterobacteriaceae, pseudomonas, anaerobes	Aspirate, rx on culture	Many pts ultimately require surgical excision.	Caused by keratinous plugging of apocrine glands of axillary and/or inguinal areas.
Burns				
Initial burn wound care	Not infected	Early excision & wound closure; shower hydrotherapy. Role of topical antimicrobics unclear.	**Silver sulfadiazine** cream, 1%, apply 1–2x/day or 0.5% **silver nitrate** solution or **mafenide acetate** cream. Apply 2x/day.	Many pts during 1st wk of sulfadiazine but resolves even if use is continued. Silver nitrate leaches electrolytes from wounds & stains everything. Mafenide inhibits carbonic anhydrase and can cause metabolic acidosis.
Burn wound sepsis Variety of skin grafts and skin substitutes, see JAMA 283:717, 2000	Strep. pyogenes, Enterobacter sp, S. aureus, S. epidermidis, E. faecalis, E. coli, P. aeruginosa. Fungi rare. Herpesvirus rare.	**(Vanco** 1.0 gm q12h IV) + (**amikacin** 10 mg/kg load then 7.5 mg/kg q12h IV) + **PIP** 4 gm q4h IV (give ½ daily dose of piperacillin into subeschar tissues with surgical eschar removal within 12 hours)		Monitor serum levels, ½ of most antibiotics ↓. Staph. aureus tend to remain localized to burn wound. If patient more toxic than expected, consider toxic shock syndrome. Candida spp. colonize but seldom invade. Pneumonia has become the major infectious complication, most often staph. Other infectious complications include septic thrombophlebitis.
Cellulitis, erysipelas: Be wary of macrolide (erythro)-resistant) S. pyogenes				
Extremities, not associated with venous catheter (see Comments): non-diabetic For diabetes, see below	Group A strep. occ. Group C, G. Staph. aureus (uncommon but difficult to exclude)	**Pen G** 1–2 mU IV q6h or (**Nafcillin or oxacillin** 2 gm q4h IV). If not severe, (**dicloxacillin** 500 mg q6h po or **cefazolin** 1 gm q8h IV). See Comment	**Erythro** or **P Ceph 1** or **clarithro** or **azithro** (Dosage, see footnote page 25) See Comment	"**Spontaneous" erysipelas of leg in non-diabetic is usually due to strep. Gps A,B,C or G.** Hence OK to start with IV **pen G 1–2 mU q6h** & observe for localized S. aureus infection. Look for tinea pedis with fissures, a common portal of entry; can mimic culture strep from between toes (CID 23:1162, 1996). For recurrent erysipelas & lymphedema & recurrent erysipelas, see prophylaxis, Table 15. Other alternatives: clinda, levo, moxi.
Facial, adult (erysipelas)	Group A strep, Staph. aureus	**Nafcillin or oxacillin** (Dosage, see erysipelas of extremity, above)	**Cefazolin** or **vanco** if not severe, **AM/CL**	**Choice of empiric therapy must have activity vs S. aureus** erysipelas of face can mimic S. pyogenes erysipelas of an extremity.
Diabetes mellitus and erysipelas (See Foot, "Diabetic", page 10)	Group A strep, Staph. aureus, Enterobacteriaceae, clostridia (rare)	Early mild: **P Ceph 2/3** or **AM/CL**. Only for severe disease: **IMP** or **MER** or **erta** IV. Dosage, see Diabetic foot.		Prompt surgical debridement indicated to rule out necrotizing fasciitis and to obtain cultures. If septic, consider x-ray of extremity to demonstrate gas. **Prognosis dependent on blood supply: assess arteries.** See Diabetic foot, page 10.
Erysipelas, recurrent 2° to congenital lymphedema (Milroy's disease)	Group A strep; Staph. aureus, Groups A; C, G.	**Benzathine pen G** 1.2 mU IM q4 wks (of minimal benefit in reducing recurrences in pts with underlying predisposing conditions)	**Azithro** or **clarithro** or **clarithro** (Dosage, see footnote page 25)	Indicated only if pt is having frequent episodes of cellulitis. Pen V 250 mg po bid should be effective but not aware of clinical trials. In pen-allergic pts: erythro 500 mg po qid, azithro 250 mg po qd, or clarithro 500 mg po qd.
Dandruff (seborrheic dermatitis)	Malassezia species	Ketoconazole shampoo 2% or selenium sulfide 2.5%		(see Page 6, chronic external otitis)
Decubitus or venous stasis or arterial insufficiency ulcers; with sepsis	Polymicrobic: S. pyogenes (Gps A,C,G), Staph. aureus, anaerobic strep, Enterobacteriaceae sp., Enterococcus sp., Pseudomonas sp., Bacteroides sp., Staph. aureus	**IMP** or **MER** or **TC/CL** or **PIP/TZ** or erta	**CIP, gati, levo,** (moxi) **PIP/TZ** or erta Dosages, see footnotes pages 10, 16, 20, 42	Without sepsis or extensive cellulitis local care may be adequate. Debride as necessary. Topical mafenide or silver sulfadiazine adjunctive. R/O underlying osteomyelitis. May need wound coverage with skin graft or skin substitute (JAMA 283:716, 2000).
Erythema multiforme	H. simplex type 1			**Rx:** Acyclovir if due to H. simplex
Erythema nodosum	Sarcoidosis, inflammatory bowel disease, M. tbc, coccidioidomycosis, yersinia, sulfonamides			**Rx:** NSAIDs; glucocorticoids if refractory.
Erythrasma	Corynebacterium minutissimum	**Erythro** 250 mg q6h po x14 d.		(Coral red fluorescence with Wood's lamp. Alt. 2% aqueous clinda topically.)
Folliculitis	Many etiologies: S. aureus, candida, P. aeruginosa, malassezia, demodex	See individual entities.	See Whirlpool folliculitis, page 88.	
Furunculosis	Staph. aureus	See Boils, page 45		

(Footnotes and abbreviations on page 45) NOTE: All dosage recommendations are for adults (unless otherwise indicated) and assume normal renal function.

TABLE 1 (36)

ANATOMIC SITE/DIAGNOSIS/ MODIFYING CIRCUMSTANCES	ETIOLOGIES (usual)	SUGGESTED REGIMENS*		ADJUNCT DIAGNOSTIC OR THERAPEUTIC MEASURES AND COMMENTS
		PRIMARY	ALTERNATIVE†	
SKIN (continued)				
Hemorrhagic bullous lesions Hx of sea water-contaminated abrasion or eating raw seafood, shock	Vibrio vulnificus, V. damsela	**Ceftazidime** 2.0 gm q8h IV + **doxy** 100 mg bid (IV or po)	Either **cefotaxan** 2.0 gm q8h IV or **CIP** 750 mg bid (IV po or 400 mg bid IV)	¾ pts have chronic liver disease with mortality in 50% (NEJM 312:343, 1985). In Taiwan, where a number of cases are seen, the impression exists that ceftazidime is superior to tetracycline (CID 15:271, 1992), hence both.
Herpes zoster (shingles). See Table 14				
Impetigo, ecthyma—usually children Group A strep impetigo: crusted lesions can be Staph. aureus + streptococci		Oral **dicloxacillin** or **cloxacillin**	**Mupirocin** ointment or **clarithro** or **erythro** or **O Ceph 2**	24% failure with pen VK (AJDC 144:1313, 1990). O Ceph 2 >90% cure (AAC 36: 1614, 1992).
			For dosages, see Table 10B for adults and Table 16, page 129 for children	
"honey-colored"-crust" lesions (nonbullous)	Staph. aureus + streptococci			
Bullous (if ruptured, thin "varnish-like" crust)	Staph. aureus impetigo	**Dicloxacillin** po or **oxacillin** po or **O Ceph 1** (not cefixime^AB)	**Mupirocin** ointment or **AM/CL** po or **azithro** or **clarithro**, see Table 10B	NOTE: Cefixime^AB not active vs Staph. aureus
		For dosages, see page 35; for post-operative, see below		
Infected wound, extremity—**Post-trauma** (for bites, see page 35; for post-operative, see below) Mild to moderate, uncomplicated	Polymicrobic: Staph. aureus, Group A & anaerobic strep, Enterobacteriaceae, Cl. perfringens, Cl. tetani. If water exposure, Pseudomonas sp., Aeromonas sp.	**AM/CL** 875/125 mg bid or 500/125 mg tid po) or **O Ceph 1** (Dosage, page 10)	**Erytho** or **clarithro** or **azithro** or **clinda** (Dosage, see page 20) or **levo** 500 mg po qd	Wound cleansing and debridement. Gram stain may enable rapid diagnosis of clostridia, staph. For **mild** S. aureus/S. pyogenes infections, could use mupirocin cream 2% tid x10 d. Antitetanus prophylaxis (See Table 20D, page 139). If freshwater exposure, Pseudomonas and Aeromonas species possible. FQ recommended therapy. NOTE: **Ertapenem** not active vs P. aeruginosa. If sea water, see hemorrhagic bullous lesions and Vibrio vulnificus, above.
Febrile with sepsis		**AM/SB** or **TC/CL** or **PIP/TZ** or **IMP** or **MER** or **erta** (Dosage, see page 16)	(**Naficillin** or **oxacillin** 2.0 gm q4h IV) + **CIP** + **clinda** or **levo** 750 mg IV/po qd	NOTE: None of treatment regimens predictably effective for MRSA. Treatment duration varies with severity, from 5–10 days.
Infected wound, post-operative—Gram stain negative				
Surgery not involving GI or female genital tract	Staph. aureus, Group A strep, Enterobacteriaceae	**O Ceph 1** or **AM/CL**	**Dicloxacillin** po ± **FQ** (Dosage, see page 16)	Gram stain exudate to guide treatment choice. Surgical drainage alone often adequate. Where MRSA prevalent, **add vanco**. Treat until sepsis after 72 hours, it can be switched to oral therapy. Treat until pt afebrile and wound granulating
Without sepsis	Staph. aureus, Group A strep, Enterobacteriaceae	**TC/CL** or **PIP/TZ**	**P Ceph 1/2/3** (Dosage, see page 16)	
With sepsis	Above + Bacteroides sp. + other anaerobes, enterococci, Group A, B, C strep.	**PIP/TZ** or **erta** (Dosage, see page 16)	**P Ceph 3** + **metro** or **erta** or **IMP** or **MER**	For all treatment options, see page 31.
Surgery involving GI tract (includes oropharynx, esophagus) or female genital tract				
Meleney's synergistic gangrene. See Necrotizing fascitis, below				
Infected wound, febrile patient—Gram stain: Gram-positive cocci in clusters	S. aureus, possibly MRSA	**Oral: TMP/SMX-DS** 1 tab po bid	**Do culture & sensitivity** **IV: Vanco** 1.0 gm IV q12h or **daptomycin** 4 mg/kg IV once daily	Apparent ↑ in community-acquired MRSA (CA-MRSA). Need culture & sensitivity to verify. Other po options for CA-MRSA include minocycline 100 mg po q12h (inexpensive) & linezolid 600 mg po q12h (expensive)
Necrotizing fascitis ("flesh-eating bacteria") Post-surgery, trauma, streptococcal skin infections See Gas gangrene, page 40, & Toxic shock, page 43	(1) S. pyogenes, (2) Clostridia sp., (3) polymicrobic: aerobic + anaerobic (if S. aureus + anaerobic then Meleney's synergistic gangrene)	For treatment of clostridia, see Muscle, gas gangrene, page 40. Meleney's synergistic gangrene, Fournier's gangrene, necrotizing fascitis is not precise: **surgical debridement** as well as antibiotics. Dx of necrotizing fascitis requires incision and probing. If no resistance to probing subcutaneous (fascial plane), dk = necrotizing fascitis. Need **Gram stain/culture** to determine if etiology is strep, clostridia or polymicrobial		(1) S. pyogenes, (2) Group A, C, G, (1) Streptococci. (Gp A, C, G streptococci. Clostridia sp. dk = necrotizing fascitis. **All require prompt** The terminology of polymicrobic wound infections is not precise. Necrotizing fascitis have a common pathophysiology. **All require prompt**
		Treatment: Pen G if strep or clostridia. **IMP** or **MER** if polymicrobial		

Footnotes and abbreviations on page 45.   NOTE: All dosage recommendations are for adults (unless otherwise indicated) and assume normal renal function

TABLE 1 (37)

ANATOMIC SITE/DIAGNOSIS/ MODIFYING CIRCUMSTANCES	ETIOLOGIES (usual)	SUGGESTED REGIMENS* PRIMARY	ALTERNATIVE*	ADJUNCT DIAGNOSTIC OR THERAPEUTIC MEASURES AND COMMENTS
SKIN *(continued)*				
Staphylococcal scalded skin syndrome Ref.: *PIDJ* 17:1088, 2000	Toxin-producing S. aureus	Nafcillin or oxacillin 2.0 gm IV q4h kg/d div. q6h) ×5-7 days	(children: 150 mg/	Toxin causes **intraepidermal split** and positive Nikolsky sign. Drugs cause epidermal/dermal split, **called toxic epidermal necrolysis**—more serious (*Ln 351: 1417, 1998*).
Warts (Hot Tub) folliculitis See Folliculitis, page 36	Pseudomonas aeruginosa	Usually self-limited, treatment not indicated		Decontaminate hot tub: drain and chlorinate. Also associated with exfoliative beauty aids (loofah sponges) (*J Clin Micro 31:480, 1993*).
SPLEEN				
Splenic abscess Endocarditis, bacteremia	Staph. aureus, streptococci	Nafcillin or oxacillin 2.0 gm q4h IV **+ Vanco** 1.0 gm q12h IV		Burkholderia (Pseudomonas) pseudomallei is common cause of splenic abscess in SE Asia.
Contiguous from intra-abdominal site	Polymicrobic	*Treat as Peritonitis, secondary, page 37*		
Immunocompromised	Candida sp.	**Amphotericin B** (dosage, see Table 11, page 76)	**Fluconazole**	

SYSTEMIC FEBRILE SYNDROMES

Spread by infected **TICK, FLEA, or LICE** (*CID 29:888, 1999*): Epidemiologic history crucial. **Babesiosis, Lyme disease, & granulocytic Ehrlichiosis** have same reservoir & tick vector

Babesiosis: see *NEJM 343: 1454, 2000.* Do not treat if asymptomatic, young, has spleen, and immunocompetent	Etiol.: B. microti et al. Vector: Usually Ixodes ticks. Host: White-footed mouse & others	(**Atovaquone** 750 mg po q12h) + **azithro** 500 mg po (day 1, then 250 mg/d) ×7-10 days **or** (**clinda** 1.2 gm bid or 600 mg tid po) **+ quinine** 650 mg po ×7 d. **Ped. dosage:** Clinda 20-40 mg/kg/d and quinine 25 mg/kg/d		Exposure endemic areas May to Sept. Can result from blood transfusion (*JAMA 1999; 1871, 1999*). Usually subclinical illness likely in asplenic pts, pts with concomitant Lyme disease, older pts, or with HIV. Dx: Giemsa-stained blood smear; antibody test available. PCR under study. Exchange transfusions successful adjunct, used early, in severe disease.
Bartonella infections: *NEJM 340:184, 1999; CID 35:684, 2002*				
Asymptomatic bacteremia	B. quintana	Doxy 100 mg po/IV ×15 d		Can lead to endocarditis &/or trench fever: found in homeless, esp. if lice/leg
Cat-scratch disease	B. henselae	Azithro if symptomatic only—see page 30; usually lymphadenitis, can involve CNS, in immunocompetent pts		**Immunocompetent Patient:** Bacteremia/endocarditis/FUO
Bacillary angiomatosis; Pelosis hepatis—pts with AIDS	B. henselae, B. quintana	**Clarithro** 500 mg bid po or **clarithro ER** 1.0 gm qd po or **azithro** 250 mg po qd or **CIP** 500-750 mg bid po	**Erythro** 500 mg po qid or **doxy** 100 mg po bid ×8 wks; if severe, combination of doxy 100 mg po/IV bid + RIF 300 mg po/IV bid (*IDC No Amer 12:37, 1998*)	**HIV/AIDS Patient:** Bacillary angiomatosis Bacillary peliosis Bacteremia/endocarditis/FUO
Endocarditis (see page 20)	B. henselae, B. quintana	**Gentamicin** 3 mg/kg IV once daily x minimum 14 d. + doxy 200 mg po once daily x28 d.		Hard to detect with automated blood culture systems. Need lysis-centrifugation and/or blind subculture onto chocolate agar at 7 & 14 days. Diagnosis often by antibody titer ≥1:800.
Trench fever (FUO)	B. quintana	Doxy 100 mg bid po		Same as Urban Trench Fever
Ehrlichiosis: CDC def. of confirmed case as one of: (1) 4× IFA antibody (2) detection of Ehrlichia DNA by PCR				
Human monocytic ehrlichiosis (HME) (*JCCP 7:252, 1998*)	Anaplasma (Ehrlichia) chaffeensis (Lone Star tick is vector)	Doxy 100 mg bid po **or** Tetracycline 500 mg po qid x7-14 d. No current recommendation for children or pregnancy		(3) visible modulae in WBC, and IFA ≥1:64 (*MMWR 46(RR-10):1-55, 1997*). 30 states: mostly SE of line from NJ to Ill. to Missouri to Texas. History of outdoor activity and tick exposure. April-Sept. Fever, rash (36%). Leukopenia and thrombocytopenia. Blood smears no help. PCR for early dx.
Human granulocytic ehrlichiosis (HGE) (*CID 31:554, 2000*)	Anaplasma phagocytophilum (Ixodes sp. ticks are vector)	Doxy 100 mg bid po **or** IV x7-14 d.	Tetracycline 500 mg 4x/d. po x7-14 d. in children or pregnancy	In endemic area (Wisc., Minn., New York), high % of adult Ixodes ticks infected. Acute febrile flu-like illness after outdoor activity. No rash. Leukopenia/thrombocytopenia common. **Dx:** Up to 80% have positive blood smear. Antibody test for confirmation. **Rx** RIF successful in pregnancy (*CID 27:213, 1998*) but worry about resistance developing (*Based on in vitro studies, no clear alternative rx—levo* activity marginal (*AAC 47:413, 2003*)).

---

¹ In endemic area (New York), high % of both adult ticks and nymphs were pointly infected with both HGE and B. burgdorferi (*NEJM 337:49, 1997*).
(*Footnotes and abbreviations on page 45*)   NOTE: All dosage recommendations are for adults (unless otherwise indicated) and assume normal renal function

TABLE 1 (38)

ANATOMIC SITE/DIAGNOSIS/ MODIFYING CIRCUMSTANCES	ETIOLOGIES (usual)	SUGGESTED REGIMENS*		ADJUNCT DIAGNOSTIC OR THERAPEUTIC MEASURES AND COMMENTS
		PRIMARY	ALTERNATIVE†	
SYSTEMIC FEBRILE SYNDROMES (continued)				
Human/dog granulocytic ehrlichiosis (NEJM 341:148 & 195, 1999)	Spread by infected TICK, FLEA or LICE/Ehrlichiosis Ehrlichia ewingii	**Doxy** 100 mg bid po or IV x7-14 d.		Previously only recognized in dogs; human cases now documented. Inclusion in granulocytes.
Lyme Disease NOTE: Think about concomitant tick-borne disease—babesiosis (JAMA 275:1657, 1996) or ehrlichiosis				Reviews: Ln ID 3:489 & 761, 2003; Ln 362:1639, 2003
Tick bites, possible Ixodes scapularis in endemic area See Comment	Borrelia burgdorferi. Urine antigen test reported unreliable (AJM 110:217 & 236, 2001)	If endemic area, if nymphal partially engorged deer tick: **doxy** 200 mg x1 with food	If not endemic area, not engorged, not deer tick: No treatment	Prophylaxis study in endemic area: erythema migrans developed in 3% of the control group and 0.4% doxy group (NEJM 345:79 & 133, 2001).
Early (erythema migrans) See Comment	Terminology ref.: AnIM 136:413, 2002. **Lyme Disease National Surveillance Case Definition** available at either NEJM 345:115, 2001 or JAMA 288:1002, 2002	**Doxy** 100 mg bid po, or **amoxicillin** 500 mg tid po or **cefuroxime axetil** 500 mg bid po, all regimens for 14-21 d. See Comment for peds doses	**Doxy** (all for 14-21 d.) with azithro & erythro (Drugs 57:157, 1999) or **erythro** 250 mg po qid x14-21 d. (10 d. as good as 20: AnIM 138:697, 2003)	High rate of clinical failure with azithro & erythro (Drugs 57:157, 1999) **Peds** (all for 14-21 d.): Amox 50 mg/kg/d in 3 div. doses or cefuroxime axetil 30 mg/kg/d in 2 div. doses or erythro 30 mg/kg/d in 3 div. doses. Lesions usually homogeneous—not target-like (AnIM 136:423, 2002).
Carditis See Comment		(**Ceftriaxone** 2.0 gm qd IV) or (**cefotaxime** 2.0 gm q8h IV) or (**pen G** 24 million u/d IV) x14-21 d. See Comment	**Doxy** (see Comment) 100 mg bid po x14-21 d. or **amoxicillin** 500 mg tid po x14-21 d.	First degree AV block: Oral regimen. IV therapy—permanent pacemaker not necessary. High degree AV block (PR >0.3 sec.): IV pen. Oral regimen OK. If normal.
Facial nerve paralysis (isolated finding, early)		**Ceftriaxone** 2.0 gm qd IV x14-21 d.		LP suggested to exclude neurologic disease. If LP neg., oral regimen OK. If abnormal or not done, suggest parenteral regimen.
Meningitis, encephalitis For encephalopathy, see Comment		(**Ceftriaxone** 2.0 gm qd IV or **cefotaxime** 2.0 gm q8h IV) or (**Pen G** 20 mil u/d in div. doses IV) x14-28 d.		Encephalopathy—memory difficulty, depression, somnolence, or headache. CSF abnormalities. 89% had objective CSF abnormalities. 18/18 pts improved with ceftriaxone 2 gm/d. x30 d. (JID 180:377, 1999).
Arthritis		(**Doxy** 100 mg bid) or (**amoxicillin** 500 mg tid po) both x30-60 d.	(**Ceftriaxone** 2 gm, qd IV) or (**cefotaxime** 2 gm x21 d. IV) or (**pen G** 20-24 mil u/d IV) x14-28 d.	
Pregnant women	[Choice should not include doxy; **amoxicillin** 500 mg tid po x21 d.]			
Asymptomatic seropositivity and symptoms post-rx		None indicated		No benefit from rx (NEJM 345:85, 2001).
Plague **As biological weapon:** JAMA 283:2281, 2000; and Table 18, page 46	Yersinia pestis Reservoir: rat Vector: rat flea	**Gentamicin** 2.0 mg/kg IV loading dose then 1.7 mg/ kg q8h IV or **streptomycin** 1.0 gm q12h IM or IV	(**Doxy** 100 mg bid po or IV) or (**chloro** 500 mg qid IV)	Reference: IV streptomycin: CID 19:1150, 1994. Septicemic form can occur without bubo. CIP effective in vitro + in animal models (JAC 41:301, 1998); success in 1 pt (CID 36:521, 2003).
Relapsing fever Can be tick-borne or louse-borne (MMWR 52:809, 2003)	Borrelia recurrentis, B. hermsii, & other borrelia sp.	**Doxy** 100 mg bid po	**Erythro** 500 mg qid po	Jarisch-Herxheimer (fever, ↑ pulse, ↑ resp., ↓ blood pressure) in 10 patients (occurs in ~2 hrs). Not prevented by prior steroids. Can relapse up to 10 times. **Dx:** Examine peripheral blood smear during fever for spirochetes.
Rickettsial diseases Spotted fevers (NOTE: Rickettsia DNA not included) **Rocky Mountain spotted fever (RMSF)** CID 27:1353, 1998; AJTMH 63:21, 2000. NOTE: Can mimic ehrlichiosis	R. rickettsii (Dermacentor ticks)	**Doxy** 100 mg bid po or (IV if vomiting)	**Chloro** use found as risk factor for RMSF (JID 184:1437, 2001)	Fever, rash (95%), petechiae 40–50%. **Rash spreads from distal extremities to trunk.** Dx: Immunohistology on skin biopsy; confirmation with antibody titers. Highest incidence in Mid-Atlantic states; also seen in Oklahoma, S. Dakota, Montana. **NOTE:** Only 3–18% of pts present with fever, rash, and hx of tick exposure; **earlier in children many early deaths and empiric doxy reasonable** (MMWR 49: 888, 2000).

(Footnotes and abbreviations on page 45)

NOTE: All dosage recommendations are for adults (unless otherwise indicated) and assume normal renal function

TABLE 1 (39)

ANATOMIC SITE/DIAGNOSIS/ MODIFYING CIRCUMSTANCES	ETIOLOGIES (usual)	SUGGESTED REGIMENS*		ADJUNCT DIAGNOSTIC OR THERAPEUTIC MEASURES AND COMMENTS
		PRIMARY	ALTERNATIVE†	
SYSTEMIC FEBRILE SYNDROMES: FLEA or LICE/Rickettsial diseases/Spotted fevers (continued)				
Other spotted fevers; e.g., R. conorii et al. 6 species. In sub-Saharan Africa, R. africae—Medical Letter 45:43. In sub-Saharan Africa, R. africae NEJM 344:1504, 2001.	Spread by infected TICK. 6 species: R. conorii et al.	**Doxy** 100 mg bid po x7 d.	Chloro 500 mg po/IV x7 d. Children 15 mg/kg/d in 2 div doses ea azithro 10 mg/kg/d x1 or 3 days equally efficacious in children with Mediterranean spotted fever (NEJM 1504, 2003; Ln 1417, 2003).	Clarithro 15 mg/d in 2 div doses and azithro 10 mg/kg/d x1 or 3 days equally efficacious in children with Mediterranean spotted fever (NEJM 344:1504, 2003; Ln 13:557, 2003; CID 34:154, 2003; Ln ID 3:557, 2003; CID 28:1417, 2003.
Typhus group—Consider in returning travelers with fever				
Louse-borne	R. prowazekii (body louse)	**Doxy** 100 mg IV/po bid x7 d.	Chloro 500 mg IV/po x7	Brill-Zinsser disease (Ln 357:1198, 2001) is a relapse of remote past infection, e.g. WW II. Truncal rash spreads centrifugally—opposite of RMSF. A winter disease
Murine typhus (cat flea typhus form)	R. typhi (rat reservoir and flea vector)	**Doxy** 100 mg IV/po bid x7 d.	Chloro 500 mg IV/po bid x7 d.	Most U.S. cases south Texas and southern Calif. "Flu-like" illness. Rash in <50%: Dx based on suspicion, confirmed serologically.
Scrub typhus	O. tsutsugamushi (rodent reservoir; vector is larval stage of mites (chiggers))	**Doxy** 100 mg IV/po bid x7 d. NOTE: Reports of doxy and chloro resistance from northern Thailand (Ln 348:86, 1996). RIF 900 mg alone 450 mg/kg po x7 d. reported effective (Ln 356:1057, 2000).		Limited to Far East (Asia, India). Cases imported into U.S. Evidence of chigger bite; flu-like illness. Louse-borne typhus.
Tularemia, typhoidal type Ref. bioterrorism: see Table 1B, page 46, & JAMA 285:2763, 2001	Francisella tularensis. (Vector depends on geography: ticks, biting flies, mosquitoes identified)	**Gentamicin** or **tobra** 5 mg/kg/d div. q8h IV x7–14 d.	Add **chloro** if evidence of meningitis. **CIP** reported effective in 12 children (PIDJ 19:449, 2000).	Typhoidal form in 5–30%, pts. No lymphadenopathy. Diarrhea, pneumonia common. Dx: blood cultures, Antibody confirmation. Antibody testing. Clinical failures with rx with P Ceph 3 (CID 17:976, 1993).
Urban trench fever (FUO)	Bartonella quintana (Vector: Body louse)	**Gentamicin** 3 mg/kg IV once daily x mos of 14 d. + **doxy** 200 mg po single daily dose x28 d.		One of many Bartonella syndromes, see page 38
Other Zoonotic Systemic Bacterial Febrile Illnesses: Obtain careful epidemiologic history				
Brucellosis Reviews: CID 21:283, 1995; E/D 3:213, 1997.	Brucella— B. abortus—cattle B. suis—pigs B. melitensis—goats B. canis—dogs	**Doxy** 100 mg po bid x6 wks + **gentamicin** 2–3 mg/kg/d (page 73) or (**doxy** x6 wks + **streptomycin** 1.0 gm IM qd x2–3 wks)	[**Doxy** + **RIF** 600–900 mg qd po, both x6 wks] or [**TMP/SMX** 1 DS tab (160 mg/800 mg) po bid + **gentamicin** 2 wks]	**Relapses:** **Doxy** 100 mg bid x6 wks + **strep** 1.0 gm IM x2 wks, relapse rate 6%. With doxy + RIF relapse rate 14%. Doxy/RIF may be less effective than doxy + SM in pts with spondylitis (AnIM 117:25, 1992). CIP alone initially effective but relapse in 25% (AAC 36:150, 1992); however, oftox + RIF reported effective. **Duration of rx:** For B. melitensis, gent for 7 d. + doxy for 45 d.—fewer relapses than gent x7 d. + doxy for 30 d. (AAC 41:80, 1997). Usual recommendation is 6 wks rx. Longer rx for spondylitis—see CID 29:1440, 1999.
Leptospirosis (CID 36:1507 & 1514, 2003)	Leptospira—in urine of domestic, livestock, dogs, small rodents	**Pen G** 1.5 MU IV q6h or **ceftriaxone** 1.0 gm qd. Duration: 7 days	**Doxy** 100 mg q12h IV or po or **AMP** 0.5–1.0 gm q6h	**Severity varies** Two-stage mild anicteric disease to severe icteric disease (Weil's disease) with renal failure and myocarditis. **Dx:** Culture slow and difficult. Sensitivity/specificity of rapid screening tests poor (J Clin Micro 40:1464, 2002).
Salmonella bacteremia (enteric fever most often caused by S. typhi)	Salmonella enteritidis—a variety of serotypes	**CIP** 400 mg IV q12h x14 d or **Chloro** 50 mg/kg/d IV or po (switch to po when clinically possible)	**Ceftriaxone** 2.0 gm qd IV x14 d, then switch to po **CIP** when possible)	Usual exposure is contaminated poultry and eggs. Many others. Mycotic aneurysm (10% of adults over age 50, AIM 110:690, 2001) seen if underlying atherosclerosis. In sickle cell, osteomyelitis, septic shock. Sporadic reports of resistance to CIP.
Miscellaneous Systemic Febrile Syndromes				
Kawasaki syndrome Usually <5 yrs. of age, peak at 1 yr of age (CID 28:169, 1999)	Unknown; syndrome of ↑ temp., rash, conjunctivitis, stomatitis, adenopathy, red hands/feet & coronary artery aneurysms (See Comment)	**IVIG** 2 gm/kg over 12 hrs + **ASA** 80–100 mg/kg/d po div. in 4 doses THEN **ASA** 3–5 mg/kg/d po 1x/d. x6-8 wks	If still febrile after 1st dose of IVIG, some give 2nd dose (PIDJ 17:1144, 1998)	IV gamma globulin (2.0 gm/kg over 10 hrs) in pts before 10th day of illness ↓ coronary artery lesions (Ln 347:1128, 1996). A current hypothesis: disease due to toxin (superantigen) production by staph or strep species (JID 29:239, 1999; PIDJ 19:91, 2000). See Table 14B, page 115 for IVIG adverse effects and expense.

(Footnotes and abbreviations on page 45)

TABLE 1 (40)

ANATOMIC SITE/DIAGNOSIS/ MODIFYING CIRCUMSTANCES	ETIOLOGIES (usual)	SUGGESTED REGIMENS*		ADJUNCT DIAGNOSTIC OR THERAPEUTIC MEASURES AND COMMENTS
		PRIMARY	ALTERNATIVE†	
SYSTEMIC FEBRILE SYNDROMES/Miscellaneous Systemic Febrile Syndromes *(continued)*				
Rheumatic Fever, acute Ref. *CID 33:806, 2001.*	Post–Group A strep pharyngitis (not Group B, C, or G).	(1) Symptom relief: **ASA** 80–100 mg/kg/d in children; 4–8 gm/d in adults. (2) Eradicate Group A strep: **Pen** x10 d. *(see Pharyngitis, page 32).* (3) Start prophylaxis; see below.		
Prophylaxis				
Primary prophylaxis		Benzathine **pen G** 1.2 mU IM *(see Pharyngitis)*		**Penicillin** for 10 days, prevents rheumatic fever even when started 7–9 days after onset of illness.
Secondary prophylaxis (previous documented rheumatic fever)		Benzathine **pen G** 1.2 mU IM q3–4 wks	Alternative: **Penicillin V** 250 mg po bid or **sulfadiazine (sulfisoxazole)** 1.0 gm/d. po or **erythro** 250 mg po bid. Duration of 2° prophylaxis varies: with carditis continue 10 yrs or until age 25; without carditis continue 5 yrs or to age 21 *(AHA JAMA 118:601, 1995)*.	
Tumor necrosis factor (TNF) blockade of Crohn's disease, rheumatoid arthritis, or other	Drugs used: Etanercept (Enbrel), infliximab (Remicade), adalimumab (Humira)			Pts at increased risk of reactivation of latent tuberculosis. Suggest: TBc history, PPD ± chest x-ray prior to starting therapy.
Typhoidal syndrome (typhoid fever / enteric fever) *(NEJM 347:1770, 2002)*	*Salmonella typhi, S. paratyphi* NOTE: 14% relapse rate with ciliated shock, assoc 5 d. of ceftriaxone *(AAC 44:450, 2000)*	**CIP** 500 mg bid po x10 d.) or **ceftriaxone** 2.0 gm (od IV x14 d.). If associated shock, use **dexamethasone** a few minutes before antibiotic *(see Comment)* In children, CIP superior to ceftriaxone *(LnID 3:537, 2003)*	**Azithro** 1 gm po day 1, then 500 mg po x6 d. *(AAC 43:1441, 1999)* or 1 gm po daily x5 d. *(AAC 44:1855, 2003)*	**Dexamethasone dose:** 3 mg/kg then 1 mg/kg q6h x8 doses ↓ mortality *(NEJM 310:82, 1984)*. **Complications:** perforation (terminal ileum & /or cecum), osteo, septic arthritis, **mycotic aneurysm** (approx. 10% over age 50, *AJM 110:62, 2001)*, meningitis. **Other rx options:** Controlled trial of CIP vs chloro. Efficacy equivalent. After 5 d. of therapy CIP shorter. Blood Culture positive chloro 36% *(AAC 47:1727, 2003)*. Sporadic reports of resistance to CIP.
Sepsis: Following assumes bacteremia; mimicked by viral, fungal, rickettsial infections and pancreatitis				
Neonatal—early onset <1 week old	Group B Strep, E. coli, klebsiella, enterobacter, Staph. aureus (uncommon), listeria (rare) in U.S.	(**AMP + APAG** 2.5 mg/kg q12h IV or IM) or (**AMP + cefotaxime** 50 mg/kg q12h)	(**AMP + APAG** 2.5 mg/kg q12h IV or IM) or (**AMP + cefotaxime** 50 mg/kg q24h IV or IM).	Blood cultures are key but only 5–10% + Discontinue antibiotics after 72 hrs if cultures and course do not support diagnosis. In Spain, listeria predominates; in S. America, salmonella. If Staph. aureus is common, add nafcillin/oxacillin or vanco (if MRSA prevalence is high). Ref. *PIDJ 16:768, 1997.*
Neonatal—late onset 1–4 weeks old	As above + H. influenzae & S. epidermidis	(**AMP + cefotaxime** 50 mg/kg q8h) or (**AMP + ceftriaxone** 75 mg/kg q24h IV)	**Nafcillin** or **oxacillin** + **cefotaxime**	
Child; not neutropenic	H. influenzae; Strep. pneumoniae, Strep. meningococci, Staph. aureus	**Cefotaxime** 50 mg/kg q8h or **ceftriaxone** 100 mg/kg q24h IV or **cefuroxime** 50 mg/kg q8h IV	(**Nafcillin** or **oxacillin**) + **cefuroxime**	AWSB and TIGCCL not currently approved for children. In children who have not received conjugate Hib vaccine, invasive Hib disease has virtually disappeared, without an increase in other organisms *(PIDJ 14:978, 1995; EJCMID 14:935, 1995)*. Meningococcemia mortality remains high *(Ln 356:961, 2000)*.
Adult; not neutropenic; NO HYPOTENSION—For Septic Shock, see page 45 Suspected nuclear; life-threatening	Aerobic Gm-neg. bacilli, Gm+ cocci; others	(**AMP** + ons of: (**P Ceph 3/4** or **PIP/TZ** or **TC/CL**) If suspect MRSA, add **vanco** If suspect VRE, add **linezolid** *Dosages in footnote 1 page 42*	**APAG** + (ons of: **P Ceph 3/4** or **PIP/TZ** or **TC/CL**) If suspect MRSA, add **vanco** If suspect VRE, add **linezolid**	Systemic inflammatory response syndrome (SIRS): 2 or more of the following: 1. Temperature >38°C or <36°C 2. Heart rate >90 beats/min 3. Respiratory rate >20 breaths/min 4. WBC >12,000/μl or >10% bands Sepsis: SIRS + a documented infection (+ culture) Severe sepsis: Sepsis + organ dysfunction, hypotension or hypoperfusion abnormalities (lactic acidosis, oliguria, ↓ mental status) **Septic shock:** Sepsis-induced hypotension (systolic BP <90 mmHg) not responsive to 500 ml IV-fluid challenge + peripheral hypoperfusion *(CCM 20:864, 1992; JAMA 273:117, 1995)*

(Footnotes and abbreviations on page 45)

NOTE: All dosage recommendations are for adults (unless otherwise indicated) and assume normal renal function

TABLE 1 (41)

ANATOMIC SITE/DIAGNOSIS/ MODIFYING CIRCUMSTANCES	ETIOLOGIES (usual)	SUGGESTED REGIMENS*		ADJUNCT DIAGNOSTIC OR THERAPEUTIC MEASURES AND COMMENTS
		PRIMARY	ALTERNATIVE¹	
SYSTEMIC FEBRILE SYNDROMES/Sepsis/Adult; not neutropenic				
If asplenic	S. pneumo, H. influ, meningococci, Capnocytophaga (DF-2)	**NO HYPOTENSION:** (Cefotaxime or ceftriaxone—footnote¹	**Source unclear; life-threatening:** (See above)	
Suspect biliary source (see p.10)	Enterococci ± aerobic Gm-neg. bacilli	**AM/SB, PIP/TZ or TC/CL**	**P Ceph 3 + metro**	
Illicit use IV drugs	S. aureus	**Naficillin/oxacillin or vanco** if high prevalence of MRSA. Some empirically use vanco ± oxacillin pending susceptibility results.		
Suspect intra-abdominal source	Mixture aerobic & anaerobic Gm-neg. bacilli		See secondary peritonitis, page 31	
Suspect urinary source	Aerobic Gm-neg. bacilli & enterococci		See pyelonephritis, page 23	
Neutropenia: Child or adult (absolute PMN count <500/mm³). Guideline: CID 34:730, 2002				
Prophylaxis—afebrile				
Post-chemotherapy	Aerobic Gm-neg. bacilli, pneumococcus (PCP)	TMP/SMX or FQ works; not recommended²	TMP/SMX ↓ number of febrile episodes and prevents PCP. ofloz also reported effective but no activity vs PCP. Problem is TMP/SMX- & FQ-resistant Gm-neg. bacilli.	
		Paradox: TMP/SMX or FQ works. to ↑ bacterial resistance		
Post-chemotherapy in AIDS patient	↑ risk pneumocystis (PCP)	TMP/SMX-DS po bid–adults; 10 mg/kg/d div bid po -children	Need TMP/SMX to prevent PCP. Hard to predict which leukemia/lymphoma/solid tumor at ↑ risk of PCP	
Allogeneic hematopoietic stem-cell transplant	↑ risk pneumocystis, herpes viruses, candida	TMP/SMX as above + (either **acyclovir or ganciclovir**) + **fluconazole**	Combined regimen justified by combined effect of neutropenia and immuno-suppression.	
Empiric therapy—febrile (≥38.3°C x1 or ≥38°C for ≥1 hr)				
Low-risk adults (Low risk in Comment)	As above	CIP 750 mg po bid + AM/CL 875 mg bid	**Treat as outpatients with 24/7 access to inpatient care if: no focal findings, no hypotension, no COPD, no fungal infection, age <60 & >16.** Neutropenic children with low blood cultures, safely switched to po cefixime⁴. 4 mg/kg q12h (CID 32:36, 2001).	
				What if severe IgE-mediated β-lactam allergy? No formal trials, but [APAG (or CIP) + aztreonam] ± vanco should work.
High-risk adults and children	Aerobic Gm-neg. bacilli; ceph-resistant viridans strep, MRSA	**Monotherapy:** CFP or ceftaz or IMP or MER	**Combination therapy:** (Gent or tobra) + (TC/CL or PIP/TZ)	Increasing resistance of viridans streptococcus to penicillins, cephalosporins & FQs (CID 34:1469 & 1524, 2002; CID 31:1126, 2000; JAC 47:67, 2001).
		Dosages: Footnote⁴ and Table 11		
		Include empiric vanco if: suspect IV access infected; colonized with DRSP or MRSA; blood culture pos. for Gm + cocci; pt hypotensive		
Persistent fever and neutropenia after 5 days of empiric antibacterial therapy—see CID 34:730, 2002	Candida species, aspergillus	Add either **ampho B** or **voriconazole** (NEJM 346:225, 2002)		Empirically adding vanco of **no benefit** (CID 37:382, 2003)

¹ **P Ceph 3 (cefotaxime** 2.0 gm q8h IV, use q4h if life-threatening; **ceftizoxime** 2.0 gm q4h IV; **ceftriaxone** 2.0 gm q12h IV; **AP Pen (piperacillin** 3.0 gm q4h IV, **ticarcillin** 3.0 gm q4h IV, **TC/CL** 3.1 gm q4h IV, **PIP/TZ** 3.375 gm q4h IV, **AM/SB** 3.0 gm q6h IV, **APAG** (see Table 9C, page 71). **AP PEN** 30 mg/kg q4h IV, **clinda** 900 mg q8h IV, **IMP** 0.5 gm q6h IV, **MER** 1.0 gm q8h IV, **Naficillin** or **oxacillin** 2.0 gm q4h IV, **aztreonam** 2.0 gm q6h IV, **metro** 1.0 gm loading dose then 0.5 gm q6h or 1.0 gm q12h IV, **vanco** 1.0 gm q12h IV, **P Ceph 3 AP (ceftazidime** 2.0 gm q8h IV), **P Ceph 4 (CFP** 2.0 gm q12h IV) (q8h if neutropenic) **cefpirome** 2.0 gm q12h IV), **P Ceph 4 (CFP** 400 mg q12h IV, **ofloxa** 400 mg q12h IV, **levo** 750 mg IV/po, **linezolid** 600 mg q12h IV). NOTE: All dosage recommendations are for adults (unless otherwise indicated) and assume normal renal function
(Footnotes and abbreviations on page 45)

TABLE 1 (42)

ANATOMIC SITE/DIAGNOSIS/ MODIFYING CIRCUMSTANCES	ETIOLOGIES (usual)	SUGGESTED REGIMENS*		ADJUNCT DIAGNOSTIC OR THERAPEUTIC MEASURES AND COMMENTS
		PRIMARY	ALTERNATIVE†	
SYSTEMIC FEBRILE SYNDROMES (continued)				
Shock syndromes				
Septic shock: Fever & hypotension Bacteremic shock, endotoxin shock *Res., 351:1501, 1998; NEJM 340:207, 1999 Activ. Protein C: Med Lett 44:17, 2002*	Bacteremia with aerobic Gm-neg. bacteria or Gm+ cocci	**Proven therapy: (1) Replete intravascular volume, (2) if possible, drain abscess & remove infected foreign body, (3) appropriate empiric antimicrobial rx: see suggestions under life-threatening disease, above. As below under activated Protein C** (drotrecogin alfa), see *Comment*. **(5) Investigational rx: reasonable: low-dose steroids** if document relative adrenal insufficiency (see *Comment* for criteria). [Hydrocortisone 50 mg IV q6h + fludrocortisone (Florinef) 50 μg via NG once daily] x 7 d. **(6) Low-dose vasopressin** reported effective for catecholamine-resistant septic shock (*Ln 359:1209, 2002*).		**Activ. Protein C: Drotrecogin (Xigris):** In a single prospective random double-blind study (*NEJM 344:699 & 759, 2001*) lowered 28-day mortality from 31 to 25% in highly selected pts. shock with multi-organ failure, DIC, & low-risk of hemorrhage. 2% inc. serious hemorrhage. [Gene-activated Protein C. Ed's comment: approx. cost 5% toxicity from hemorrhage.] **Dose: 24 μg/kg/hr over 96 hrs by continuous IV infusion. Stop 2 hrs before & restart 12 hrs after surgery. cost of drug: 4-day course: $6800.** **Low-dose steroids:** Based on one controlled random double-blind trial. Treat if low baseline cortisol & 9 μg/dl response to 250 mg IV cosyntropin. 28-day mortality 63% placebo & 53% steroid group (*JAMA 288:862 & 886, 2002*).
Toxic shock syndrome, staphylococcal. Superantigen review. *Ln 2:156, 2002*	Colonization by toxin-producing Staph. aureus of: vagina (tampon-assoc.), surgical/traumatic wounds, endometrium, burns	[**Nafcillin** or **oxacillin** 2.0 gm q4h IV or (if MRSA, **vanco** 1.0 gm q12h) + **IVIG**]	[**Cefazolin** 1–2 gm q8h IV or (if MRSA, **vanco** 1.0 gm q12h) + **IVIG**]	Nafcillin/oxacillin/cefazolin have no effect on initial syndrome, but ↓ recurrences. Seek occult abscess. TSS may occur with "clean" colonized post-op wounds. Case fatality 5–15%. **IVIG reasonable** (see *Streptococcal TSS*)—dose 1.0 gm/kg day 1, then 0.5 gm/kg days 2 & 3.
Toxic shock syndrome, streptococcal [Ref. *JID 179(Suppl 2):S366–374, 1999*]. NOTE: For necrotizing fasciitis without toxic shock, *see page 9*	Group A, B, C, & G Strep. Associated with invasive disease, i.e., erysipelas, necrotizing fasciitis, secondary strep infection via, e.g. varicella. Secondary cases TSS reported *NEJM 335:547 & 590, 1996; CID 27:150, 1998).*	[**Pen G** 24 mU/d IV in div. doses] + **clinda** 900 mg + IVIG associated with ↓ in sepsis-related organ failure	[**Ceftriaxone** 2.0 gm q24h IV + **clinda** 900 mg q8h IV]	**Definition:** Isolation of Group A strep, hypotension and ≥2 of: renal impairment, coagulopathy, liver involvement, ARDS, generalized rash, soft tissue necrosis (*JAMA 269:390, 1993*). Associated with invasive disease. **Surgery usually required.** Mortality with early rx 30%, even with late rx 80%. **IVIG** 2 gm/kg x1 dose + repeat at 48h if necessary (*CID 14:2, 1992*). Clinda ↓ toxin production. Use of NSAID may predispose to TSS. For discussion of possible reasons pen G may fail in fulminant S. pyogenes infections, *see JID 167:1401, 1993*).
		IVIG associated with ↓ in sepsis-related organ failure *(CID 28:800, 1999, 37:333 & 341, 2003)*. IVIG dose 1 gm/kg day 1, then 0.5 gm/kg days 2 & 3.		
Other Toxin-Mediated Syndromes—no fever unless complicated				
Botulism *(AnIM 129:221, 1998; CID 31:1018, 2000*. *and Table 1B, page 46)*	C. botulinum	**Biologic weapon:** *JAMA 285:1059, 2001; and Table 1B, page 46)* Follow vital capacity; other supportive care.		**Biologic weapon:** Obtain from State Health Depts. or CDC (404-639-2206 M-F OR 404-639-2888 evenings/weekends). Skin test first & desensitize if necessary.
Food-borne		Trivalent (types A, B, E) equine serum antitoxin—State Health Dept. or CDC (*See Comment*)		One vial IV and one vial IM. **Antimicrobials:** May make infant botulism worse. Untested in wound botulism. When used, pen G the usual drug. If complications (pneumonia, UTI) occur, avoid antimicrobials with assoc. neuromuscular blockade, i.e., aminoglycosides, tetracycline
Infant		Human botulinum immunoglobulin (BIG) IV for single dose. Call 510-540-2646. Do not use equine antitoxin.		No antibiotics; may lyse "C. botulinum in gut and ↑ load of toxin
Wound		Debridement & anaerobic cultures. Role of antitoxin unclear.		Trivalent equine antitoxin Can result from spore contamination of tar heroin.
Tetanus	C. tetani	[**Pen G** 24 mU IV in div. dose or **doxy** 100 mg q12h IV]	[**Metro** 500 mg q6h or 1.0 gm q12h IV xM-10 d. (See *Comment*)]	Primary rx is control of muscle spasms. Diazepam agent of choice. Morbidity less with metro than pen G (*BMJ 291:648, 1985*). Tetanus toxin and pen G both GABA antagonists (*NEJM 332:812, 1995*).

(Footnotes on page 45)   NOTE: All dosage recommendations are for adults (unless otherwise indicated) and assume normal renal function

TABLE 1 (43)

ANATOMIC SITE/DIAGNOSIS/ MODIFYING CIRCUMSTANCES	ETIOLOGIES (usual)	SUGGESTED REGIMENS* PRIMARY	ALTERNATIVE¹	ADJUNCT DIAGNOSTIC OR THERAPEUTIC MEASURES AND COMMENTS
VASCULAR				
Cavernous sinus thrombosis	Staph. aureus, Group A strep, H. influenzae, asper-gillus/peribranchis/aspergillus/mucor/rhizopus	**(Nafcillin or oxacillin** 2.0 gm q4h IV) **+ P Ceph 3 AP (ceftazidime** 2.0 gm q8h IV or IMP 0.5 gm q6h IV)	**Vanco** 1.0 gm q12h IV plus nafcillin/oxacillin 1.0 gm q12h IV or **MER** 1.0 gm q8h IV	CT or MRI scan for diagnosis. Heparin indicated (Ln 338:597, 1991). If patient diabetic with ketoacidosis or post-desferoxamine rx or neutropenic, consider fungal: aspergillus, mucor, rhizopus, see Table 11A, pages 74 & 80.
IV line infection (see IDSA Guidelines: CID 32:1249, 2001): **Treatment** Heparin lock, midline catheter, non-tunneled central venous catheter (subclavian, internal jugular), peripherally inserted central catheter (PICC) Avoid femoral vein if possible. ↑ risk of infection and/or thrombosis (JAMA 286:700, 2001)	Staph. epidermidis, Staph. aureus	**Vanco** 1.0 gm q12h IV. Other (x and z) and duration: **(1)** If **S. aureus**: remove catheter. Can use TEE result to determine if 2 or 4 wks of rx. **(2)** If **S. epidermidis**, can try to "save" catheter. 80% cure after 7-10 d. of rx. Catheter-hub/lumen: Infections may respond to antibiotic lock rx & allow salvage of catheter (JAC 48:597, 2001). Drug (**vanco, gent, CIP**) at 1-5 mg/ml mixed with 50-100 units heparin (or saline) in 2-5 ml volume; fill catheter when not in use. Continue 2 wks. **For S. aureus, need full course of parenteral therapy.**	**Linezolid alternative—see Comment.**	**Linezolid has predictable bacteriostatic activity vs most S. aureus and S. epidermidis isolates—including MRSA/MRSE. Authors prefer vanco in order to ↑ longevity of linezolid activity. If MRSA/MRSE and either failure or allergy, linezolid dose 600 mg IV/po q12h.** If MRSE or MRSA rare in hospital, nafcillin/oxacillin for vanco. Culture removed catheter. With "roll" method, >15 colonies (NEJM 312:1142, 1985) suggests infection. Lines do not require "routine" changing when not infected. When infected, do not insert new catheter over a wire. If antibiotic-coated catheters and other technologies may ↓ infection risk (EID 7:197, 2001; CID 34:1232, 2002).
Tunnel type indwelling venous catheters and ports (Broviac, Hickman, Groshong, Quinton), dual lumen hemodialysis catheters (Perma-cath)	Staph. epidermidis, Staph. aureus, (Candida sp.). Rarely, leuconostoc or lactobacillus-sen resistant to vanco (see Table 2)	If candida, see Hyperalimentation and Table 11A pages 75–77.		If **S. epidermidis & catheter left in**, **vanco can cure 80%** of infections limited to exit site but only 25% cure if infection in subcutaneous tunnel between skin and subclavian vein. If **S. aureus & catheter left in, vanco cure rate 10% at exit site & 0% with tunnel infection** (AJM 89:137, 1990). Similar statistics for infected "ports" (CID 29:102, 1999). Infected hemodialysis access catheters should be removed (AVM 127:275, 1997).
Impaired host (burn, neutropenic)	As above + Pseudomonas sp., Enterobacteriaceae, Corynebacterium jeikeium, aspergillus, rhizopus			Usually have associated septic thrombophlebitis. Biopsy of vein to rule out fungi. If fungal, surgical excision + amphotericin B. Surgical drainage, ligation or removal often indicated.
Hyperalimentation	Staph. aureus + Candida sp. (Candida/torula and resistant Candida species)	If candida, **amphotericin B** 0.5–0.6 mg/kg qd IV, total dose 3 mg/kg, **or voriconazole** 3 mg/kg bid IV or **caspofungin** 70 mg IV day 1, then 50 mg IV qd		Remove venous catheter and discontinue antimicrobial agents if possible. If Candida isolated on blood culture, ophthalmologic consultation recommended. **Rx all patients with + blood cultures.** See Table 11A, Candidiasis.
Intravenous lipid emulsion	Staph. epidermidis Malassezia furfur	**Vanco** 1.0 gm q12h IV. **Amphotericin B**		Discontinue intralipid
IV line infection: Prevention (CID 35:1281, 2002; NEJM 348:1123, 2003): To minimize risk of infection: 1. Maximal sterile barrier precautions during catheter insertion 2. Use 2% chlorhexidine for skin antisepsis 3. If infection rate high despite #1 & 2, use either chlorhexidine/silver sulfadiazine or minocycline/rifampin-impregnated catheters				Use heparin during antibiotic regimen. Continued oral anticoagulation not recommended. Cefotetan less active than cefoxitin vs more fragile bacteroides. Cefotetan and cefmetazole have methyltetrazole side-chain which is associated with hypoprothrombinemia (prevent with vitamin K).
Septic pelvic vein thrombophlebitis Postpartum or postabortion or postpelvic surgery	Streptococci, bacteroides, Enterobacteriaceae	**Metro + P Ceph 3 cefoxitin, TC/CL, PIP/TZ, or AM/SB**	**IMP or MER** or **erta** or **(aztreonam or clinda) + APAG**)	

TABLE 1 (44): FOOTNOTES AND ABBREVIATIONS

* **Dosages suggested are for adults** (unless otherwise indicated) with clinically severe (often life-threatening) infections. Dosages also assume normal renal function, and not severe hepatic dysfunction. See Table 16, page 129, for pediatric dosages.

§ **Alternative therapy** includes these considerations: allergy, pharmacology/pharmacokinetics, compliance, costs, local resistance profiles.

AG = aminoglycoside
AHA = American Heart Association
AM/CL = amoxicillin (Augmentin), **AM/CL-ER** (Augmentin XR)
AM/SB = ampicillin/sulbactam (Unasyn)
Amox = amoxicillin
AMP = ampicillin
APAG = antipseudomonal aminoglycosidic antibiotics
AP Pen = antipseudomonal penicillin, β-lactamase susceptible penicillins, e.g. piperacillin. See Table 4, page 52 for details.
ARDS = adult respiratory distress syndrome
ARF = acute rheumatic fever
ASA = acetylsalicylic acid (aspirin)
ATS = antistreptolysin O
Azithro = azithromycin
Ceftaz = ceftazidime
CFP = cefepime
Chlor = chloramphenicol
CIP = ciprofloxacin; **CIP-ER** = ciprofloxacin extended release
Clarithro = clarithromycin; **Clarithro ER** = clarithromycin extended release
Clinda = clindamycin
C&S = culture and sensitivities
CSD = cat-scratch disease (see page 30)
Doxy = doxycycline
DRSP = drug-resistant Streptococcus pneumoniae
DS = double-strength
EBV = Epstein-Barr virus
EDC = expected date of confinement
EES = erythromycin ethyl succinate
Era = ertapenem
Erythro = erythromycin

ETB = ethambutol;**FQ** = fluoroquinolone
GAS = Group A streptococcus
Gati = gatifloxacin
GC = gonorrhea (N. gonorrhoeae)
Gemi = gemifloxacin
GNB = Gram-negative bacilli
HHV-2 = human herpesvirus type 2
HIV-1 = human immunodeficiency virus type 1
HLGR = high-level gentamicin resistance
HLR = high-level resistance
IMP = imipenem cilastatin (Primaxin)
INH = isoniazid
IVDU = intravenous drug users
IVIG = intravenous immune globulin
LCM = lymphocytic choriomeningitis virus
LCR = ligase chain reaction
Levo = levofloxacin
LRTI = lower respiratory tract infection
Macrolides = erythro, azithro, clarithro, dirithro
Metro = metronidazole
Moxi = moxifloxacin
MOTT = mycobacteria other than M. tuberculosis
MRI = magnetic resonance imaging
MRSA/MRSE = methicillin-sensitive/methicillin-resistant Staph. aureus
MSSE/MRSE = methicillin-sensitive/methicillin-resistant Staph. epidermidis
MTb = Mycobacterium tuberculosis
NF = nitrofurantoin

NSAIDs = nonsteroidal anti-inflammatory drugs
NUS = not available in the United States
O Ceph 1, 2, 3 = oral cephalosporins—see Table 9B, page 65
Oflox = ofloxacin
P Ceph 1, 2, 3 = parenteral cephalosporins—see Table 9B, pages 65
P Ceph 3 AP = third generation with enhanced antipseudomonal activity
P Ceph 4 = third generation with antistaphylococcal and antipseudomonal activity
PCR = polymerase chain reaction
Peflox = pefloxacin
PIP/TZ = piperacillin/tazobactam
PVE = prosthetic valve endocarditis
Q/D = quinupristin/dalfopristin
Rick = rickettsia (spotted fever, Q fever)
RIF = rifampin
R/O = rule out
SA = Staph. aureus
Skin/SC = skin and related skin structures
Strep = streptomycin
STD = sexually transmitted diseases
TBc = tuberculosis
TC/CL = ticarcillin/clavulanate (Timentin)
TEE = transesophageal echocardiography
Telithro = telithromycin
TMP/SMX = trimethoprim/sulfamethoxazole
Tobra = tobramycin
Toxo = toxoplasmosis
UTI = urinary tract infection
Vanco = vancomycin

ABBREVIATIONS OF JOURNAL AND TEXT TITLES

AAC: Antimicrobial Agents & Chemotherapy
Adv PID: Advances in Pediatric Infectious Diseases
Adv Par: Advances in Parasitology
AIDS: AIDS
AIDS Clin Care: AIDS Clinical Care
AJG: American Journal of Gastroenterology
AJM: American Journal of Medicine
AJRCCM: American Journal of Respiratory Critical Care Medicine
AJTMH: American Journal of Tropical Medicine & Hygiene
AnEM: Annals of Emergency Medicine
AnIM: Annals of Internal Medicine
AnSurg: Annals of Surgery
AIM: Archives of Internal Medicine
ARRD: American Review of Respiratory Disease
CCM: Critical Care Medicine
CID: Clinical Infectious Diseases

COID: Current Opinion in Infectious Disease
CTID: Clinical Topics in Infectious Disease
EMID: Emerging Microbiology and Infectious Disease
EID: Emerging Infectious Disease
EJCMID: European Journal of Clin. Micro. & Infectious Diseases
Gastro: Gastroenterology
ICHE: Infection Control and Hospital Epidemiology
IDC No. Amer: Infectious Disease Clinics of North America
IDCP: Infectious Diseases in Clinical Practice
J Clin Micro: Journal of Clinical Microbiology
J Ped: Journal of Pediatrics
JAC: Journal of Antimicrobial Chemotherapy
JAMA: Journal of the American Medical Association
JAVMA: Journal of the American Veterinary Medical Association
JID: Journal of Infectious Diseases
JNS: Journal of Neurosurgery
JTMH: Journal of Tropical Medicine and Hygiene

JTP: Journal of Tropical Pediatrics
Ln: Lancet
Ln ID: Lancet Infectious Disease
Med Lett: Medical Letter
MMWR: Morbidity & Mortality Weekly Report
NEJM: New England Journal of Medicine
Peds: Pediatrics
PIDJ: Pediatric Infectious Disease Journal
QJM: Quarterly Journal of Medicine
SGO: Surgery, Gynecology and Obstetrics
SMJ: Southern Medical Journal
Tr RSTM: Transactions of the Royal Society of Medicine
Tr RSTMH: Transactions of the Royal Society of Tropical Medicine & Hygiene
WJM: Western Journal of Medicine

TABLE 1B: PROPHYLAXIS AND TREATMENT OF ORGANISMS OF POTENTIAL USE AS BIOLOGICAL WEAPONS

DISEASE	ETIOLOGY	SUGGESTED EMPIRIC TREATMENT REGIMENS		SPECIFIC THERAPY AND COMMENTS
		PRIMARY	**ALTERNATIVE**	
Anthrax **Cutaneous, inhalational, gastrointestinal** Refs. JAMA 286: 2549, 2554 & 2556, 2001; N/EJM 345:1607 & 1621, 2001; CID 35:851, 2002; www.bt.cdc.gov Also see Table 1, pages 28 & 34	Bacillus anthracis Post-exposure prophylaxis Ref.: Med Lett 43:91, 2001	**Adults (including pregnancy):** CIP 500 mg po bid x60 d. **Children:** CIP 20-30 mg/kg/div q12h po x60 d.	**Adults (including pregnancy): Doxy** 100 mg po bid x60 d. (see Comment) **Children: Doxy** >8 y/o & >45 kg: 100 mg po bid; >8 y/o & ≤45 kg: 2.2 mg/kg po bid; ≤8 y/o: 2.2 mg/kg po bid. All for 60 days.	1. Once organism shows susceptibility to penicillin, switch children to **amoxicillin** 80 mg/kg/d div q8h (max. 500 mg q8h); switch pregnant to **Amox** 500 mg po q8h. 2. Do not use cephalosporins or TMP/SMX. 3. Other **FQs** (gati, levo, moxi) should work but no clinical experience.

	Treatment—**inhalational**
	See Comment
		Adults (including pregnancy): CIP 400 mg IV q12h or (**doxy** 100 mg IV q12h) + **clinda** 900 mg IV q8h + **RIF** 300 mg IV q12h. Switch to po when able & CIP 500 mg po bid, or **doxy** 100 mg po bid. See Table 2, page 15. Treat x60 days. See Table 16, page 28 for oral dosage.	**Adults (including pregnancy): Doxy** >8 y/o & >45 kg: 100 mg IV q12h; >8 y/o & ≤45 kg: 2.2 mg/kg IV q12h; ≤8 y/o: 2.2 mg/kg IV q12h.
			plus clindamycin 7.5 mg/kg IV q6h
			plus RIF 20 mg/kg IV q24h qd. Treat x60 d. See Table 16, page 28 for oral dosage.
				1. Clinda may block toxin production.
				2. Rifampin penetrates CSF & intracellular sites.
				3. If isolate shown penicillin-susceptible:
				  a. **Adult: Pen G** 4 mU IV q4h
				  b. **Child: Pen G** <12 y/o: 50,000 U/kg IV q6h; >12 y/o: 4 mU IV q4h
				  c. Constitutive & inducible β-lactamases—do not use pen or amp alone.
				4. Do not use cephalosporins or TMP/SMX.
				5. Erytho, azithro should work. clarithro active.
				6. No person-to-person transmission.

	Cutaneous anthrax N/EJM 345:1611, 2001			
	Characteristic signs & symptoms—**Fever, Dyspnea, N/V, Abdominal pain, hemorrhea, sore throat** (AnIM 139:337, 2003)			
To report bioterrorism event: 770-488-7100				
Botulism Ref: JAMA 285:1059, 2001 Food-borne¹ See Table 1, page 43	Clostridium botulinum	Purge GI tract if ileus absent. Trivalent antitoxin (types A, B, E): single 10 ml vial/pt. diluted in saline IV (slowly)	Antibiotics have no effect on toxin	Supportive care for all types. Follow vital capacity. Submit suspect food for toxin testing.
Hemorrhagic fever viruses Ref: JAMA 287:2391, 2002	Ebola, Lassa, Hanta, yellow fever, & others	Fluid/electrolyte balance. Optimize circulatory volume.	For Lassa & Hanta: **Ribavirin** (dose same as for Hantavirus) 2 gm IV x1, then 16 mg/kg (max. 1 gm) IV q6h x4 d, then 8 mg/kg IV q8h x6 d.	Ribavirin active in vitro, not FDA-approved for this indication. NOTE: Ribavirin contraindicated in pregnancy. However, in this setting, the benefits outweigh the risks.
Plague Ref: JAMA 283:2281, 2000 Inhalation pneumonic plague¹ See Table 1, page 39	Yersinia pestis **Treatment**	**Gentamicin** 5 mg/kg IV qd or **streptomycin** 1 gm q12h IV bid. Tobramycin should work.	(**Doxy** 200 mg IV x1, & then 100 mg IV q12h) or (**CIP** 500 mg po bid or 400 mg IV q12h)	1. **Chloro** also active. 25 mg/kg IV qid. 2. In mass casualty situation, may have to treat po. 3. Pregnancy: As for non-pregnant adults 4. Isolate during first 48 hrs of treatment For community/pneumonic plague epidemic: Pediatric doses: see Table 16, page 129.
	Post-exposure prophylaxis	**Doxy** 100 mg po bid x7 d.	CIP 500 mg po bid x7 d.	Pediatric doses: see Table 16, page 129. Pregnancy: As for non-pregnant adults
Smallpox Ref: N/EJM 346:1300, 2002 Government	Variola virus	Smallpox vaccine up to 4 days after exposure: isolation; gloves, gown, & N95 respirator	Cidofovir protected mice against aerosol cowpox (JID 181:10, 2000)	**Immediately notify State Health Dept. & State notifies CDC (770-488-7100).** Vaccinia immune globulin (if avail.) for vaccine complications. See JAMA 288:1901, 2002
Tularemia Ref: JAMA 285:2763, 2001 See Table 1, page 40	Francisella tularensis **Treatment**	**Doxy** 100 mg IV bid x14-21 d. or (**gentamicin** 5 mg/kg/d qd) x10 d.	**Doxy** 100 mg bid (or 750 mg po) bid x14-21 d.	For pediatric doses, see Table 16, page 129. **Streptomycin** should work. **Tobramycin** should work.
	Post-exposure prophylaxis	**Doxy** 100 mg bid x14 d.	CIP 500 mg bid x14 d.	For pediatric doses, see Table 16, page 129. Pregnancy: As for non-pregnant adults

¹ There are other clinical forms of botulism, plague, and tularemia, but the inhalation form seems most probable in bioterrorism.

TABLE 1C
TEMPORAL APPROACH TO DIFFERENTIAL DIAGNOSIS OF INFECTION AFTER ORGAN TRANSPLANTATION*

USUAL HOSPITAL-ACQUIRED INFECTIONS	OPPORTUNISTIC INFECTIONS	COMMUNITY-ACQUIRED OR CHRONIC INFECTIONS

VIRAL:
— HSV
— CMV
— Onset of Hepatitis B or C
— EBV, VZV, Influenza, RSV, Adenovirus
— CMV retinitis or colitis...‡
— Papillomavirus, PTLD[1]...‡

BACTERIAL:
— Pneumonia, IV line, UTI, Wound...
— Nocardia
— Listeria, Tuberculosis

FUNGAL:
— Pneumocystis
— Aspergillus
— Cryptococcus
— Coccidioidomycosis, Histoplasmosis

PARASITIC
— Candida
— Leishmania
— Strongyloides
— Toxoplasma
— Trypanosoma cruzi

MONTHS AFTER TRANSPLANTATION
1 2 3 4 5 6

[1] **PTLD** = Post-transplant lymphoproliferative disease. * Adapted from Fishman and Rubin, *NEJM* 338:1741, 1998. For hematopoietic stem cell transplant recipients, see *MMWR* 49:RR-10, 2000. ‡ Solid lines indicate usual time period for onset of infection; dotted lines indicate risk at reduced level

TABLE 2: RECOMMENDED ANTIMICROBIAL AGENTS AGAINST SELECTED BACTERIA

BACTERIAL SPECIES	ANTIMICROBIAL AGENT (See footnote[2] for abbreviations)		
	RECOMMENDED	ALTERNATIVE	ALSO EFFECTIVE[3] (COMMENTS)
Alcaligenes xylosoxidans (Achromobacter xylosoxidans)	IMP, MER, AP Pen	TMP/SMX. Some strains susc. to ceftaz (AAC 32:276, 1988)	Resistant to APAG; P Ceph 1, 2, 3, 4; aztreonam; FQ (AAC 40:772, 1996)
Acinetobacter calcoaceticus–baumannii complex	IMP or MER or [FQ + (amikacin or ceftaz)]	AM/SB (CID 24:932, 1997). Sulbactam[NUS] also effective (JAC 42: 793, 1998); colistin (CID 36: 1111, 2003)	Polymyxin B; up to 5% isolates resistant to IMP; resistance to FQs, amikacin increasing. Ceftaz + amikacin effective in animal model (JAC 45: 493, 2000). (See Table 5, page 56)
Actinomyces israelii	AMP or Pen G	Doxy, ceftriaxone	Clindamycin, erythromycin
Aeromonas hydrophila	FQ	TMP/SMX or (P Ceph 3, 4)	APAG; erta; IMP; MER; tetracycline (some resistant to carbapenems)
Arcanobacterium (C.) haemolyticum	Erythromycin	Benzathine Pen G	Sensitive to most drugs, resistant to TMP/SMX (AR 38:142, 1994)
Bacillus anthracis (anthrax): Inhalation *See Table 1B, page 46*	CIP or doxy. For systemic infections, add 1 or 2 of: (RIF, clinda)	If Pen G susceptible: Pen G or amox	Also active: IMP, MER, vanco, chloramphenicol, clindamycin. Resistant to expanded-spectrum cephalosporins (MMWR 50: 909, 2001; NEJM 345: 1621, 2001; JAMA 287:2236, 2002).
Bacillus cereus, B. subtilis	Vancomycin, clindamycin	FQ, IMP	
Bacteroides fragilis (ssp. fragilis) "DOT" group of bacteroides[a]	Metronidazole	Clindamycin	Cefoxitin, erta, IMP, MER, TC/CL, PIP/TZ, AM/SB, cefotetan, AM/CL (not cefotetan)
Bartonella (Rochalimaea) henselae, quintana *See Table 1, pages 30, 34, 38*	Erythro or doxy (bacillary angiomatosis) or azithro (cat-scratch) (PIDJ 17:447, 1998)	Clarithro or CIP	Other drugs: TMP/SMX (CID No. Amer 12:137, 1998). Consider doxy + RIF for severe bacillary isolates (IDC N-Amer 12:137, 1998)
Bordetella pertussis	Erythromycin	TMP/SMX	An erythro-resistant strain reported in Arizona (MMWR 43:807, 1994)
Borrelia burgdorferi, B. afzelii, B. garinii *(See Comments)*	Ceftriaxone, cefuroxime axetil, doxy, amox	Penicillin G (HD), cefotaxime	Clarithro. Choice depends on stage of disease, Table 1, page 39
Borrelia sp.	Doxy	Erythromycin	Penicillin G
Brucella sp.	Doxy + either gentamicin or streptomycin	(Doxy + RIF) or (TMP/SMX + gentamicin)	FQ + RIF (AAC 41:80, 1997; Emerg ID 3:213, 1997; CID 21:283, 1995)
Burkholderia (Pseudomonas) cepacia	TMP/SMX or MER or CIP	Minocycline or chloramphenicol	(Usually resistant to APAG, IMP) (AAC 37: 123, 1993 & 43:213, 1999) (Some resistant to carbapenems). Combination rx may be necessary (AJRCCM 161:1206, 2000).
Burkholderia (Pseudomonas) pseudomallei *See Table 1, page 27, & Ln 361:1715, 2003*	Initially, IV ceftaz or IMP (CID 29:381, 1999)	Then, combination of po chloro, doxy, & TMP/SMX	(In Thailand, 12–80% strains resistant to TMP/SMX). FQ active in vitro. Combination of chloro, TMP/SMX, doxy more effective than doxy alone for maintenance rx (CID 29:375, 1999).
Campylobacter jejuni	Erythromycin	FQ (↑ resistance, NEJM 340:1525,1999)	Clindamycin, doxy, azithro, clarithro (see Table 5, page 56)
Campylobacter fetus	IMP	Gentamicin	AMP, chloramphenicol, erythromycin
Capnocytophaga ochracea (DF-1) and canimorsus (DF-2)	Clindamycin or AM/CL	CIP, Pen G	P Ceph 3, IMP, cefoxitin, FQ. (Resistant to APAG, TMP/SMX). C. hemolytica & C. granulosa are often more resistant to β-lactams & aminoglycosides [CID 35(Suppl.1):S17, 2002].
	AM/CL		
Chlamydophila pneumoniae	Doxy	Erythromycin, FQ	Azithro, clarithro, telithro
Chlamydia trachomatis	Doxy or azithro	Erythromycin or ofloxacin	Levofloxacin
Chryseobacterium (Flavobacterium) meningosepticum	Vancomycin ± RIF (CID 26:1169, 1998)	CIP, levofloxacin	In vitro susceptibilities may not correlate with clinical efficacy (AAC 41: 1301, 1997; CID 26:1169, 1998)
Citrobacter diversus (koseri), C. freundii	CARB	FQ	APAG
Clostridium difficile	Metronidazole (po)	Vancomycin (po)	Bacitracin
Clostridium perfringens	Pen G ± clindamycin	Doxy	Erythromycin, chloramphenicol, cefazolin, cefoxitin, AP Pen, CARB
Clostridium tetani	Metronidazole or Pen G	Doxy	CARB
Corynebacterium jeikeium	Vancomycin	Pen G + APAG	
C. diphtheriae	Erythromycin	Clindamycin	RIF. Penicillin reported effective (CID 27:845, 1998)
Coxiella burnetii (Q fever) acute disease	Doxy (see Table 1, page 20)	Erythromycin	In meningitis consider FQ (CID 20:489, 1995)
chronic disease	(CIP or doxy) + RIF	FQ + doxy x3 yrs (CID 20:489, 1995)	Chloroquine + doxy (AAC 37:1773, 1993). ? gamma interferon (Ln 20:546, 2001)
Ehrlichia chaffeensis, Ehrlichia ewingii, Anaplasma (Ehrlichia) phagocytophilum	Doxy	Tetracycline, RIF (CID 27:213, 1998)	CIP, oflox, chloramphenicol also active in vitro. Resistant to clinda, TMP/SMX, IMP, AMP, erythro, azithro (AAC 41: 76, 1997)
Eikenella corrodens	Penicillin G or AMP or AM/CL	TMP/SMX, FQ	Doxy, cefoxitin, cefotaxime, IMP (Resistant to clindamycin, cephalexin, erythromycin, and metronidazole)

TABLE 2 (2)

BACTERIAL SPECIES	ANTIMICROBIAL AGENT (See footnote² for abbreviations)		
	RECOMMENDED	ALTERNATIVE	ALSO EFFECTIVE¹ (COMMENTS)
Enterobacter spp. (aerogenes, cloacae)	CARB or (AP Pen + APAG)	TC/CL or PIP/TZ or CIP	P Ceph 4. As many as 40% strains from ICUs may be ceftaz-resistant
Enterococcus faecalis	Penicillin G or AMP Add gentamicin for endocarditis or meningitis	Vancomycin	Linezolid. For UTI, nitrofurantoin, fosfomycin effective. High-level gentamicin, vancomycin resistance increasing (see footnote page 19). (See Table 5, p. 55)
Enterococcus faecium, β-lactamase +, high-level aminoglycoside resist., vancomycin resist.	No regimen of proven efficacy. Consultation recommended if pt has endocarditis or other life-threatening infection. (See Endocarditis, Table 1, page 19, & Table 5, page 55)		See discussion, page 19, page 64, and Table 5, page 55; quinu/dalfo, linezolid
Erysipelothrix rhusiopathiae	Penicillin G or AMP	P Ceph 3, FQ	IMP, AP Pen (vancomycin, APAG, TMP/SMX resistant)
Escherichia coli	Sensitive to BL/BLI, cephalosporins, FQ, TMP/SMX, APAG, nitrofurantoin, CARB. Selection of drug depends on site of infection, i.e., UTI multiple po agents; meningitis P Ceph 3 or MER. See Table 1 for infections due to E. coli O157:H7 & related strains.		
Francisella tularensis (tularemia) See Table 1B, page 46	Gentamicin, tobramycin, or streptomycin	Doxy or CIP	Chloramphenicol, RIF. Doxy/chloro bacteriostatic → relapses
Gardnerella vaginalis (bacterial vaginosis)	Metronidazole	Clindamycin	See Table 1, page 17 for dosage
Hafnia alvei	Same as Enterobacter spp.		
Helicobacter pylori	See Table 1, page 13		Drugs effective in vitro often fail in vivo.
Hemophilus aphrophilus	((Penicillin or AMP) + gentamicin) or [AM/SB + gentamicin)	P Ceph 2, 3 ± gentamicin	(Resistant to vancomycin, clindamycin, methicillin)
Hemophilus ducreyi (chancroid)	Azithro or ceftriaxone	Erythromycin, CIP	Most strains resistant to tetracycline, amox, TMP/SMX
Hemophilus influenzae Meningitis, epiglottitis & other life-threatening illness	Cefotaxime, ceftriaxone	TMP/SMX, CARB, FQs (AMP if β-lactamase negative) (U.S. 25-30% AMP resistance, Japan 35%)	Chloramphenicol (downgraded from 1st choice because of hematotoxicity). 9% of U.S. strains resistant to TMP/SMX (AAC 41:292, 1997).
non-life threatening illness	AM/CL, O Ceph 2/3, TMP/SMX, AM/SB		Azithro, clarithro, telithro
Klebsiella pneumoniae, Klebsiella oxytoca	P Ceph 3, FQ, CARB	APAG, TC/CL, AM/SB, PIP/TZ, erta	AP Pen, aztreonam, AM/CL (extended release). Outbreaks of ceftaz-resistance reported (AnIM 119:353, 1993) (See Table 4, page 56)
Klebsiella ozaenae/rhinoscleromatis	FQ	RIF + TMP/SMX	(Lancet 342:122, 1993)
Lactobacillus sp.	(Pen G or AMP) ± gentamicin	Clindamycin, erythromycin	**May be resistant to vancomycin**
Legionella sp. (42 species & 60 serotypes recognized) (Sem Resp Inf 13:90, 1998)	FQ, or azithro, or (erythromycin ± RIF)	Clarithro, telithro	TMP/SMX, doxy. Most active FQs in vitro: gemi, gati, levo, moxi. See AnIM 129:328, 1998
Leptospira interrogans	Penicillin G	Doxy	Ceftriaxone (CID 36:1507, 2003)
Leuconostoc	Pen G or AMP	Clindamycin, erythromycin, minocycline	APAG **NOTE: Resistant to vancomycin**
Listeria monocytogenes	AMP	TMP/SMX	Erythromycin, penicillin G (high dose), APAG may be synergistic with β-lactams. **Cephalosporin-resistant!**
Moraxella (Branhamella) catarrhalis	AM/CL or O Ceph 2/3, TMP/SMX	Azithro, clarithro, dirithromycin, telithro	Erythromycin, doxy, FQs
Morganella sp.	CARB or P Ceph 3 or 4 or FQ	Aztreonam, BL/BLI	APAG
Mycoplasma pneumoniae	Erythro, azithro, clarithro, dirithro, or FQ	Doxy	(Clindamycin and β lactams NOT effective)
Neisseria gonorrhoeae (gonococcus)	Ceftriaxone, cefixime[NUS], cefpodoxime	Ofloxacin & other FQs (Table 1, page 15), spectinomycin	Kanamycin (used in Asia). FQ resistance in Asia: rare in U.S. (MMWR 47:405, 1998)
Neisseria meningitidis (meningococcus)	Penicillin G	Ceftriaxone, cefuroxime, cefotaxime	Sulfonamide (some strains), chloramphenicol. Chloro-resistant strains found in SE Asia (NEJM 339:868, 1998) (Prophylaxis: page 6)
Nocardia asteroides	TMP/SMX, sulfonamides (high dose)	Minocycline	Amikacin + (IMP or ceftriaxone or cefuroxime) for brain abscess
Nocardia brasiliensis	TMP/SMX, sulfonamides (high dose)	AM/CL	Amikacin + ceftriaxone
Pasteurella multocida	Pen G, AMP, amox	Doxy, AM/CL, P Ceph 2, ceftriaxone	Ceftriaxone, cefpodoxime, FQ (active in vitro), azithro (active in vitro) (DMID 30:99, 1998; AAC 43:1475, 1999)
Plesiomonas shigelloides	CIP	TMP/SMX	AM/CL, P Ceph 1,2,3,4, IMP, MER, tetracycline, aztreonam
Proteus mirabilis (indole–)	AMP	TMP/SMX	Most agents except nafcillin/oxacillin. β-lactamase (including ESBL) production now being described in P. mirabilis (JCM 40:1549, 2002)
vulgaris (indole +)	P Ceph 3 or FQ	APAG	CARB, aztreonam, BL/BLI
Providencia sp.	Amikacin or P Ceph 3 or FQ	TMP/SMX	AP Pen + amikacin, IMP

TABLE 2 (3)

BACTERIAL SPECIES	ANTIMICROBIAL AGENT (See footnote[2] for abbreviations)		
	RECOMMENDED	ALTERNATIVE	ALSO EFFECTIVE[1] (COMMENTS)
Pseudomonas aeruginosa	AP Pen, AP Ceph 3, IMP, MER, tobramycin, CIP, aztreonam. For serious inf., use AP β-lactam + tobramycin or CIP	For UTI, single drugs usually effective: AP Pen, AP Ceph 3, cefepime, IMP, MER, APAG, CIP, aztreonam.	Resistance to β-lactams (IMP, ceftaz) may emerge during rx. β-lactam inhibitor adds nothing to activity of TC or PIP against P. aeruginosa. Clavulanic acid has been shown to antagonize TC in vitro (AAC 43:882, 1999). (See also Table 5)
Rhodococcus (C. equi)	IMP, APAG, erythromycin, vancomycin, or RIF (consider 2 agents)	CIP (variable) [resistant strains SE Asia (CID 27: 370, 1998)], TMP/SMX, tetracycline, or clindamycin	Vancomycin active in vitro but intracellular location of R. equi may impair efficacy (Sem Resp Inf 12:57, 1997; CID 34:1379, 2002)
Rickettsiae species	Doxy	Chloramphenicol	FQ
Salmonella typhi	FQ, ceftriaxone	Chloramphenicol, amox, TMP/SMX, azithro (for uncomplicated disease) AAC 43:1441, 1999)	Multi drug resistant strains (chloramphenicol, AMP, TMP/SMX) common in many developing countries, more in immigrants. FQ resistance now being reported (AJTMH 61:163, 1999).
Serratia marcescens	P Ceph 3, erta, IMP, MER, FQ	Aztreonam, gentamicin	TC/CL, PIP/TZ
Shigella sp.	FQ or azithro	TMP/SMX and AMP (resistance common in Middle East, Latin America). Azithro ref.: AnIM 126:697, 1997	
Staph. aureus, methicillin-susceptible	Oxacillin/nafcillin	P Ceph 1, vancomycin, clindamycin	Erta, IMP, MER, BL/BLI, FQ, erythromycin, clarithro, dirithromycin, azithro, quinu/dalfo, linezolid
Staph. aureus, methicillin-resistant	Vancomycin	Teicoplanin[NUS], TMP/SMX (some strains resistant), quinu/dalfo, linezolid, daptomycin	Fusidic acid[NUS], >60% CIP-resistant in U.S. (Fosmomycin + RIF), novobiocin. Partially vancomycin-resistant strains isolated (MMWR 57:624, 1997)
Staph. aureus, methicillin-resistant [community-acquired (CA-MRSA)]	(TMP/SMX or doxy) ± RIF	Clinda (if susceptible to erythro & clinda); linezolid	CA-MRSA usually not multiply-resistant (Ln 359:1819, 2002; JAMA 286:1201, 2001). Often resist. to erythro & variably to FQ. Vanco, teico[NUS], or daptomycin can be used in pts requiring hospitalization.
Staph. epidermidis	Vancomycin ± RIF	RIF + (TMP/SMX or FQ)	Cephalothin or nafcillin/oxacillin if sensitive to nafcillin/oxacillin but 75% are resistant. FQs. (See Table 5)
Staph. haemolyticus	TMP/SMX, FQ, nitrofurantoin	Oral cephalosporin	Recommendations apply to UTI only.
Staph. saprophyticus (UTI)	Oral cephalosporin or AM/CL	FQ	Susceptible to most agents used for UTI; occ. failure of sulfonamides, nitrofurantoin reported (JID 155:170, 1987).
Stenotrophomonas (Xanthomonas, Pseudomonas) maltophila	TMP/SMX	TC/CL or (aztreonam + TC/CL) (AAC 41:2612, 1997)	Minocycline, doxy, ceftaz. [In vitro synergy (TC/CL + TMP/SMX) and (TC/CL + CIP), (AAC 39:2220, 1995; CMR 11:57, 1998)]
Streptobacillus moniliformis	Penicillin G or doxy	Erytho, clindamycin	
Streptococcus, anaerobic (Peptostreptococcus)	Penicillin G	Clindamycin	Erythromycin, doxy, vancomycin
Streptococcus pneumoniae penicillin-susceptible	Penicillin G	Multiple agents effective, e.g., amox	See footnote, page 4
penicillin-resistant (MIC ≥2.0)	(Vancomycin ± RIF) + (cefo or mero) See footnote page 4 and Table 5, page 55		For non-meningeal infections: P Ceph 3/4, CARB, quinu/dalfo, linezolid
Streptococcus pyogenes, Groups A, B, C, G & F, **Strep. milleri** (constellatis, intermedius, anginosus)	Penicillin G or V (some add gentamicin for serious Group B strep infections)	Erythro, azithro, clindamycin, clarithro, telithro	In France, Finland & Japan, resistance to macrolides over 50%, but 1 in Japan to <1% (Arch Ped 148:67, 1994)
Vibrio cholerae	Doxy, FQ	TMP/SMX	Strain 0139 is resistant to TMP/SMX
Vibrio parahaemolyticus	Antibiotic rx does not ↓ course		Sensitive in vitro to FQ, doxy
Vibrio vulnificus, alginolyticus, damsela	Doxy + ceftaz	Cefotaxime, FQ (e.g., levo, AAC 46:3580, 2002)	APAG often used in combination with ceftaz
Yersinia enterocolitica	TMP/SMX or FQ	P Ceph 3 or APAG	CID 19:655, 1994
Yersinia pestis (plague) See Table 1B, page 46	Streptomycin, gentamicin, or tobramycin	Chloramphenicol, doxy, or CIP	Susceptible to FQ, TMP/SMX in vitro (AAC 44:1995, 2000). Despite in vitro activity, AMP, cephalosporins, & RIF were not active in mouse model (caused enhanced mortality) (AAC 42:675, 1998).

[1] These agents are more variable in effectiveness than the "Recommended" or "Alternative" or "Also Effective" agents. Selection of "Alternative" or "Also Effective" agents is based on in vitro susceptibility testing, pharmacokinetics, host factors such as auditory, renal, hepatic function, and cost.

[2] **AM/CL:** amoxicillin clavulanate; **Amox:** amoxicillin; **AMP:** ampicillin; **AM/SB:** ampicillin sulbactam; **APAG:** antipseudomonal aminoglycosides; **AP Pen:** antipseudomonal penicillin (see page 52); **Azithro:** azithromycin; **BL/BLI:** β-lactam/β-lactamase inhibitor (AM/CL, TC/CL, AM/SB, or PIP/TZ); **CARB:** carbapenems (ertapenem, imipenem, or meropenem); **Ceftaz:** ceftazidime; **CIP:** ciprofloxacin; **Clarithro:** clarithromycin; **DOT group**: B. distasonis, B. ovatus, B. thetaiotaomicron, B. vulgatus; **Doxy:** doxycycline; **Erta:** ertapenem; **FQ:** fluoroquinolone (ciprofloxacin, ofloxacin, lomefloxacin, enoxacin, pefloxacin, levofloxacin); **IMP:** imipenem + cilastatin; **MER:** meropenem; **NUS:** not available in the U.S.; **P Ceph**: parenteral cephalosporins; **PIP/TZ:** piperacillin/tazobactam; **Quinu/dalfo**: quinupristin/dalfopristin; **RIF:** rifampin; **TC/CL:** ticarcillin clavulanate; **Telithro:** telithromycin; **TMP/SMX:** trimethoprim/sulfamethoxazole

TABLE 3: SUGGESTED DURATION OF ANTIBIOTIC THERAPY IN IMMUNOCOMPETENT PATIENTS[1,2]

SITE	CLINICAL SITUATION / CLINICAL DIAGNOSIS	DURATION OF THERAPY (Days)
Bacteremia	Bacteremia with removable focus (no endocarditis)	10–14 *(Clin Inf Dis 14:75, 1992) (See Table 1)*
Bone	Osteomyelitis, adult; acute	42
	adult; chronic	Until ESR normal (often > 3 months)
	child; acute; staph. and enterobacteriaceae[3]	21
	child; acute; strep., meningococci, hemophilus[3]	14
Ear	Otitis media with effusion	10 (or 1 dose ceftriaxone)
	Recent metanalysis suggests 5 days of "short-acting" antibiotics effective for uncomplicated otitis media *(JAMA 279:1736, 1998).*	
Endocardium	Infective endocarditis, native valve	
	Viridans strep	14 or 28 *(See Table 1, pages 18–19)*
	Enterococci	28 or 42 *(See Table 1, page 19)*
	Staph. aureus	14 (R-sided only) or 28 *(See Table 1, page 19)*
Gastrointestinal *Also see Table 1*	Bacillary dysentery (shigellosis)/traveller's diarrhea	3
	Typhoid fever (S. typhi): Ceftriaxone	14*
	FQ[6]	5–7
	Chloramphenicol	14
		*[Short courses less effective *(AAC 44:450, 2000)*]
	Helicobacter pylori	10–14
	Pseudomembranous enterocolitis (C. difficile)	10
Genital	Non-gonococcal urethritis or mucopurulent cervicitis	7 days doxy[6] or single dose azithro[6]
	Pelvic inflammatory disease	14
Heart	Pericarditis (purulent)	28
Joint	Septic arthritis (non-gonococcal) Adult	14–28 *(Ln 351:197, 1998)*
	Infant/child	Rx as osteomyelitis above
	Gonococcal arthritis/disseminated GC infection	7 *(See Table 1, page 15)*
Kidney	Cystitis (bladder bacteriuria)	3
	Pyelonephritis	14 (7 days if CIP used)
	Recurrent (failure after 14 days rx)	42
Lung	Pneumonia, pneumococcal	Until afebrile 3–5 days (minimum 5 days)
	Pneumonia, enterobacteriaceae or pseudomonal	21, often up to 42
	Pneumonia, staphylococcal	21–28
	Pneumocystis carinii, in AIDS;	21
	other immunocompromised	14
	Legionella, mycoplasma, chlamydia	14–21
	Lung abscess	Usually 28–42[4]
Meninges[5]	N. meningitidis	5–7 *(IDCP 7:370, 1998)*
	H. influenzae	7
	S. pneumoniae	10–14
	Listeria meningoencephalitis, gp B strep, coliforms	14–21 (longer in immunocompromised)
Multiple systems	Brucellosis *(See Table 1, page 40)*	42 (add SM[6] or GM[6] for 1st 7–14 days)
	Tularemia *(See Table 1, pages 29, 30, 40)*	7–14
Muscle	Gas gangrene (clostridial)	10
Pharynx *Also see Pharyngitis, Table 1, page 32*	Group A strep pharyngitis	10 (O Ceph 2/3, azithromycin effective at 5 d.) *(JAC 45, Topic T123, 2000)*
	Diphtheria (membranous)	7–14
	Carrier	7
Prostate	Chronic prostatitis (TMP/SMX)[6]	30–90
	(FQ)	28–42
Sinuses	Acute sinusitis	10–14[7]
Skin	Cellulitis	Until 3 d. after acute inflammation disappears
Systemic	Lyme disease	*See Table 1, page 39*
	Rocky Mountain spotted fever *(See Table 1, page 39)*	Until afebrile 2 days

[1] It has been shown that early change from parenteral to oral regimens (about 72 hours) is cost-effective with many infections, i.e., intra-abdominal *(AJM 91:462, 1991)*

[2] The recommended duration is a minimum or average time and should not be construed as absolute

[3] These times are with proviso: sx & signs resolve within 7 days and ESR[6] is normalized *(J.D. Nelson, APID 6:59, 1991)*

[4] After patient afebrile 4-5 days, change to oral therapy

[5] In children relapses seldom occur until 3 days or more after termination of rx. Practice of observing in hospital for 1 or 2 days after rx is expensive and non-productive. For meningitis in children, *see Table 1, page 4.*

[6] **Azithro** = azithromycin; **CIP** = ciprofloxacin; **Doxy** = doxycycline; **ESR** = erythrocyte sedimentation rate; **FQ** = fluoroquinolones; **GM** = gentamicin; **rx** = treatment; **SM** = streptomycin; **TMP/SMX** = trimethoprim/sulfamethoxazole

[7] If pt not sx-free at 10 d., sinus puncture and/or rx for 7 more days *(NEJM 326:319, 1992)*. One study reports 3 days of TMP/SMX effective *(JAMA 273:1015, 1995)*. Therapy with azithro for 3 & 6 days as effective as 10 days of AM/CL *(AAC 47:2770, 2003)*.

TABLE 4
COMPARISON OF ANTIMICROBIAL SPECTRA*
(These are generalizations; there are major differences between countries, areas and hospitals depending upon antibiotic usage patterns—verify for individual location. See Table 5 for resistant bacteria)

Organisms	Penicillin G	Penicillin V	Methicillin	Nafcillin/Oxacillin	Cloxacillin/Dicloxacillin	Amp/Amox	Amox/Clav	Amp/Sulb	Ticarcillin	Ticar/Clav	Pip/Tazo	Piperacillin	Ertapenem	Imipenem	Meropenem	Aztreonam	Ciprofloxacin	Ofloxacin	Lomefloxacin	Perfloxacin	Levofloxacin	Moxifloxacin	Gemifloxacin	Gatifloxacin
GRAM-POSITIVE:																								
Strep, Group A,B,C,G	+	+	+	+	+	+	+	+	+	+	+	+	+	+	+	0	±	+	±		+	+	+	+
Strep. pneumoniae	+	+	+	+	+	+	+	+	+	+	+	+	+	+	+	0	±	±	±		+	+	+	+
Viridans strep	±	+	±	±	±	±	+	+	±	+	+	+	+	+	+	0	±	±	±		+	+	+	+
Strep. milleri	±	+	±	±	±	±	+	+	±	+	+	+				0	0	0	0					
Enterococcus faecalis	+	+	+	0	0	+	+	+	±	+	+	+	±	+	±	0	**	**		0				
Enterococcus faecium	±	±	±	0	0	+	+	±	±	±	±		0	±	0	0	0			0	0		±
Staph. aureus (MSSA)	0	0	+	+	+	0	+	+	0	+	+	0	+	+	+	0	+	+	+		+	+	+	+
Staph.aureus (MRSA)	0	0	0	0	0	0	0	0	0	0	0	0	0	0	0	0	0				0	±		±
Staph. epidermidis	0	0	±	±	±	0	±	±	0	±	±	0	±	±	±	0	±				±			±
C. jeikeium	0	0	0	0	0	0	0	0	0	0	0	0		±		0	+				+			+
L. monocytogenes	+	0	0	0	0	+	+	+	0				+	+	+	0	±	±			±	±	±	+
GRAM-NEGATIVE:																								
N. gonorrhoeae	0	0	0	0	0	±	±	+		+	+	+	+	+	+	+	+	+	+		+	+	+	+
N. meningitidis	+	0	0	0	0	+	+		+			+	+	+	+	+	+	+	+		+		+	+
M. catarrhalis	0	0	0	0	0	+	+	+	+	+	+	+	+	+	+	+	+	+	+		+	+	+	+
H. influenzae	0	0	0	0	0	±	+	±	+	+	+	+	+	+	+	+	+	+	+		+	+	+	+
E. coli	0	0	0	0	0	±	+	+	+	+	+	+	+	+	+	+	+	+	+		+	+	+	+
Klebsiella sp.	0	0	0	0	0	0	+	+	0	+	+	+	+	+	+	+	+	+	+		+	+	+	+
Enterobacter sp.	0	0	0	0	0	0	0	±	0	±	+	+	+	+	+	+	+	+	+		+	+	+	+
Serratia sp.	0	0	0	0	0	0	0	0	±	±	+	+	+	+	+	+	+	+	+		+	±		+
Salmonella sp.	0	0	0	0	0	±	+	+	+	+	+	+	+	+	+	+	+	+	+		+	+	+	+
Shigella sp.	0	0	0	0	0	±	+	+	+	+	+	+	+	+	+	+	+	+	+		+	+	+	+
Proteus mirabilis	0	0	0	0	0	+	+	+	+	+	+	+	+	+	+	+	+	+	+		+	+	+	+
Proteus vulgaris	0	0	0	0	0	0	+	+	±	+	+	+	+	+	+	+	+	+	+		+	+	+	+
Providencia sp.	0	0	0	0	0	0	+	+	+	+	+	+	+	+	+	+	+	+	+		+	±		+
Morganella sp.	0	0	0	0	0	0	+	+	+	+	+	+	+	+	+	+	+	+	+		+	±		+
Citrobacter sp.	0	0	0	0	0	0	0	±	+	+	+	+	+	+	+	+	+	+	+		+	+		+
Aeromonas sp.	0	0	0	0	0	0	±	±	+	+	+	+		+	+	+	+	+	+		+	+		+
Acinetobacter sp.	0	0	0	0	0	0	±	+	±	+	+	+		+	+	0	±	+	+		±	+		+
Ps. aeruginosa	0	0	0	0	0	0	0	0	+	+	+	+	0	+	+	+	+	±			±	0	0	±
S. (Ps.) cepacia§	0	0	0	0	0	0	0	0	±	±	±	±	0	±	±	0	±	±			±			±
S. (X.) maltophilia§	0	0	0	0	0	0	0	0	±	±	0	0	0	0	0	0	±				±	±		±
Y. enterocolitica	0	0	0	0	0	0	0	0	+	+	+	+		+	+	+	+	+	0		+			0
Legionella sp.	0	0	0	0	0	0	0	0	0	0	0	0	0	0	0	0	+	+	+		+	+	+	+
P. multocida	+		0	0	0	+	+	+	+	+	+	+		+	+	+	+				+	+		+
H. ducreyi	+					0	+	+		+	+	+					+				+	+		+
MISC.:																								
Chlamydia sp.	0	0	0	0	0	0	0	0	0	0	0	0		0		0	+	+	+		+	+	+	+
M. pneumoniae	0	0	0	0	0	0	0	0	0	0	0	0	0	0	0	0	+	+	+		+	+	+	+
ANAEROBES:																								
Actinomyces	+					+	+	+	+	+	+	+		+	+		±	±			+	+		+
Bacteroides fragilis	0	±	0	0	0	0	+	+		+	+	±	+	+	+	0	0	0	0	0	0	±		±
P. melaninogenica§	+	0	0	0	0	±	+	+	+	+	+	+		+	+	0	±	±			±	±		+
Clostridium difficile (not difficile)	+¹						+¹				+¹	+¹	+¹	+¹	0	0				0	0		±¹
Clostridium (not difficile)	+	+				+	+	+	+	+	+	+		+	+		±	±			0	±		±¹
Peptostreptococcus sp.	+	+				+	+	+	+	+	+	+		+	+		±	±	0		±	+		+

+ =usually effective clinically or >60% susceptible; ± = clinical trials lacking or 30–60% susceptible; blank = data not available
*** effective clinically or <30% susceptible; 0 = not
§ B. melaninogenicus → Prevotella melaninogenica, Pseudomonas cepacia → Burkholderia cepacia, Xanthomonas → Stenotrophomonas
*** Most strains ±, can be used in UTI, not in systemic infection
Ticar/Clav = ticarcillin clavulanate; **Amp/Sulb** = ampicillin sulbactam; **Amox/Clav** = amoxicillin clavulanate; **MSSA** = methicillin-sensitive Staph. aureus; **MRSA** = methicillin-resistant Staph. aureus; **Pip/Tazo** = piperacillin/tazobactam;
¹ No clinical evidence that penicillins or fluoroquinolones are effective for C. difficile enterocolitis (but they may cover this organism in mixed intra-abdominal and pelvic infections)

TABLE 4 (2)

Organisms	Cefazolin	Cefotetan	Cefoxitin	Cefuroxime	Cefotaxime	Ceftizoxime	Ceftriaxone	Ceftazidime	Cefepime	Cefadroxil	Cephalexin	Cefaclor/Loracarbef*	Cefprozil	Cefuroxime axetil	Cefixime[AUS]	Ceftibuten	Cefpodox/Cefdinir/Cefditoren
GRAM-POSITIVE:																	
Strep, Group A,B,C,G	+	+	+	+	+	+	+	+	+	+	+	+	+	+	+	+	+
Strep. pneumoniae[1]	+	+	+	+	+	+	+	+[1]	+	+	+	+	+	+	+	±	+
Viridans strep	+	+	+	+	+	+	+	+[1]	+	+	+	+	0	+	+	0	+
Enterococcus faecalis	0	0	0	0	0	0	0	0	0	0	0	0	0	0	0	0	0
Staph. aureus (MSSA)	+	+	+	+	+	+	+	±	+	+	+	+	+	+	0	0	+
Staph. aureus (MRSA)	0	0	0	0	0	0	0	0	0	0	0	0	0	0	0	0	0
Staph. epidermidis	±	±	±	±	±	±	±	±	±	±	±	±	±	±	0	0	±
C. jeikeium	0	0	0	0	0	0	0	0	0	0	0	0	0	0	0	0	0
L. monocytogenes	0	0	0	0	0	0	0	0	0	0	0	0	0	0	0	0	0
GRAM-NEGATIVE:																	
N. gonorrhoeae	+	±	±	±	±	±	±	±	+	0	0	±	±	±	+	±	+
N. meningitidis	0	±	±	+	+	±	+	±	+	0	0	±	±	±	+	±	
M. catarrhalis	±	±	+	+	+	+	+	+	+	0	0	±	+	+	+	+	+
H. influenzae	+	+	+	+	+	+	+	+	+	0	0	+	+	+	+	+	+
E. coli	+	+	+	+	+	+	+	+	+	+	+	+	+	+	+	+	+
Klebsiella sp.	+	+	+	+	+	+	+	+	+	+	+	+	+	+	+	+	+
Enterobacter sp.	0	±	0	0	+	+	+	+	+	0	0	0	0	0	0	±	0
Serratia sp.	0	±	0	0	+	+	+	+	+	0	0	0	0	0	0	±	0
Salmonella sp.					+					0							
Shigella sp.										0							
Proteus mirabilis	+	+	+	+	+	+	+	+	+	+	+	+	+	+	+	+	+
Proteus vulgaris	0	±	±	+	+	+	+	+	+	0	0	0	0	0	+	+	+
Providencia sp.	0	±	+	0	+	+	+	+	+	0	0	0	0	0	+	+	0
Morganella sp.	0	±	±	±	+	+	+	+	+	0	0	0	0	0	+	+	0
C. freundii	0	0	0	0	+	+	+	0	+	0	0	0	0	0	+	+	0
C. diversus	0	±	±	±	+	+	+	+	+	0	0	0				+	
Citrobacter sp.	0	±	±	±	+	+	+	+	+	0	±	0	±		+	+	+
Aeromonas sp.	0	±	±	±	+	+	+	+	+	0	0	0			+	+	+
Acinetobacter sp.	0	0	0	0	±	±	±	+	±	0	0	0	0	0	0	0	0
Ps. aeruginosa	0	0	0	0	±	±	±	+	+	0	0	0	0	0	0	0	0
B. (Ps.) cepacia[§]	0	0	0	0	±	±	0	±	0	0	0	0	0	0	0	+	0
S. (X.) maltophilia[§]	0	0	0	0	0	0	0	0	0	0	0	0	0	0	0		
Y. enterocolitica	0	±	±	±	+	+	+	±	+	0	0						
Legionella sp.	0	0	0	0	0	0	0	0	0	0	0	0	0	0	0	0	0
P. multocida					+	+				0						+	+
H. ducreyi			+		+	+	+									+	
ANAEROBES:																	
Actinomyces						+	+										
Bacteroides fragilis	0	+[2]	+	0	0	±	0	0	0		0	0	0	0	0	0	0
P. melaninogenica[§]		+	+	+	+	±	+	0				+	+	+			
Clostridium difficile			0		0	0	0										
Clostridium (not difficile)		+	+	+	+	+	+	+					+	+	0		
Peptostreptococcus sp.	+	+	+	+	+	+	+	+	+		+	+	+	+			

+ = usually effective clinically or >60% susceptible; ± = clinical trials lacking or 30–60% susceptible; 0 = not effective clinically or <30% susceptible; blank = data not available.

[§] B. melaninogenicus → Prevotella melaninogenica, P. cepacia → Burkholderia cepacia, Xanthomonas → Stenotrophomonas

* A 1-carbacephem best classified as a cephalosporin

[1] Ceftaz 8–16x less active than cefotax/ceftriax, effective only vs Pen-sens. strains (AAC 39:2193, 1995). Oral cefuroxime, cefprozil, cefpodoxime most active in vitro vs resistant S. pneumo (PIDJ 14:1037, 1995).

[2] Cefotetan is less active against B. ovatus, B. distasonis, B. thetaiotamicron

[3] **Cefpodox** = Cefpodoxime proxetil

MSSA = methicillin-sensitive Staph. aureus; **MRSA** = methicillin-resistant Staph. aureus

TABLE 4 (3)

Organisms	AMINOGLYCOSIDES				Chloramphenicol	MACROLIDES				Ketolide	TETRACYCLINES		GLYCOPEPTIDES		Fusidic Acid	Trimethoprim	TMP/SMX	URINARY TRACT AGENTS		MISCELLANEOUS					
	Gentamicin	Tobramycin	Amikacin	Netilmicin[AUS]	Chloramphenicol	Clindamycin	Erythro/Dirithro	Azithromycin	Clarithromycin	Telithromycin	Doxycycline	Minocycline	Vancomycin	Teicoplanin	Fusidic Acid	Trimethoprim	TMP/SMX	Nitrofurantoin	Fosfomycin	Enoxacin	Rifampin	Metronidazole	Quinupristin/dalfopristin	Daptomycin	Linezolid
GRAM-POSITIVE:																									
Strep Group A,B,C,G	0	0	0	0	+	+	+	+	+	+	±	+	+	+	±	±	+[2]		0	+	0	+	+	+	+
Strep. pneumoniae	0	0	0	0	+	+	+	+	+	+	±	+	+	+	±	±	+[2]	±	0	+	0	+	+	+	+
Enterococcus faecalis	S	S	S	S	±	0	0	0	0	±	0	0	+	+	±	+	+[2]	+	±	+	0	0	+	+	+
Enterococcus faecium	S	0	0	0	±	0	0	0	0	0	0	0	±	±		0	0	+	0	0	0	0	+	+	+
Staph.aureus (MSSA)	+	+	+	+	±	±	±	+	+	+	±	+	+	+	+	±	+	+	0	+	+	0	+	+	+
Staph.aureus (MRSA)	0	0	0	0	0	0	0	0	0	0	±	±	+	+	+	±	±	+	0	+	+	0	+	+	+
Staph. epidermidis	±	±	±	±	0	0	±	0	0	0	0	±	+	+	+	±	+	+		+	+	0	+	+	+
C. jeikeium	0	0	0	0	0	0	0	0	0	0	0	0	+	+	0	0	0	+	0	0	+	0	+	+	+
L. monocytogenes	S	S	S	S	+		+	+	+	+	±	+				+	+				+	0	+	+	+
GRAM-NEGATIVE:																									
N. gonorrhoeae	0	0	0	0	+	0	±	±	±		±	±	0			+	0	+		±	0		+	0	+
N. meningitidis	0	0	0	0	+	0	+	+		+	+	+	0	0		0	±	±			+	0	0	0	0
M. catarrhalis[§]	+	+	+	+	+	0	+	+	+	+	+	+	0			+	+				+	0	±	±	±
H. influenzae	+	+	+	+	+	0	±	+	±	+	±	±	0			+	+		±	±	+	0	±	±	±
Aeromonas	+	+	+	+	+						+	+			0		+	+			0	0			
E. coli	+	+	+	+	+	0	0	0	0	0		0	0	0		+	+	+	+	+	0	0	0	0	0
Klebsiella sp.	+	+	+	+	+	0	0	0	0	0	±	±	0			±	+	±	±	+	0	0	0	0	0
Enterobacter sp.	+	+	+	+	0	0	0	0	0	0	±	±	0			±	+	±	±	+	0	0	0	0	0
Salmonella sp.	0	0	0	0	+	0	0	0	0	0	0	0	0			+	+	0		+	0	0	0	0	0
Shigella sp.	+	+	+	+	+	0	+	0	0	0	±	±	0			+	+	+		+	0	0	0	0	0
Serratia marcescens	+	+	+	+	0	0	0	0	0	0	0	0	0			±	+	0		+	0	0	0	0	0
Proteus vulgaris	+	+	+	+	±	0	0	0	0	0	0	0	0			+	+	0		+	0	0	0	0	0
Acinetobacter sp.	0	0	0	0			0				+	+				±	+	0		±	0	0	0	0	0
Ps. aeruginosa	+	+	+	+	0	0	0	0	0	0	0	±	0			0	0	0	0	+	0	0	0	0	0
B. (Ps.) cepacia[§]	0	0	0	0	+	0	0	0	0	0	0	0	0			+	+			+		0			
S. (X.) maltophilia[§]	0	0	0	0	+	0	0	0	0	0	0	±	0			0	+	0		0		0			
Y. enterocolitica	+	+	+	+	+	0	0	0	0	0	0	0	0			0	+	0		0		0			
F. tularensis	+				+						+											+			
Brucella sp.	+				+						+					0	+				+	0			
Legionella sp.					+	0	+	+	+	+	+	+	0			±	±			+	+	0			
H. ducreyi					+		0	+	+	+						0	±				±	0			
V. vulnificus	±	±	±		+						+	+			0							0			
MISC.:																									
Chlamydophila sp.	0	0	0	0	+	±	+	+	+	+	+	+				0	0				+	0	+	+	+
M. pneumoniae	0	0	0	0	+	0	+	+	+	+	+	+				0	0				0	+	0	0	0
Rickettsia sp.	0	0	0	0	+		±				+	+					0				+	0	0	0	0
Mycobacterium avium			+				+	+	+												+	0			
ANAEROBES:																									
Actinomyces	0	0	0	0	+	+	±	+	+	+	+	+				0					0				
Bacteroides fragilis	0	0	0	0	+	+	0	0	0		±	±	0		+		+	0			0	+	±		
P. melaninogenica[§]	0	0	0	0	+	+	0	0	0		±	±	0		+		0				+	+	+		
Clostridium difficile	0	0	0	0	±								+	+							0	+	±	±	
Clostridium (not difficile)**					+	+	±	±	+		+	+	+	+	+						+	+	+	+	
Peptostreptococcus sp.					+	+	+	+	+		+	+	+								+	+	+		

+ = usually effective clinically or >60% susceptible; ± = clinical trials lacking or 30–60% susceptible; 0 = not effective clinically or <30% susceptible; S = synergistic with penicillins (ampicillin); blank = data not available. Antimicrobials such as azithromycin have high tissue penetration and some such as clarithromycin are metabolized to more active compounds, hence in vivo activity may exceed in vitro activity.

[1] In vitro results discrepant, + in one study, 0 in another [JAC 31(Suppl. C):39, 1993].

[2] Although active in vitro, TMP/SMX is not clinically effective for Group A strep pharyngitis or for infections due to E. faecalis.

§ B. melaninogenicus → Prevotella melaninogenica, P. cepacia → Burkholderia cepacia, Xanthomonas → Stenotrophomonas

** Vancomycin, metronidazole given po active vs C. difficile; IV vancomycin not effective

Dirithro = dirithromycin; **Erythro** = erythromycin; **TMP/SMX** = trimethoprim/sulfamethoxazole; **MSSA** = methicillin-sensitive Staph. aureus; **MRSA** = methicillin-resistant Staph. aureus; **S** = potential synergy in combination with penicillin, ampicillin, vancomycin, or teicoplanin

TABLE 5: TREATMENT OPTIONS FOR SELECTED HIGHLY RESISTANT BACTERIA*

ORGANISM/RESISTANCE	THERAPEUTIC OPTIONS	COMMENT[1]
E. faecalis. Resistant to:		
Vanco + strep/gentamicin (MIC >500 µg/ml), β-lactamase neg. (JAC 40:161, 1997).	Penicillin G or AMP (systemic infections); Nitrofurantoin, fosfomycin (UTI only). Usually resistant to Synercid	Non BL+ strains of E. faecalis resistant to penicillin and AMP recently described in Spain, but unknown (except BL+ strains) so far in U.S. and elsewhere (AAC 40:2420, 1996). Linezolid also effective in 60–70% of cases (Ln 358:135, 2003). Daptomycin active in vitro (AAC 52:123, 2003).
Penicillin (β-lactamase producers)	Vanco, AM/SB	Appear susceptible to AMP and penicillin by standard in vitro methods. Must use direct test for β-lactamase with chromogenic cephalosporin (nitrocefin) to identify in lab (JCM 31:1965, 1993). Rarely seen since early 1990s
E. faecium. Resistant to:		
Vanco and high level (MIC >500 µg/ml) of streptomycin and gentamicin	Penicillin G or AMP (systemic infections); fosfomycin, nitrofurantoin (UTI only)	For strains with pen/AMP MICs of >8 ≤64 µg/ml there is anecdotal evidence that high-dose (300 mg/kg/day) AMP rx may be effective. Daptomycin active in vitro (AAC 52:123, 2003).
Penicillin, AMP, vanco, & high-level resist. to streptomycin and gentamicin (NEJM 342:710, 2000)	Linezolid 600 mg po or IV q12h may be effective (AAC 44:625, 2000); quinu/dalfo 7.5 mg/kg IV q8h are bacteriostatic against most strains of E. faecium. Can try combinations of cell wall-active antibiotics with vanco &/or high levels (including FQ, chloramphenicol, RIF, or doxy). Chloramphenicol alone effective in some cases of bacteremia (CMI 7:17, 2001). Nitrofurantoin or fosfomycin may work for UTI.	For strains with Van B phenotype (vanco R, teico S), teicoplanin[NUS] preferably in combination with streptomycin or gentamicin if not highly AG resistant, may be effective. Synercid roughly 70% effective in clinical trials (CID 30:790, 2000, & 33:816, 2001). Linezolid shows similar efficacy. Emergence of resistance to linezolid during monotherapy with either quinu/dalfo or linezolid (CID 30:790, 2000; Ln 357:1179, 2001). Nosocomial spread of linezolid-resistant E. faecium possible (CID 30:790, 2000; 33:816, 2001). Daptomycin active in vitro against most strains (AAC 52:123, 2003).
S. aureus. Resistant to:		**Infectious disease consultation imperative**
Methicillin (Ln 349:1901, 1997; Clin Micro Rev 10:781, 1997; CID 32:108, 2001)	Vanco	Other alternatives include teicoplanin[NUS], linezolid (Chest 124:1789, 2003), TMP/SMX (test susceptibility first), minocycline & doxy (some strains), daptomycin, or quinu/dalfo (CID 34:1481, 1993). Fusidic acid[NUS] & fosfomycin, RIF, novobiocin, FQ are active but must be used in combination regimens to prevent in vivo emergence of resistance. **Investigational drugs with activity against MRSA include oritavancin (LY333328), and dalbavancin.**
Vanco (VISA or VRSA) (AAC 43:1449, 1999; JID 179:1536, 1998; CID 32:108, 2001; MMWR 51:902, 2002; NEJM 348:1342, 2003)	Unknown, but even high-dose vanco may fail. Linezolid, quinu/dalfo active in vitro.	Most clinical isolates of VRMRSA have had only low levels (MIC ≤16 µg/ml) of vanco resistance (MMWR 27:624, 1997; AAC 40:135, 1997). Some call these strains VISA or GISA. Only anecdotal data on therapeutic regimens. Most susceptible to TMP/SMX, minocycline, doxycycline, RIF and AG (CID 32:108, 2001). RIF should always be combined with a 2ⁿᵈ therapeutic agent to prevent emergence of RIF resistance during therapy. Two clinical isolates of truly vancomycin-resistant (MIC >64 MRSA described; strains still susceptible to TMP/SMX, chloro, linezolid, minocycline, quinu/dalfo (MMWR 51:902, 2002; NEJM 348:1342, 2003).
S. epidermidis. Resistant to:		
Methicillin.	Vanco (± RIF and gentamicin for prosthetic valve endocarditis)	
Methicillin, glycopeptides	Quinu/dalfo (see comments on E. faecium) active in vitro as is linezolid	Vanco more active than teicoplanin[NUS] (Clin Microbiol Rev 8:585, 1995). New FQs (levofloxacin, gatifloxacin, moxifloxacin) active in vitro, but development of resistance is a potential problem.
S. pneumoniae. Resistant to:		
Penicillin G (MIC ≤1.0)	Ceftriaxone or cefotaxime. High-dose penicillin (≥10 million units/day) or AMP (amox) likely effective for non-meningeal sites of infection (e.g., pneumonia)	IMP, erta, cefepime, cefpodoxime, cefuroxime also active (IDCP 3:75, 1994). MER less active than IMP (AAC 38:898, 1994). Gati, gemi, levo, moxi also have good activity (AAC 38:898, 1994; DMID 31:45, 1998; Exp Opin Invest Drugs 8:123, 1999).
Penicillin G (MIC ≥2.0)	Vanco ± RIF. Alternatives if (non-meningeal infection: ceftriaxone/cefotax, high-dose AMP, erta, IMP, MER, or an active FQ: gati, gemi, levo, moxi.	High-dose cefotaxime (300 mg/kg/day, max. 24 gm/day) effective in meningitis due to strains with cefotaxime MICs as high as 2 µg/ml (AAC 40:218, 1996). Review: IDCP 6(Suppl 2):S21, 1997.
Penicillin, erythro, tetracycline, chloramphenicol, TMP/SMX	Vanco ± RIF	60–80% of strains susceptible to clindamycin (Diag Microbiol Inf Dis 25:201, 1996). Levo, gemi, gati, moxi active in vitro (AAC 40:2431, 1996).

* Footnotes on next page

TABLE 5 (2)

ORGANISM/RESISTANCE	THERAPEUTIC OPTIONS	COMMENT[1]
Acinetobacter baumannii. Resistant to: IMP, AP Ceph 3, AP Pen, APAG, FQ	AM/SB (sulbactam alone is active against some A. baumannii, JAC 42:793, 1998)	6/8 patients with A. baumannii meningitis (7 organisms resistant to IMP cured with AM/SB (CID 24:932, 1997). Various combinations of FQs and AGs, IMP and AGs, or AP Ceph 3s with AGs may show activity against **some** multiresistant strains (AAC 41:881, 1997; AAC 41:1073, 1997; CID 36:1268, 2003). N. colistin also shown activity (CID 28:1008, 1999; CID 36:1111, 2003)
Campylobacter jejuni. Resistant to: FQs	Erythro, azithro, clarithro, doxy, clindamycin	Strains resistant to **both** FQs & macrolides have been reported from Thailand (CID 22:868, 1996) & elsewhere (EID 7:24, 2002; AAC 47:2358, 2003)
Klebsiella pneumoniae (producing ESBL) **Resistant to:** Ceftazidime, P Ceph 3, aztreonam	IMP, MER, FQ	P Ceph 4, TC/CL, PIP/TZ show in vitro activity, but have not been proven entirely effective in animal models (JAA 8:37, 1997) and some strains which hyperproduce ESBLs are primarily resistant to TC/CL and PIP/TZ (JCM 34:358, 1996). Note that there are strains of ESBL-producing klebsiella for which in vitro tests suggest susceptibility to P Ceph 2, 3 but resistance to ceftazidime. Infections due to such strains do not respond to P Ceph 2 or 3 (CID 39:206, 2001).
Pseudomonas aeruginosa. Resistant to: IMP, MER	CIP (check susceptibility). APAG (check susceptibility).	Many strains remain susceptible to aztreonam & ceftazidime or AP Pens (AAC 36:1037, 1995). Combinations of (AP Pen & APAG) or (AP Ceph 3 + APAG) may show in vitro activity (AAC 39:2411, 1995). N. colistin may have some utility (CID 28:1008, 1999).

[1] Guideline on prevention of resistance: CID 25:584, 1997. **Abbreviations: AGs** = aminoglycosides, **Amox** = amoxicillin, **AMP** = ampicillin, **AM/SB** = ampicillin/sulbactam, **AP Pen** = antipseudomonal penicillin, **AP Ceph 3** = third generation parenteral cephalosporin with enhanced antipseudomonal activity, **APAG** = antipseudomonal aminoglycoside antibiotic, **Azithro** = azithromycin, **BL** = beta-lactamase, **Clarithro** = clarithromycin, **CIP** = ciprofloxacin, **Erythro** = erythromycin, **ESBL** = extended spectrum β-lactamases, **Eta** = ertapenem, **Doxy** = doxycycline, **FQ** = fluoroquinolone, **Gemi** = gemifloxacin, **Gati** = gatifloxacin, **Levo** = levofloxacin, **Moxi** = moxifloxacin, **IMP** = imipenem cilastatin, **MER** = meropenem, **P Ceph** = parenteral cephalosporin, **PIP/TZ** = piperacillin/tazobactam, **R** = resistant, **RIF** = rifampin, **S** = sensitive, **TC/CL** = ticarcillin/clavulanate, **Vanco** = vancomycin, **VISA** = vancomycin-intermediately-resistant Staph. aureus, **Quinu/dalfo** = quinupristin/dalfopristin, **VRMRSA** = vancomycin-resistant, methicillin-resistant Staph. aureus.

TABLE 6A: METHODS FOR PENICILLIN DESENSITIZATION

[Penicillin Allergy Reviews: CID 35:26, 2002 & MMWR 51 (RR-6):28-30, 2002]

Perform in ICU setting. Discontinue all β-adrenergic antagonists. Have IV line, ECG and spirometer (Curr Clin Topics Inf Dis 13:131, 1993). Once desensitized, rx must not lapse or risk of allergic reactions ↑. A history of Stevens-Johnson syndrome, exfoliative dermatitis, erythroderma are nearly absolute contraindications to desensitization (use only as an approach to IgE sensitivity).

Oral Route: If oral prep available and pt has functional GI tract, oral route is preferred. 1/3 pts will develop transient reaction during treatment, usually mild.

Step	1	2	3	4	5	6	7	8	9	10	11	12	13	14
Drug (mg/ml)	0.5	0.5	0.5	0.5	0.5	5.0	5.0	5.0	5.0	5.0	50	50	50	50
Amount (ml)	0.1	0.2	0.4	0.8	1.6	0.32	0.64	1.2	2.4	4.8	1.0	2.0	4.0	8.0

* Interval between doses: 15 min. After Step 14, observe for 30 minutes, then 1.0 gm IV

Parenteral Route:

Step**	1	2	3	4	5	6	7	8	9	10	11	12	13	14	15	16	17
Drug (mg/ml)	0.1	0.1	0.1	0.1	1.0	1.0	1.0	10	10	10	100	100	100	100	1000	1000	1000
Amount (ml)	0.1	0.2	0.4	0.8	0.16	0.32	0.64	0.12	0.24	0.48	0.1	0.2	0.4	0.8	0.16	0.32	0.64

** Interval between doses: 15 min. After Step 17, observe for 30 minutes, then 1.0 gm IV

[Adapted from Sullivan, TJ, in Allergy: Principles and Practice, Middleton, E., et al., Eds. C.V. Mosby, 1993, with permission]

TABLE 6B: RAPID ORAL TMP/SMX DESENSITIZATION*

Hour	Dose TMP/SMX (mg)	Comment
0	0.004/0.02	Perform in hospital or clinic. Use oral suspension [40mg TMP/200 mg SMX per 5 ml (tsp)]. Take 6 oz. water after each dose. Corticosteroids, antihistamines NOT used. Refs: CID 20:849, 1995; AIDS 5:311, 1991
1	0.04/0.2	
2	0.4/2	
3	4/20	
4	40/200	
5	160/800	

TABLE 7: RISK CATEGORIES OF ANTIMICROBICS IN PREGNANCY

DRUG	FDA PREGNANCY RISK CATEGORIES*
Antibacterial Agents	
Aminoglycosides:	
Amikacin, gentamicin, isepamicin[N.6];	
netilmicin, streptomycin & tobramycin	D
Beta Lactams *(CPh 27:49, 1994)*	
Penicillins; pens + BLI; cephalosporins; aztreonam	B
Imipenem/cilastatin	C
Meropenem, ertapenem	B
Chloramphenicol	C
Ciprofloxacin, ofloxacin, levoflox, gatiflox, gemiflox, moxiflox	C
Clindamycin	B
Colistin	?
Daptomycin	B
Fosfomycin	B
Linezolid	C
Macrolides:	
Erythromycins/azithromycin	B
Clarithromycin	C
Metronidazole	B
Nitrofurantoin	B
Sulfonamides/trimethoprim	C
Tetracyclines	D
Vancomycin	C

DRUG	FDA PREGNANCY RISK CATEGORIES*
Antifungal Agents: *(CID 27:1151, 1998)*	
Amphotericin B preparations	B
Caspofungin	C
Fluconazole, itraconazole, ketoconazole,	C
Terbinafine	B
flucytosine	C
Voriconazole	D
Antiparasitic Agents:	
Albendazole/mebendazole	C
Atovaquone/proguanil	C
Chloroquine, eflornithine	C
Ivermectin	C
Mefloquine	C
Miltefosine	X
Nitazoxanide	B
Pentamidine	C
Praziquantel	B
Pyrimethamine/pyrisulfadoxine	C
Quinidine	C
Quinine	X
Antimycobacterial Agents:	
Capreomycin	B
Clofazimine/cycloserine	C
Dapsone	C
Ethambutol	B
Rifampin	C
Thalidomide	X

DRUG	FDA PREGNANCY RISK CATEGORIES*
Antimycobacterial Agents *(continued)*	
Ethionamide	"do not use"[1]
INH, pyrazinamide, rifampin	C
Rifabutin	B
Antiviral Agents:	
Abacavir	C
Acyclovir, famciclovir, valacyclovir	B
Adefovir	C
Amantadine, rimantadine	C
Amprenavir, fosamprenavir, indinavir	C
Atazanavir	B
Cidofovir	C
Delavirdine, efavirenz, nevirapine	C
Didanosine (ddl)	B
Enfuvirtide	B
Foscarnet	C
Ganciclovir, valganciclovir	C
Interferons	C
Lamivudine/stavudine	C
Lopinavir/ritonavir	C
Nelfinavir, ritonavir, saquinavir	B
Oseltamivir	C
Ribavirin	X
Tenofovir	B
Valacyclovir	B
Zalcitabine/zidovudine	C

* **FDA Pregnancy Categories: A**—studies in pregnant women, no risk. **B**—animal studies no risk, but human not adequate or animal toxicity but human studies show toxicity. **C**—animal studies show toxicity, human studies inadequate but benefit of use may exceed risk. **D**—evidence of human risk, but benefits may outweigh. **X**—fetal abnormalities in humans, risk > benefit.
Abbreviations: BLI = b-lactamase inhibitor; **FQ** = fluoroquinolones

1 From CDC: TB Core Curriculum, 3rd Ed., 1994

TABLE 8: ANTIMICROBIAL AGENTS ASSOCIATED WITH PHOTOSENSITIVITY

The following drugs are known to cause photosensitivity in some individuals. There is no intent to indicate relative frequency or severity of reactions.

Source: 2003 Drug Topics Red Book, Medical Economics, Montvale, NJ. Listed in alphabetical order:

Amantadine, azithromycin, benznidazole, ciprofloxacin, dapsone, doxycycline, enoxacin, erythromycin ethyl succinate, flucytosine, ganciclovir, griseofulvin, interferons, levofloxacin, lomefloxacin, ofloxacin, pefloxacin, pyrazinamide, saquinavir, sparfloxacin, sulfonamides, tetracyclines, tretinoins, trimethoprim.

The approximate photoxic potential among fluoroquinolones (from *CID 28:352, 1999)* is: lomefloxacin, fleroxacin > sparfloxacin > enoxacin >pefloxacin[N.6] > ciprofloxacin, gemifloxacin, levofloxacin, moxifloxacin, ofloxacin

TABLE 9. SELECTED PHARMACOLOGIC FEATURES OF ANTIMICROBIAL AGENTS

DRUG	DOSE, ROUTE OF ADMINISTRATION	FOR PO DOSING—Take Drug[7]			% AB[1]	PEAK SERUM LEVEL μg/ml[6]	PROTEIN BINDING, %	SERUM T½, HOURS[2]	BILIARY EXCRETION, %[3]	CSF[5]/BLOOD, %	CSF LEVEL POTENTIALLY THERAPEUTIC[6]
		WITH FOOD	WITHOUT FOOD[4]	WITH OR WITHOUT FOOD							
PENICILLINS: Natural											
Benzathine Pen G	1.2 MU IM					0.15					
Penicillin G	2 MU IV					20	65		500	5-10	Yes for Pen-sens S. pneumo
Penicillin V	500 mg po		X		60-73	5-6	65	0.5			
PEN'ASE-RESISTANT PENICILLINS											
Clox/Diclox	500 mg po		X		50	10-15	95-98	0.5			
Nafcillin/Oxacillin	500 mg po		X		Erratic	10-15	90-94	0.5	>100/25	9-20	Yes-high-dose IV therapy
AMINOPENICILLINS											
Amoxicillin	250 mg po			X	75	4-5	17	1.2	100-3000	13-14	Yes
AM/CL	875/125 mg po			X		11.6/2.2	20/30	1.4/1.1	100-3000		
AM/CL-ER		X				17/2.1	18/25	1.3/1.0			Yes
Ampicillin	2.0 gm IV					47	18-22	1.2	100-3000	13-14	
AM/SB	3 gm IV					109-150	28/38	1.2			
ANTIPSEUDOMONAL PENICILLINS											
Indanyl carb.	382 mg po		X		35	6.5	50	1.0		30	Not for P. aeruginosa; marginal for coliforms
Piperacillin	4 gm IV					400	16-48	1.0	100-6000		
PIP/TZ	3.375 gm IV					209	16-48	1.0	>100		
Ticarcillin	3.0 gm IV					260	45	1.2		40	Not for P. aeruginosa; marginal for coliforms
TC/CL						324	45/30	1.2			
CEPHALOSPORINS—1st Generation											
Cefadroxil	500 mg po			X	90	16	20	1.5	22		
Cefazolin	1.0 gm IV					188	73-87	1.9	29-300	1-4	No
Cephalexin	500 mg po			X	90	18-38	5-15	1.0	216		
CEPHALOSPORINS—2nd Generation											
Cefaclor	500 mg po	X			93	9.3	22-25	0.8	>60		
Cefaclor-CD	500 mg po	X				8.4	22-25	0.8	>60		
Cefotetan	1.0 gm IV					124	78-91	4.2	2-21		
Cefoxitin	1.0 gm IV					110	65-79	0.8	280		
Cefprozil	500 mg po			X	95	10.5	36	1.5		3	±
Cefuroxime	1.5 gm IV					100	33-50	1.5	35-80	17-88	Yes
Cefuroxime axetil	250 mg po	X			52	4.1	50	1.2			
Loracarbef	250 mg po			X	90	8	25	1.2			

See page 62 for all footnotes

TABLE 9 (2)

DRUG	DOSE, ROUTE OF ADMINISTRATION	FOR PO DOSING—Take Drug[7] WITH FOOD	WITHOUT FOOD[8]	WITH OR WITHOUT FOOD	% AB[1]	PEAK SERUM LEVEL µg/ml[s]	PROTEIN BINDING, %	SERUM T½, HOURS[2]	BILIARY EXCRETION, %[3]	CSF[f]/BLOOD, %	CSF LEVEL POTENTIALLY THERAPEUTIC[c]
CEPHALOSPORINS—3rd Generation											
Cefdinir	300 mg po		X		25	1.6	60–70	1.7			
Cefditoren	400 mg po	X			16	4	88	1.6			
Cefixime[s]	400 mg po		X		50	3–5	65	3.1	800		
Cefotaxime	1.0 gm IV					100	30–51	1.5	15–75	10	Yes
Cefpodoxime proxetil	200 mg po	X			46	2.9	40	2.3	115		
Ceftazidime	1.0 gm IV					60	<10	1.8	13–54	20–40	Yes
Ceftibuten	400 mg po		X		80	15	65	2.4			
Ceftizoxime	1.0 gm IV					132	30	1.7	34–82	8–16	
Ceftriaxone	1.0 gm IV					150	85–95	8	200–500	10	Yes
CEPHALOSPORIN—4th Generation											
Cefepime	2.0 gm IV					193	20	2.0	∝ 5	10	Yes
CARBAPENEMS											
Ertapenem	1.0 gm IV					154	95	4	10	21	Yes
Imipenem	500 mg IV					40	15–25	1	minimal	8.5	+[9]
Meropenem	1.0 gm IV					49	2	1	3–300	Approx. 2	+
MONOBACTAM											
Aztreonam	1.0 gm IV					125	56	2	115–405	3–52	±
AMINOGLYCOSIDES	Amikacin, gentamicin, kanamycin, tobramycin—see Table 10C, page 73, for dose & serum levels										
Neomycin	po				<3	0		2.5	10–60	0–30	No: intrathecal: 5–10 mg
FLUOROQUINOLONES[10]	**po**										
Ciprofloxacin	750 mg po			X	70	1.8–2.8	20–40	4	2800–4500	26	1 µg/ml: Inadequate for Strep. species (CID 31:1131, 2000).
	400 mg IV			X		4.6	20–40	4	2800–4500		
	500 mg ER po			X		1.6	20–40	6.6			
	1000 mg ER po			X		3.1	20–40	6.3			
Gatifloxacin	400 mg po/IV			X	96	4.2–4.6	20	7–8		36	
Gemifloxacin	320 mg po			X	71	0.7–2.6	55–73	7			
Levofloxacin	500 mg po/IV			X	98	5.7	24–38	7		30–50	
	750 mg po/IV			X	98	8.6	24–38	7			
Moxifloxacin	400 mg po/IV			X	89	4.5	50	10–14			
Ofloxacin[s]	400 mg po/IV			X	98	4.4/6.2	24–38	7			

See page 62 for all footnotes

TABLE 9 (3)

DRUG	DOSE, ROUTE OF ADMINISTRATION	FOR PO DOSING—Take Drug WITH FOOD	WITHOUT FOOD[3]	WITH OR WITHOUT FOOD	% AB[1]	PEAK SERUM LEVEL μg/ml	PROTEIN BINDING, %	SERUM T½, HOURS[2]	BILIARY EXCRETION, %[2]	CSF/ BLOOD, %	CSF LEVEL POTENTIALLY THERAPEUTIC[2]
MACROLIDES, AZALIDES, LINCOSAMIDES											
Azithromycin	500 mg po / 500 mg IV				37	0.4 / 3.6	7-51 / 7-51	68 / 12/68	High		
Clarithromycin	500 mg po / ER-500 mg po	X			50 / ∞ 50	3-4 / 2-3	65-70 / 65-70	5-7	7000		No
Dirithromycin	500 mg po	X			10	0.4	15-30	8			
Erythromycin Oral (various)	500 mg po		X		18-45	0.1-2 / 3-4	70-74 / 70-74	2-4 / 2-4			
Lacto/glucep	500 mg IV										
Telithromycin	400 mg po			X	57	2.3	60-70	10		2-13	
Clindamycin	150 mg po / 600 mg IV			X / X	90	2.5 / 10	85-94 / 85-94	2.4 / 2.4	250-300 / 250-300		No
MISCELLANEOUS ANTIBACTERIALS											
Chloramphenicol	1.0 gm po		X		High	11-18	25-50	4.1			
Colistin	150 mg IV					5-7.5	93	2-3			No
Doxycycline	100 mg po		X			1.5-2.1	<10	18	200-3200		
Fosfomycin	3.0 gm po	X				26	31	5.7		60-70	
Linezolid	600 mg po/IV	X			100	15-20	20	5	100		
Metronidazole	500 mg po/IV	X				20-25	20	6-14	200-3200		
Minocycline	200 mg po	X				2.0-3.5	76	16			
Polymyxin B	20,000 U/kg IV					1-8		4.3-6			No
Quinu/Dalfo	7.5 mg/kg IV					5		1.5			
Rifampin	600 mg po		X		70-90	4-32	80	2-5	10,000		Most meningococci resistant. Static vs coliforms
Sulfamethoxazole (SMX)	2 gm po					50-120		7-12			
Trimethoprim (TMP)	100 mg po				80	1		8-15			
TMP/SMX-DS	160/800 mg po / 160/800 mg IV	X			85	1-2/40-60 / 9/105			100-200 / 40-70	50/40	60-70
Tetracycline	250 mg po		X			1.5-2.2	<10-55	4-6	50	7-14	Need high doses. See Meningitis, Table 1, page 4
Vancomycin	1.0 gm IV					20-50					
ANTIFUNGALS											
Amphotericin B Standard: 0.4-0.7 mg/kg IV						0.5-3.5		24		0	
Ampho B lipid complex (ABLC): 5 mg/kg IV						1-2.5		24			
Ampho B cholesteryl complex: 4 mg/kg IV						2.9		39			
Liposomal ampho B: 5.0 mg/kg IV						58 ± 21		7-10/100			

See page 62 for all footnotes

TABLE 9 (4)

DRUG	DOSE, ROUTE OF ADMINISTRATION	FOR PO DOSING—Take Drug			% AB[1]	PEAK SERUM LEVEL μg/ml[4]	PROTEIN BINDING, %	SERUM T½, HOURS[5]	BILIARY EXCRETION, %[3]	CSF[6]/BLOOD, %	CSF LEVEL POTENTIALLY THERAPEUTIC[5]
		WITH FOOD	WITHOUT FOOD[3]	WITH OR WITHOUT FOOD							
ANTIFUNGALS (continued)											
Caspofungin	70 mg IV x1, then 50 mg IV qd						97	9-11			22-100 (CID 37:728, 2003)
Fluctyosine	2.5 gm po			X	78-90	30-40		3-6		60-100	Yes
Azoles											
Fluconazole	400 mg/IV po			X	90	6.7		20-50		50-94	Yes
	800 mg po/IV				90	Approx. 14		20-50			
Itraconazole	Oral soln 200 mg po		X		Low	0.3-0.7	99.8	35		0	
Voriconazole	200 mg po		X		96	3	58				
ANTIMYCOBACTERIALS											
Ethambutol	25 mg/kg po	X			80	2-6	10-30	4		25-50	No
Isoniazid	300 mg po		X		100	3-5		0.7-4		20-90	Yes
Pyrazinamide	20-25 mg/kg po			X	95	30-50	5-10	10-16		100	Yes
Rifampin	600 mg po		X		70-90	4-32	80	1.5-5	10,000	7-56	Yes
Streptomycin	1.0 gm IV (see Table 10C, page 73)					25-50	0-10	2.5	10-60	0-30	No. Intrathecal: 5-10 mg
ANTIPARASITICS											
Albendazole	400 mg po	X				0.5-1.6	70	4		25-50	No
Atovaquone suspension:	750 mg po	X			47	15	99.9	67		<1	No
Dapsone	100 mg po		X		100	1.1		10-50			
Ivermectin	12 mg po		X			0.05-0.08					
Mefloquine	1.25 gm po	X				0.5-1.2	98	**13-24 days**			
Nitazoxanide	200 mg po	X				3	99				
Proguanil[11]							75				
Pyrimethamine[11]	25 mg po	X			"High"	0.1-0.3	87	96			
Praziquantel	20 mg/kg po	X			80	0.2-2.0		0.8-1.5			
ANTIVIRAL DRUGS—NOT HIV											
Acyclovir	400 mg po			X	10-20	1.21	9-33	2.5-3.5			
Adefovir	10 mg po			X		0.02	<20	2-3			
Famciclovir	500 mg po			X	77	3-4	<20	2-3			
Foscarnet	60 mg/kg IV					155		4		<1	
Ganciclovir	5 mg/kg IV					8.3	1-2	3.5			No
Oseltamivir	75 mg po			X	75	0.65/3.5[12]	3	1-3			
Ribavirin	600 mg po			X	64	0.8		44			
Rimantadine	100 mg po			X		0.1-0.4		25			
Valacyclovir	1000 mg po			X	55	5.6	13-18	3			
Valganciclovir	900 mg po	X			59	5.6	1-2	4			

See page 62 for all footnotes

TABLE 9 (5)

DRUG	DOSE, ROUTE OF ADMINIS-TRATION	FOR PO DOSING—Take Drug			% AB[1]	PEAK SERUM LEVEL µg/ml[3]	PROTEIN BINDING, %	INTRACELLULAR T½, HOURS[4]	SERUM T½, HOURS[2]	CYTOCHROME P450
		WITH FOOD	WITHOUT FOOD[5]	WITH OR WITHOUT FOOD						
ANTI-HIV VIRAL DRUGS										
Abacavir	300 mg po			X	83	2.9	50	3.3	1.5	
Amprenavir	1200 mg po			X	No data	6-9	90		7-11	Inhibitor
Atazanavir	400 mg po	X			"Good"	2.5	86		7	
Delavirdine	400 mg po			X	85	19 ± 11	98		5.8	Inhibitor
Didanosine	400 mg EC[13] po		X		30-40	?	<5	25-40	1.4	
Efavirenz	600 mg po		X		42	13 µM	99		40-55	Inducer/inhibitor
Enfuvirtide	90 mg sc				84	5	92		4	
Fosamprenavir	700 mg + 100 ritonavir po			X	No data	6	90	No data	7.7	
Indinavir	800 mg po		X		65	12.6 µM	60		1.2-2	Inhibitor
Lamivudine	300 mg po			X	86	2.6	<36	16	3.6	
Lopinavir	400 mg po	X			No data	9.6	98-99		5-6	Inhibitor
Nelfinavir	750 mg po	X			20-80	3-4	98		3.5-5	Inhibitor
Nevirapine	625 mg po			X	>90	2	60		25-30	Inducer
Ritonavir	300 mg po	X			65	7.8	98-99		3-5	Potent inhibitor
Saquinavir (gel)	400 mg po (with ritonavir)	X			?	?	97		1-2	Inhibitor
Stavudine	100 mg XR[14] po			X	86	1.4	"Low"[7]	3.5	1	
Tenofovir	300 mg po	X			39	0.12	<7	10-50	17	
Zalcitabine	0.75 mg po			X	85	0.03		3	1.2	
Zidovudine	300 mg po			X	60	1-2	<38	3	1.1	

FOOTNOTES:

1. % absorbed under optimal conditions
2. Assumes CrCl >80 ml/min.
3. Peak concentration in bile/peak concentration in serum x 100. If blank, no data.
4. CSF levels with inflammation
5. Judgment based on drug dose & organ susceptibility. CSF concentration ideally ≥10 above MIC.
6. Total drug; adjust for protein binding to determine free drug concentration.
7. For adult oral preps; not applicable for peds suspensions.
8. Food decreases rate and/or extent of absorption
9. Concern over seizure potential; see Table 10
10. Take all po FQs 2-4 hours before sucralfate or any multivalent cations: Ca^{++}, Fe^{++}, Zn^{++}
11. Given with atovaquone as Malarone for malaria prophylaxis.
12. Oseltamivir/oseltamivir carboxylate
13. EC = enteric coated
14. XR = extended release

TABLE 10A
SELECTED ANTIBACTERIAL AGENTS—ADVERSE REACTIONS—OVERVIEW

Adverse reactions in individual patients represent all-or-none occurrences, even if rare. After selection of an agent, the physician should read the manufacturer's package insert [statements in the product labeling (package insert) must be approved by the FDA].

Numbers = frequency of occurrence (%); **+** = occurs, incidence not available; **++** = significant adverse reaction; **0** = not reported; **R** = rare, defined as <1%. NOTE: Important reactions in bold print.

PENICILLINS, CARBAPENEMS, MONOBATAMS, AMINOGLYCOSIDES

ADVERSE REACTIONS	Penicillin G,V	PENICILLINASE-RESISTANT ANTI-STAPH. PENICILLINS — Cloxacillin	Dicloxacillin	Nafcillin	Oxacillin	AMINO-PENICILLINS — Amoxicillin	Amox/Clav	Ampicillin	Amp/Sulb	AP PENS — Piperacillin	Pip/Taz	Ticarcillin	Ticar/Clav	CARBAPENEMS — Ertapenem	Imipenem	Meropenem	Aztreonam	AMINO-GLYCOSIDES — Amikacin, Gentamicin, Kanamycin, Netilmicin[NUS], Tobramycin	MISC — Linezolid	Telithromycin
Local, phlebitis	+			++					3	4	1	3		4	3	1	4			
Hypersensitivity	+																			
Fever	+	+	+	+	+	+	+	+	+	+		2		+	+		2			+
Rash	**3**	**4**	**4**	**4**	**4**	**5**	**3**	**5**	**2**	**1**	**4**	**3**	**2**	**++**	**+**		**2**			
Photosensitivity	0	0	0	0	0	0	0	0	0	0	0	0	0	0			0			
Anaphylaxis	R	0	0	R	R	0	R	R	+	0	0	0	+		+		+			
Serum sickness	4									+	+	+	+		+		+			
Hematologic																				
+ Coombs	3	0	0	R	R	+	0	+	0	+	+	0	+		2	+	R			
Neutropenia	R	0	0	+	R	+	0	+	0	+	+	0	+		+	+	+		1.1	
Eosinophilia	+	+	+	22	22	2	+	22	22	+	+	+	5	1	+		8			
Thrombocytopenia	R	0	0	R	R	R	R	R	R	+	+	R	R		+	+	R		3–10 (see 10B)	
↑ PT/PTT	R	0	0	+	0	+	0	+	0	+	+	+	+		R		R			
GI																				
Nausea/vomiting		+	+	0	0	2	3	2	+	+	7	+	1	3	2	4	R		3/1	6/2
Diarrhea		+	+	0	0	**5**	**9**	**10**	2	2	11	3	1	**6**	2	5	R		4	8
C. difficile colitis	R	R	R	R	R	R	+	R	+	+	+	+	+	+	+	+	+		+	+
Hepatic, LFTs	R	R	R	0	+	R	+	R	6	+	+	0	+	6	4	4	2		1.3	
Hepatic failure	0	0	0	0	0	0	0	0	0	0	0	0	0	0						
Renal: ↑ BUN, Cr	R	0	0	0	0	R	0	R	R	+	+	0	0		+	0	0	**5–25†**		
CNS																				
Headache	R	0	0	R	R	0	+	R	R	R	8	R	R	2	+	3	+		2	1.5
Confusion	R	0	0	R	R	0	0	R	R	R	R	R	R		+		+			
Seizures	R	0	0	R	0	0	R	R	0	R	R	R	+	See footnote² →			+			
Special Senses																				
Ototoxicity	0	0	0	0	0	0	0	0	0	0	0	0	0		R		0	**3–14†**		
Vestibular	0	0	0	0	0	0	0	0	0	0	0	0	0	0			0	**4–6†**		
Cardiac																				
Dysrhythmias	R	0	0	0	0	0	0	0	0	0	0	0	0	0			0			
Miscellaneous, Unique (Table 10B)	+		+	+	+	+	+	+	+	+					+	+	+			+
Drug/drug interactions, common (Table 22)	0	0	0	0	0	0	0	0	0	0	0	0	0	0			0	+	+	+

¹ Varies with criteria used

² **All β-lactams in high concentration can cause seizures** (JAC 45:5, 2000). In rabbit, IMP 10x more neurotoxic than benzylpenicillin (JAC 22:687, 1988). In clinical trial of IMP for pediatric meningitis, trial stopped due to seizures in 7/25 IMP recipients; hard to interpret as purulent meningitis causes seizures (PIDJ 10:122, 1991). Risk with IMP less with careful attention to dosage (Epilepsia 42:1590, 2001).

    Postulated mechanism: Drug binding to $GABA_A$ receptor. IMP binds with greater affinity than MER. Package insert, percent seizures: ertapenem 0.5, IMP 0.4, MER 0.7. However, in 3 clinical gtrials of MER for bacterial meningitis, no drug-related seizures (Scand J Inf Dis 31:3, 1999; Drug Safety 22:191, 2000). In febrile neutropenic cancer pts, IMP-related seizures reported at 2% (CID 32:381, 2001; Peds Hem Onc 17:585, 2000).

TABLE 10A (2)

ADVERSE REACTIONS	Cefazolin	Cefotetan	Cefoxitin	Cefuroxime	Cefotaxime	Ceftazidime	Ceftizoxime	Ceftriaxone	Cefepime	Cefpirome[NUS]	Cefaclor/Cef.ER[1]/Loracarb	Cefadroxil	Cefdinir	Cefixime[NUS]	Cefpodoxime	Cefprozil	Ceftibuten	Cefditoren pivoxil	Cefuroxime-axetil	Cephalexin
Local, phlebitis	+	R	R	2	5	1	4	2	1											
Hypersensitivity	5	1			2				+	+	2									
Fever	+	+	+			R	+	R	+	+					R	+			R	R
Rash	+		2	R	2	2	2	2	2	1	1	+	R	1	1	1	R	R	R	1
Photosensitivity	0	0	0	0	0	R	0	0												
Anaphylaxis	R	+			R						R								R	
Serum sickness											≤0.5[2]	+								+
Hematologic																				
Anemia				10	R						+							2	R	
+ Coombs	3	+	2	R	6	8			14	3	R							R	R	+
Neutropenia	+		2	R	+	1	+	2	1		+		+	R	R	R	R	R	R	3
Eosinophilia		+	3	7	1	8	4	6	1				R	R	3	2	5	R	1	9
Thrombocytopenia	+					+	+		+		2				R	R	+	R		
↑ PT/PTT		++	+		+	+	+	+	+											
GI			2																	
Nausea/vomiting		1		R	R	R		R	1	+	3		3	13		6			2	2
Diarrhea			4	R	1	1		3	1	+	1-4			15	16	7	3	3	1.4	4
AAC	+	+	+	+	**+**	**+**	**+**	**+**	+	+	+	+	+	+	+	+	+	+	+	+
Hepatic, ↑ LFTs	+	1	3	4	1	6	4	3	+	+	3	+	1	R	4	2	R	R	2	+
Hepatic failure		0	0	0	0	0	0	0	0	0	0									
Renal: ↑ BUN, Cr	+			3				R	1		+		R	4	R	R	R			
CNS																				
Headache	0						2	R	2		3		2	1	R	R		2	R	+
Confusion	0										+				R					
Seizures	0																			
Special Senses																				
Ototoxicity	0	0	0		0	0	0	0				0	0	0	0	0	0		0	0
Vestibular	0	0	0		0	0	0	0				0	0	0	0	0	0		0	0
Cardiac																				
Dysrhythmias	0	0	0		0	0	0	0				0	0	0	0	0	0		0	0
Miscellaneous, Unique (Table 10B)								+			+[2]							+		
Drug/drug interactions, common (Table 22)	0	0	0	0	0	0	0	0			0	0		0	0	0			0	0

[1] Cefaclor extended release tablets

[2] Serum sickness requires biotransformation of parent drug plus inherited defect in metabolism of reactive intermediates (Ped Pharm & Therap 125:805, 1994)

* See note at head of table, page 63

TABLE 10A (3)

ADVERSE REACTIONS (AE)	MACROLIDES				QUINOLONES[1]						OTHER AGENTS									
	Azithromycin	Clarithromycin, Reg. & ER*	Dirithromycin	Erythromycin	Ciprofloxacin/Cipro XR	Gatifloxacin	Gemifloxacin	Levofloxacin	Moxifloxacin	Ofloxacin	Chloramphenicol	Clindamycin	Daptomycin	Metronidazole	Minocycline	Quinupristin/dalfopristin[2]	Rifampin	Tetracycline/Doxycycline	TMP/SMX	Vancomycin
Rx stopped due to AE	1	3	3		3.5	2.9	2.2	4	3.8	4			2.8							
Local, phlebitis			+		5							+	6			++		+		13
Hypersensitivity																	1	R	++	8
Fever					R	R					+	+	2				+	+	+	1
Rash	R		R	+	3	R	1-22[a]	1.7	R	2	+	+	4	+	+	R	+	+	3	
Photosensitivity	R				R	R	R	R	R	R			4					+	+	0
Anaphylaxis				+	R		R	R		R										R
Serum sickness												+								
Hematologic					R											R				
Anemia											++		2							+
Neutropenia	R	1			R	R				1	+	+		+	+			+	2	2
Eosinophilia					R					1		+			R	+		+	+	+
Thrombocytopenia	R	R	R		R						+	+			R	+		+	+	
↑ PT/PTT		1																		0
GI																			3	
Nausea/vomiting	3	3[a]	8	25	5	8/2	2.7	7/2	7/2	7		+	6.3	12	+		+		3 +	+
Diarrhea	5	3-6	8	8	2	4	3.6	1.2	6	4	+	7	5	+	+		+		3	
AAC		+		+	R	R	R	R		R	++	+						R	+	+
Hepatic, LFTs	R	R	R	+	2	R		1.5	+	2		+					2	+	+	0
Hepatic failure	0	0	0														+	+		
Renal																				
↑ BUN, Cr	+	4	1		1					R	0		R				+	+	+	5
CNS														++						
Dizziness, lightheadedness					R	3	0.8	2.5	3	3										
Headache	R	2		4	1	4	1.2	5.4	2		+	+	5		+			+	+	
Confusion				+	+			+	R	2	+	+			+		+	+	+	
Seizures				+	+				R		+	+		+						
Special senses																				
Ototoxicity	+			+			0			R					+					R
Vestibular															21					
Cardiac																				
Dysrhythmias			+	+	R	+[3]	+[3]	+[3]	+[3]	+[3]		R								0
Miscellaneous, Unique (Table 10B)	+			+	+	+	+	+	+	+	+	+	+	+	+	+	+	+	+	+
Drug/drug interactions, common (Table 22)	+	+	+	+	+	+	+	+	+	+						+		++	+	+

[1] Concern expressed that quinolones may be associated with episodes of tendonitis.

[2] Quinupristin/dalfopristin = Synercid

[3] Fluoroquinolones as class assoc. **with QT$_c$ prolongation**; ↑ QT$_c$ can cause torsades de pointes which can lead to ventricular fibrillation. ↑ risk with concomitant ↓ K$^+$, ↓ Mg^{++}, or concomitant class Ia or IIIa antiarrhythmic agents. Ref.: CID 34:861, 2002.

[4] Regular and extended-release formulations

[5] Less GI upset/abnormal taste with ER formulation

[6] **Highest frequency:** females <40 years of age after 14 d. of rx

* See note at head of table, page 63

TABLE 10B: SUMMARY OF CURRENT ANTIBIOTIC DOSAGE* AND SIDE-EFFECTS

CLASS, AGENT, GENERIC NAME (TRADE NAME)	USUAL ADULT DOSAGE (Cost)	ADVERSE REACTIONS, COMMENTS (See Table 10A for Summary)
NATURAL PENICILLINS		**Most common adverse reactions are hypersensitivity.** Anaphylaxis in up to 0.05%, 5–10% total. Commercially available skin test antigen (penicilloyl polylysine) does not predict anaphylactoid reactions. Hematologic, renal, CNS (seizures) reactions usually seen with high dose (>20 million units/day) and renal failure. With procaine pen G and
Benzathine penicillin G (Bicillin)	600,000–1.2 million u IM q2–4 wks Cost: 1.2 mU $30.90 Low: 600,000–1.2 million u/d IM High: ≥20 million u u/d IV (≈12 gm) Cost: 5 mU $5.66	benzathine pen G, an immediate but transient (5–30 min. after injection) toxic reaction with bizarre behavior and neurologic reactions can occur (Hoigne syndrome). Coombs test positive (high dose) rarely causes hemolytic anemias are rare but typically severe; in contrast, the Coombs test is often positive with cephalosporin therapy, but clinically significant hemolysis is rare.
Penicillin G		
Penicillin V	0.25–0.5 gm bid, tid, qid before meals & hs Cost: 500 mg G $0.23	Penicillin allergy ref.: JAMA 278:1895, 1997
PENICILLINASE-RESISTANT PENICILLINS		
Cloxacillin (Cloxapen)	0.25–0.5 gm q6h ac, po. Cost: 250 mg G $0.60	Blood levels ~2x greater than cloxacillin. Acute hemorrhagic cystitis reported. Acute abdominal pain with GI bleeding without antibiotic-associated colitis also reported.
Dicloxacillin (Dynapen)	0.125–0.5 gm q6h ac, po. Cost: 500 mg G $1.20	In Australia, cholestatic hepatitis [women predominate, age >65, rx mean 2 weeks, onset 3 weeks from starting rx (Ln 339:679, 1992)]. 16 deaths since 1980. recommendation: use only in severe infection (Ln 344:676, 1994).
Flucloxacillin^NUS (Floxapen, Lutropin, Staphcil)	0.25–0.5 gm q6h po 1.0–2.0 gm q6h IV	Extravasation can result in tissue necrosis. ↑ LFTs usually ↑ in severe infection (Ln 344:676, 1994). **Reversible neutropenia (over 10% with ≥21-day rx, occasionally WBC <1000/mm³).**
Nafcillin (Unipen, Nafcil)	1.0–2.0 gm q4h IV, IM. Cost: 1.0 gm IV $3.35	**Hepatic dysfunction with ≥12 gm/d.** LFTs usually ↑ 2–24 days after start of rx, reversible. ↑ SGOT in 9/11 HIV+ pts
Oxacillin (Prostaphlin)	1.0–2.0 gm q4h IV, IM. Cost: 2.0 gm IV $6.53	(AVIM 118:1048, 1994). In children, more rash and liver toxicity with nafcillin (CID 34:50, 2002).
AMINOPENICILLINS		
Amoxicillin (Amoxil, Polymox)	250 mg–1.0 gm tid po Cost: 500 mg G $0.58 NB $0.55	IV available in UK, Europe. IV amoxicillin rapidly converted to ampicillin. Rash with infectious mono—see Ampicillin. 500–875 mg po bid listed in past, may be inadequate due to ↑ resistance.
Amoxicillin/clavulanate (Augmentin) AM/CL extra-strength peds suspension and tabs	See Comment for adult products Peds susp: 600/42.9 per 5 ml. Dose: 90/6.4 mg div bid.	With bid regimen, less diarrhea & less diarrhea. Clavulanate assoc. with rare reversible cholestatic hepatitis, esp. men >60 yrs, on rx >2 weeks (AVIM 156:1327, 1996). 2 cases anaphylactoid reaction to clavulanic acid (J All Clin Immun 96:748, 1995). Comparison adult Augmentin product dosage regimens: Cost for 10 days rx:
AM/CL—extended release adult tabs	See Comment for adult products Cost: 75 mg $38.00	Augmentin 500/125 1 tab po tid $106
Ampicillin (Principen)	0.25–0.5 gm q6h po. Cost: 500 mg G $0.34 150–200 mg/kg/d IV. Cost: 1.0 gm IV G $2.80	Augmentin 875/125 1 tab po bid $106 Augmentin-XR 1000/62.5 2 tabs po bid $109 A maculopapular rash occurs (not urticarial), **not true penicillin allergy,** in 65–100% pts with infectious mono, 90% with chronic lymphocytic leukemia, and 15–20% with allopurinol therapy.
Ampicillin/sulbactam (Unasyn)	1.5–3.0 gm q6h IV. Cost: 3.0 gm NB $15.35 (see Comment)	Supplied in vials: ampicillin 1.0 gm, sulbactam 0.5 gm or amp 2.0 gm, sulbactam 1.0 gm. Antibiotic is not active vs pseudomonas. Total daily dose sulbactam ≤4 gm.
ANTIPSEUDOMONAL PENICILLINS NOTE: Piperacillin has better activity vs enterococci & klebsiella than ticarcillin		
Piperacillin (Pipracil)	3.0–4.0 gm q4–6h IV (200–300 mg/kg/d up to 500 mg/kg/d) IV. **For urinary tract infection: 2.0 gm q6h IV.** Cost: 3.0 gm NB $22.12	1.85 mEq Na⁺/gm
Piperacillin/tazobactam (Zosyn)	3.375 gm q6h IV. Cost: 3.375 gm NB $16.52 4.5 gm q8h available 4.5 gm NB $20.63	Supplied in vials: piperacillin 3.0 gm, tazobactam (TZ) 0.375 gm. In Europe, studied mostly as 4.0 gm pip/0.5 gm tazo. TZ is similar to clavulanate and more active than sulbactam as β-lactamase inhibitor. Has ↑ activity over pip alone vs gram-negatives and anaerobes. PIP/TZ 3.375 gm q6h as monotherapy **not adequate for serious pseudomonas infections.** OK when this dose combined with an aminoglycoside (tobramycin).

*NOTE: all dosage recommendations are for adults (unless otherwise indicated) and assume normal renal function.

TABLE 10B (2)

CLASS, AGENT, GENERIC NAME (TRADE NAME)	USUAL ADULT DOSAGE (Cost)	ADVERSE REACTIONS, COMMENTS (See Table 10A for Summary)
ANTIPSEUDOMONAL PENICILLINS (continued)		
Ticarcillin disodium (Ticar)	3.0 gm q4-6h IV. Cost: 3.0 gm NB $13.43	Coagulation abnormalities common with large doses, interferes with platelet function, ↑ bleeding times; may be clinically significant in pts with renal failure. (4.5 mEq Na⁺/gm)
Ticarcillin/clavulanate (Timentin)	3.1 gm q4-6h IV. Cost: 3.1 gm NB $17.41	Supplied in vials: ticarcillin 3.0 gm, clavulanate 0.1 gm/vial. 4.5–5.0 mEq Na⁺/gm. Diarrhea due to clavulanate. Rare reversible cholestatic hepatitis secondary to clavulanate (AHM 156:1327, 1996).
CARBAPENEMS		
Ertapenem (Invanz)	1.0 gm qd IV/IM. Cost: 1.0 gm $49.97	Lidocaine diluent for IM use; ask about lidocaine allergy.
Imipenem + cilastatin (Primaxin)	0.5 gm q6h IV. Cost: 500 mg NB $33.10	For seizure comment, see footnote 2, Table 10A, page 63. In pts with history of pen allergy & pos. pen skin tests, ⅓ had pos. IMP skin tests (J All Clin Imm 82:213, 1988). Resistance of P. aeruginosa reported (see Table 5).
Meropenem (Merrem)	0.5–1.0 gm q8h IV. Up to 2.0 gm q8h IV for menin- gitis. Cost: 1.0 gm NB $52.00	For seizure incidence comment, see Table 10A, page 63. Comments: Does not require a dehydropeptidase inhibitor (cilastatin). Activity vs aerobic gm-neg, slightly ↑ over IMP, activity vs staph & strep slightly ↓, anaerobes = to IMP. B. ovatus, B. distasonis more resistant to meropenem.
MONOBACTAMS		
Aztreonam (Azactam)	1.0 gm q8h–2.0 gm q6h IV. Cost: 1.0 gm NB $21.61	Can be used in pts with allergy to penicillins/cephalosporins. Animal data and a letter raise concern about cross-reactivity with ceftazidime (Rev Inf Dis 7:613, 1985); side-chains of aztreonam and ceftazidime are identical.
CEPHALOSPORINS (1st parenteral, then oral drugs).		NOTE: Prospective data demonstrate correlation between use of cephalosporins (esp. 3rd generation) and ↑ risk of C. difficile toxin-induced diarrhea. May also ↑ risk of colonization with vancomycin-resistant enterococci.
1st Generation, Parenteral		
Cefazolin (Ancef, Kefzol)	0.25 gm q8h–1.5 gm q6h IV, IM. Cost: 1.0 gm G $2.74, NB $4.38	Do not give into lateral ventricles—seizures!
2nd Generation, Parenteral		
Cefotetan (Cefotan)	1–3 gm q12h IV, IM. (Max. dose not >6 gm qd). Cost: 1.0 gm NB $13.15	Increasing resistance of B. fragilis, Prevotella bivius, Prevotella disiens (most common in pelvic infections). Methylthiotetrazole (MTT) side chain can inhibit vitamin K activation.
Cefoxitin (Mefoxin)	1.0 gm q8h–2.0 gm q4h IV, IM. Cost: 1.0 gm G $11.23, NB $15.29	In vitro may induce ↑ β-lactamase, esp. in Enterobacter sp.: clinical significance ?.
Cefuroxime (Kefurox, Zinacef)	0.75–1.5 gm q8h IV,IM. Cost: 1.5 gm IV NB $13.90	More stable vs staphylococcal β-lactamase than cefazolin.
3rd Generation, Parenteral	One study correlated use of P Ceph 3 drugs with incidence of C. difficile toxin diarrhea (Am J Gastro 89:519, 1994).	
Cefotaxime (Claforan)	1.0 gm q8-12h to 2.0 gm q4h IV. Cost: 2.0 gm NB $26.38	Maximum daily dose: 12 gm.
Ceftazidime (Ceptaz, Fortaz, Tazicef, Tazidime)	1.0–2.0 gm q8-12h IV, IM. Cost: 2.0 gm NB $28.45–43.30	Excessive use may result in ↑ incidence of C. difficile-assoc. diarrhea and/or selection of vancomycin-resistant E. faecium. Ceftaz is susceptible to extended-spectrum cephalosporinases (CID 27:76 & 81, 1998).
Ceftizoxime (Cefizox)	1.0 gm q8-12h to 4.0 gm q8h IV. Cost: 2.0 gm NB $24.64	Maximum daily dose: 12 gm.

(See page 72 for footnotes and abbreviations)   * NOTE: all dosage recommendations are for adults (unless otherwise indicated) and assume normal renal function.

TABLE 10B (3)

CLASS, AGENT, GENERIC NAME (TRADE NAME)	USUAL ADULT DOSAGE (Cost)	ADVERSE REACTIONS, COMMENTS (See Table 10A for Summary)
CEPHALOSPORINS, 3rd Generation, Parenteral *(continued)*		
Ceftriaxone (Rocephin)	**Commonly used IV dosage in adults:** **≥ Age 65: 2.0 gm once daily** **> Age 65: 1.0 gm once daily** **Purulent meningitis: 2.0 gm q12h.** Can give IM in 1% lidocaine. Cost: 1.0 gm NB $0.24	Dosage: 2.0 gm IV q12 gives better tissue levels than 1.0 gm q12h (overcomes protein binding). (see footnote[1]) "Pseudocholelithiasis:" 2° to sludge in gallbladder by ultrasound (50%), symptomatic (9%) (*NEJM* 322:1821, 1990). More likely with ≥2 gm/d with pt on total parenteral nutrition and not eating (*AnIM* 115:712, 1991). Clinical significance still unclear but has led to cholecystectomy (*JID* 17:356, 1995) and gallstone pancreatitis (*Ln* 17:662, 1998)
4th Generation, Parenteral		
Cefepime (Maxipime)	1.0–2.0 gm q12h IV. Cost: 2.0 gm NB $35.86	Active vs P. aeruginosa and many strains of Enterobacter, serratia, S. freundii resistant to ceftazidime, cefotaxime, aztreonam (*CID* 20:56, 1995). More active vs S. aureus than 3rd generation cephalosporins.
Cefpirome[A,B] (HR 810)	1.0–2.0 gm q12h IV	Similar to cefepime; ↑ activity vs enterobacteriaceae, P. aeruginosa, Gm + organisms. Anaerobes: less active than cefoxitin, more active than cefotax or cefta.
Oral Cephalosporins		The oral cephalosporins are generally safe. **Patients with a history of IgE-mediated allergic reactions to a penicillin (e.g., anaphylaxis, angioneurotic edema, immediate urticaria) should not receive a cephalosporin.** If the history is a "measles-like" rash to a penicillin, available data suggest a 5–10% risk of rash in such patients; there is no enhanced risk of anaphylaxis.
1st Generation, Oral		
Cefadroxil (Duricef)	0.5–1.0 gm q12h po. Cost: 0.5 gm G $3.32, NB $4.65	Any of the cephalosporins can result in **C. difficile toxin**-mediated diarrhea/enterocolitis.
Cephalexin (Keflex, Keftab, generic)	0.25–0.5 gm q6h po. Cost: 0.5 gm NB $3.43, G $0.44	The reported frequency of nausea/vomiting and non-C. difficile toxin diarrhea is summarized in Table 10A. There are few drug-specific adverse effects.
2nd Generation, Oral		
Cefaclor (Ceclor)	0.25–0.5 gm q8h po. Cost: 0.25 gm NB $2.33, G $0.66	**Cefaclor:** Serum sickness-like reactions 0.1–0.5%—arthralgia, rash, multiforme but no adenopathy, proteinuria or demonstrable immune complexes. Anecdotal reports of similar reaction to loracarbef. Appear due to mixture of drug biotransformation and genetic susceptibility (*Ped Pharm & Therap* 125:805, 1994).
Cefaclor-ER (Ceclor CD)	0.375–0.5 gm q12h po. Cost: 0.5 gm $4.40	
Cefprozil (Cefzil)	0.25–0.5 gm q12h po. Cost: 0.5 gm NB $8.26	**Cefdinir:** Drug-drug complex causes red stools in roughly 1% of pts.
Cefuroxime axetil po (Ceftin)	0.125–0.5 gm q12h po. Cost: 0.5 gm NB $8.05	**Cefditoren pivoxil:** Hydrolysis yields pivalate. Pivalate absorbed (70%) & becomes pivaloylcarnitine which is renally excreted, 39–63%. In several wash/wear cycles, serum carnitine ↓. Carnitine involved in fatty acid (FA) metabolism & FA transport into mitochondria. Effect transient & reversible. No clinical events documented to date (*Med Lett* 44:5, 2002).
Loracarbef (Lorabid)	0.4 gm q12h po. Cost: 0.4 gm NB $6.37	Also contains casinate (milk protein); **avoid if milk allergy** (not same as lactose intolerance). Need gastric acid for optimal absorption.
3rd Generation, Oral		
Cefdinir (Omnicef)	300 mg q12h or 600 mg qd Cost: 300 mg $4.45	**Cefpodoxime:** There are rare reports of acute liver injury, bloody diarrhea, pulmonary infiltrates with eosinophilia.
Cefditoren pivoxil (Spectracef)	0.2–0.4 gm q12–24h po Cost: 200 mg $1.57	
Cefixime[A,B] (Suprax)	0.2–0.4 gm q12–24h po Cost: 0.4 gm NB $8.83, G $1.00	
Cefpodoxime proxetil (Vantin)	0.1–0.2 gm q12h po Cost: 0.2 gm NB $3.17	
Ceftibuten[A] (Cedax)	0.4 gm qd po Cost: 0.4 gm NB $7.11	
AMINOGLYCOSIDES AND RELATED ANTIBIOTICS—See Table 10C, page 73, and Table 17, page 130		

[1] The age-related dosing of ceftriaxone is based on unpublished pharmacokinetic data that show an age-related reduction in hepatic clearance of ceftriaxone; hence, there is possible underdosing in younger pts, therefore the suggested 2 gm/day dose.   * NOTE: all dosage recommendations are for adults (unless otherwise indicated) and assume normal renal function.
(See page 72 for footnotes and abbreviations)

TABLE 10B (4)

CLASS, AGENT, GENERIC NAME (TRADE NAME)	USUAL ADULT DOSAGE (Cost)	ADVERSE REACTIONS, COMMENTS (See Table 10A for Summary)
GLYCOPEPTIDES		
Teicoplanin[AUS] (Targocid)	**For septic arthritis—maintenance dose 12 mg/kg/d; S. aureus endocarditis—trough serum levels >20 µg/ml required (12 mg/kg x3 loading dose, then 12 mg/kg qd).**	Hypersensitivity: fever (at 3 mg/kg) 2.2%, at 24 mg/kg 8.2%); skin reactions 2.4%; Marked ↓ platelets (high dose ≥15 mg/kg/d). Red neck syndrome less common than with vancomycin (JAC 32:792, 1993).
Vancomycin (Vancocin)	15 mg/kg q12h IV; 125 mg q6h po; intrathecal 5–10 mg q48–72h. Cost: 1.0 gm IV ($ 6.00, NB $16.00. Oral "Pulvule" 125 mg. Cost $7.05 For other uses, see Comment. One report of safety & efficacy of once-daily vanco, 30 mg/kg (JAC 49:155, 2002).	**Measure serum levels** if: planned dose ≥2.0 gm/d, rapidly changing renal function, chronic renal failure, or on hemodialysis. Target levels: peak 20–50 µg/ml; trough 5–10 µg/ml. Rapid infusion (over <1 hr) can cause non-specific histamine release manifest as angioneurotic edema, flushed skin ("red neck syndrome") or hypotension. Can continue vanco but infuse over 1–2 hrs. **Ototoxicity and nephrotoxicity now rare** unless vanco given with other ototoxic/nephrotoxic drugs, e.g. aminoglycoside. Rarely, association with linear IgA bullous dermatosis (AnIM 129:507, 1998) Neutropenia, rash occur. Rarely, association with meningitis and/or ventriculitis/shunt infections. **Initial dosing ranges from 5–10 mg/d (infants) to 10–20 mg/d (children/adults) adjusted to achieve trough CSF conc. of 10–20 µg/ml (AnPharmacotherapy 27:912, 1993). **Intrathecal Vanco:** used for meningitis and/or ventriculitis/shunt infections. **Critically ill pts:** Safe & reasonable to give loading dose of 25 mg/kg and 500 mg/hr (AJC 47:246, 2001).
CHLORAMPHENICOL, CLINDAMYCIN(S), ERYTHROMYCIN GROUP, KETOLIDES, OXAZOLIDINONES, QUINUPRISTIN/DALFOPRISTIN (SYNERCID)		
Chloramphenicol (Chloromycetin)	0.25–1 gm po/IV q6h po, max. of 4 gm/day Cost: 1.0 gm IV $7.60; po $0.86.	No oral drug distributed in the US. Hematologic: (↓ RBC – 1/3 pts, aplastic anemia 1:21,600 courses). Gray baby syndrome in premature infants, anaphylactoid reactions, optic atrophy or neuropathy (very rare), digital paresthesias, minor disulfiram-like reactions.
Clindamycin (Cleocin)	0.15–0.45 gm q6h po. 600–900 mg q8h IV, IM.	0.5 gm q6–8h po, 0.6 gm q8h IV, IM. Cost: 500 mg po $2.00, 300 mg IV $3.97	Based on number of exposed pts, these drugs are the most frequent cause of **C. difficile toxin-mediated diarrhea**. In most severe form can cause pseudomembranous colitis/toxic megacolon.
Lincomycin (Lincocin)		0.5 gm q6–8h po, 0.6 gm q8h IV, IM. Cost: 500 mg po $2.00, 300 mg IV $3.97	
Erythromycin Group (Review drug interactions before use) Ref.: Mayo Proc 74:613, 1999		**Motilin** is gastric hormone that activates duodenal/jejunal receptors to initiate peristalsis. Erythro (E) and E. esters, both po and IV, activate motilin receptors and hence produce nausea/vomiting, diarrhea, and abdominal cramping, with resultant 20–25% incidence of anorexia, nausea or vomiting (Gut 33:397, 1992). Less binding and GI distress with azithromycin/clarithromycin.
Azithromycin (Zithromax)	po: 0.5 gm on day 1, then 0.25 gm qd on days 2–5 or 0.5 gm po qd x 3 d Cost: 250 mg IV $7.58 IV: 0.5 gm/d. Cost: $26.90		**Systemic erythro** in 1st 2 wks of life associated with **infantile hypertrophic pyloric stenosis** (J Peds 139:380, 2001). **Frequent drug-drug interactions:** see Table 21, page 138. Ex.: Amiodarone (or haloperidol) + erythro (or clarithro) can result in ↑ Q-T intervals, torsades de pointes, ↑ V tachycardia. Erythro alone can prolong QT[c] interval (Chest 115:983, 1999), esp. in women (JAMA 280:1774, 1998). Erythro/clarithro most common prescribed drugs with potential to ↑ Q-T (AnJM 114:135, 2003).
Base and esters (Erythrocin, Ilosone) IV name: E. lactobionate	0.25 gm q6h–0.5 gm q6h po. IV: 15–20 mg/kg up to 4.0 gm qd. Infuse over 30 or more minutes. Cost: po 250 mg base GG $0.18, stearate $0.18, estolate $0.31. ESS 400 $0.23. IV 1.0 gm NB $7.64		Cholestatic hepatitis in approx. 1:1000 adults (not children) given E. estolate. **Transient hearing loss or deafness** with 24 gm/d of erythro IV in pts with renal or hepatic impairment. Reported with >600 mg/d of azithro (CID 24:76, 1997).
Clarithromycin (Biaxin) or clarithro extended release (Biaxin XL)	0.5 gm q12h po. Cost: 500 mg $4.55 Extended release: Two 0.5 gm tabs po/d. Cost 500 mg ER $4.66		Dosages of oral erythro preparations expressed as base equivalents. With differences in absorption/biotransformation, variable amounts of erythro esters required to achieve same free erythro serum level, e.g. 400 mg E ethyl succinate = 250 mg E base. Macrolide-induced Churg-Strauss syndrome reported in an atopic pt (LN 350:563, 1997).
Dirithromycin (Dynabac)	0.5 gm po qd. Cost: 250 mg $4.25		**Dirithromycin** available as once-daily macrolide. **Very low serum levels; do not use if potential for bacteremic disease.**
Ketolide Telithromycin (Ketek)	**Two 400 mg tabs po qd—anticipated dose** 400 mg tabs.		First ketolide antimicrobial. Diarrhea, nausea/vomiting. Drug-drug common side-effects. Drug-drug interactions with itraconazole, itraconazole, and ketoconazole—see Table 22, page 145. No dosage adjustment necessary for age or hepatic insufficiency; dose reduction for severe renal insufficiency (see Table 17).

NOTE: all dosage recommendations are for adults (unless otherwise indicated) and assume normal renal function.

(See page 72 for footnotes and abbreviations.)

TABLE 10B (5)

CLASS, AGENT, GENERIC NAME (TRADE NAME)	USUAL ADULT DOSAGE (COST)	ADVERSE REACTIONS, COMMENTS (See Table 10A for Summary)
CHLORAMPHENICOL, CLINDAMYCIN(S), ERYTHROMYCIN GROUP, KETOLIDES, OXAZOLIDINONES, QUINOLDINONES, QUINUPRISTIN/DALFOPRISTIN (SYNERCID) *(See Table 10A for Summary)* (continued)		
Linezolid (Zyvox)	PO or IV dose: 600 mg q12h all indications **except uncomplicated skin infections**, 400 mg q12h for uncomplicated skin infections Available as 400 & 600 mg tabs, oral suspension (100 mg/5 ml), & IV solution. 600 mg po $57, 600 mg IV $77.50	First oxazolidinone. Nausea/vomiting & diarrhea most common adverse effects. **Rx duration-dependent reversible thrombocytopenia, neutropenia, & anemia: monitor blood counts if rx beyond 2 weeks** (CID 34:695, 2002). Tongue discoloration. **Inhibitor of monoamine oxidase**: risk of severe hypertension if taken with foods rich in tyramine. Be careful with drugs containing pseudoephedrine, phenylpropanolamine or if taking SSRIs.[1] **Serotonin syndrome** (fever, agitation, mental status changes, tremors) reported (CID 34:1651, 2002 & 37:1274, 2003).
Quinupristin + dalfopristin (Synercid)	7.5 mg/kg q8h IV via central line x21–72 d. Cost: 500 mg IV $150 mg IV $120.60	Venous irritation (5%); none with central venous line. Asymptomatic ↑ in unconjugated bilirubin. **Arthralgia** 2%. Asymptomatic ↑ in conjugated bilirubin, many more—see Table 22.
TETRACYCLINES *(Mayo Clin Proc 74:727, 1999)*		Similar to other tetracyclines. ↑ nausea on empty stomach. Erosive esophagitis, esp. if taken hs. Phototoxicity + but less than with tetracycline. Deposition in teeth less. Can be used in patients with renal failure.
Doxycycline (Vibramycin, Doryx, Monodox)	**0.1 gm po or IV q12h.** Cost: 100 mg po G $0.08–0.11, IV NB $4.50. 100 mg IV NB $14.16	
Minocycline (Minocin)	**0.1 gm q12h po.** Cost: 100 mg G $0.60, NB $3.68	**Comments:** Effective in treatment and prophylaxis for malaria, leptospirosis, typhus fevers. **Vestibular symptoms** (30–90% in some groups; none in others); vertigo 33%; ataxia 43%; nausea 50%, vomiting 3%, women more frequently than men. Hypersensitivity pneumonitis, reversible, ~34 cases reported (BMJ 310:1520, 1995). **Comments:** More effective than other tetracyclines vs staph in prophylaxis of meningococcal disease. P. acnes: many resistant to other tetracyclines, not to mino. Active vs Nocardia asteroides. Mycobacterium marinum.
Tetracycline, Oxytetracycline (Terramycin)	**0.25–0.5 gm q6h po, 0.5–1.0 gm q12h IV** Cost: 250 mg po $0.06	SE (oxy 19%, tetra 4), anaphylactoid reaction (rare), deposition in teeth, negative N balance, hepatotoxicity, enamel agenesis, pseudotumor cerebri/emesis reported. Outdated drug: Fanconi syndrome. See drug-drug interactions, Table 22. **Contraindicated in pregnancy, hepatotoxicity in mother, transplacental to fetus.** *Comments:* IV dosage over 2.0 gm/d may be associated with fatal hepatotoxicity
FLUOROQUINOLONES (FQs)		**Children:** No FQ approved for use under age 16 based on joint cartilage injury in immature animals. Articular SEs in children est. at 2–3% *(Ln ID 3:537, 2003).*
Ciprofloxacin (Cipro) and ciprofloxacin-extended release (Cipro XR)	**500–750 mg bid po.** Urinary tract infection: **250 mg bid po or Cipro XR 500 mg qd** **Parenteral** rx 200–400 mg q12h. Cost: 500 mg po $5.47, Cipro XR 500 mg $8.66, 400 mg IV $30.00	**CNS toxicity:** Poorly understood. Varies from mild (lightheadedness) to moderate (confusion) to severe (seizures). May be aggravated by NSAIDs. **Gemi skin rash:** Macular rash after 8–10 d. of rx. Frequency highest females, < age 40, treated 14 d. (22.6%). In men, < age 40, treated 14 d., frequency 7.7%. Mechanism unclear. Indication to DC therapy. **Hypoglycemia/hyperglycemia** (Med Lett 45:64, 2003): Data based on case reports only. Various FQs ↑ insulin release in rats. No known drug-drug interactions; most pts reported to have type 2 diabetes. No interaction with oral hypoglycemic drugs found. No data to allow comparative frequency between FQs.
Gatifloxacin (Tequin)	**200–400 mg IV/po qd** Cost: 400 mg po $99.00, 400 mg IV $98.20	**Opiate screen false-positives:** FQs can cause **false-positive urine assay for opiates** (JAMA 266:3115, 2001).
Gemifloxacin (Factive)	**320 mg qd po** Cost: Pending 11/03	**Photosensitivity:** See Table 8, page 57
Levofloxacin (Levaquin)	**250–750 mg qd po or IV** Cost: $11.79–500 mg IV $43.82	*(Continued on next page—QT, interval prolongation & Tendinopathy)*

(Continued on next page—QT, interval prolongation & Tendinopathy)

[1] **SSRI** = selective serotonin reuptake inhibitors, e.g., fluoxetine (Prozac).
(See page 72 for footnotes and abbreviations) * NOTE: all dosage recommendations are for adults (unless otherwise indicated) and assume normal renal function.

TABLE 10B (6)

CLASS, AGENT, GENERIC NAME (TRADE NAME)	USUAL ADULT DOSAGE (Cost)	ADVERSE REACTIONS, COMMENTS (See Table 10A for Summary)
FLUOROQUINOLONES (continued)		
Moxifloxacin (Avelox)	400 mg po or IV qd Cost: 400 mg po @ 9.00, IV @ 44	**(Continued from previous page)** **QT$_c$ (corrected QT) interval prolongation:** ↑ QT$_c$ (>500 msec or >60 msec from baseline) can lead to torsades de pointes and ventricular tachycardia. Risk varies with specific FQ (data limited): greatest with sparfloxacin, least with ciprofloxacin. (Pharmacother 21:1468, 2001; JAC 49:593, 2002; CID 34:861, 2002). Risk ↑ in women, ↓ K⁺, ↓ Mg²⁺, bradycardia.
Ofloxacin (Floxin)	200–400 mg po or IV q12h. Cost: 400 mg po @ 5.44	**Avoid concomitant drugs with potential to prolong QT$_c$:**

Antiarrhythmics:	Anti-Infectives:	CNS Drugs:	Misc.
Amiodarone	Clarithro	Fluoxetine	Salmeterol
Disopyramide	Erythro	Sertraline	Naratriptan
Dofetilide	Foscarnet	Tricyclics	Sumatriptan
Flecainide	Mefloquine	Venlafaxine	Dolasetron
Ibutilide	Pentamidine	Haloperidol	Droperidol
Procainamide	**Anti-Hypertensives:**	Phenothiazines	Fosphenytoin
Quinidine	Bepridil	Pimozide	Indapamide
Risperidone	Isradipine	Quetiapine	Tamoxifen
Sotalol	Nicardipine	Ziprasidone	Tizanidine
	Moxipril		

Updates online: **www.qtdrugs.org**; **www.torsades.org.**
Tendinopathy: Over age 60, approx. 2-6% of all Achilles tendon ruptures attributable to use of FQ. ↑ risk with concomitant steroid or renal disease (CID 36:1404, 2003).

MISCELLANEOUS AGENTS		
Colistin (Coly-Mycin)	2.5–5.0 mg/kg/d div. into 2–4 doses. **Dose based on ideal body weight** (see formula top of Table 1, page 73). Cost 150 mg @ 64.65	Transient reversible neuro. disturbances: circumoral paresthesia, tingling of extremities, pruritus, vertigo; may resolve with reduced dosage.
Daptomycin (Cubicin)	**Skin/soft tissue: 4 mg/kg qd IV** **Bacteremia/endocarditis: 6 mg/kg qd IV** (see Comment). Cost 500 mg @ 134.00	Dose-dependent nephrotoxicity. Respiratory arrest reported. ↑DA approved skin/soft tissue infections. Endocarditis trials ongoing. **Potential muscle toxicity:** ↑↑ A4 mg/kg q.d., ↑ CPK in 2.8% dapto pts & 1.8% comparator-treated pts. In very small study, no CPK ↑ in pts taking a statin drug given daptomycin.
Fosfomycin (Monurol)	3.0 gm mixed with water po x1 dose. Cost 35.50	Generally well-tolerated. Diarrhea in 9% of study population compared to 6% of pts given nitrofurantoin and 2.3% given TMP/SMX. If given with metoclopramide (Reglan), ↓ serum levels.
Fusidic acid⁺⁺ (Fucidin)	500 mg tid po, IV (Leo Laboratories, Denmark)	Mild GI, occ. skin rash, jaundice (17% with IV, 6% with po). (None in CSF, <1% in urine.)
Immune globulin IV therapy	**Dosage, frequency vary with the indication.** At least **6 FDA-approved indications:** primary immune-def., immune thrombocytopenia, Kawasaki syndrome, recent bone marrow transplant, B-cell lymphocytic leukemia, pediatric HIV. Many other endorsed uses. Cost by trade name: Sandoglobulin 12 gm 697; Gammar 10 gm 1000; Gammune-N 10 gm 900; Gammagard S/D 10 gm 1009; Panglobulin 12 gm 990; Venoglobulin 10 gm 1150; Iveegam 10 gm 824	Reported adverse rates range from 1–15%. Fever, headache, myalgia, N/V relate to rate of infusion, mild, & self-limited. **More serious:** anaphylactoid reactions, thromboembol, aseptic meningitis, & renal injury (in 6.7%, QJM 93:751, 2000).
Methenamine hippurate (Hiprex, Urex)	1.0 gm q6h po. Cost: 1.0 gm @ 1.49 1.0 gm = 480 mg methenamine	Nausea and vomiting, skin rash or dysuria. Overall ~3%. Methenamine requires (pH ≤5) urine to liberate formaldehyde. Limited place in therapy; useful in suppressive therapy when original infecting organisms have been cleared. Do not use for pyelonephritis or with renal insufficiency. As concentrations of formaldehyde may fall below inhibitory concentrations. Of no value in pts with continuously draining urethral catheter. If urine pH >5.0, co-administer ascorbic acid (1–2 gm q4h) to acidify the urine. Cranberry juice (1200–4000 ml/day) has been used, results ±.
Methenamine mandelate (Mandelamine)	1.0 gm q6h po (480 mg methenamine) Cost: 1.0 gm NB @ 0.69	

(See page 72 for footnotes and abbreviations.)

* NOTE: all dosage recommendations are for adults (unless otherwise indicated) and assume normal renal function.

TABLE 10B (7)

CLASS, AGENT, GENERIC NAME (TRADE NAME)	USUAL ADULT DOSAGE (Cost)	ADVERSE REACTIONS, COMMENTS (See Table 10A for Summary)
MISCELLANEOUS AGENTS (continued)		
Metronidazole (Flagyl) Ref: Mayo Clin Proc 74:825, 1999	**Anaerobic infections:** usually IV, 7.5 mg/kg (~500 mg) q6h (not to exceed 4.0 gm qd). **With long T½, can use IV at 15 mg/kg q12h.** If life-threatening, use loading dose of 15 mg/kg. Oral dose: 500 mg qid. Cost: 500 mg tab G $0.21, NB $4.11; 500 mg IV G $2.80, NB $14.83; IV 15 mg/kg. Ext. release 750 mg $8.30	Can be given rectally (enema or suppository). In pts with **decompensated liver disease** (manifest by ≥2↑ of ascites, encephalopathy, ↑ prothrombin time, ↓ serum albumin) **½ prolonged; unless dose ↓ by approx. ½, side-effects ↑**. Absorbed into serum from vaginal gel. **Neurol.:** headache, rare paresthesias or peripheral neuropathy, ataxia, seizures, aseptic meningitis, report of reversible metro-induced cerebellar lesions (NEJM 346:68, 2002). **Avoid alcohol during & 48 hrs after (disulfiram-like reaction)** Very dark urine (common but harmless). Skin: urticaria. Mutagenic in Ames test. Tumorigenic in animals (high dose over lifetime). No evidence of risk in man. No teratogenicity.
Mupirocin (Bactroban cream)	Skin cream 2%: Apply tid. 15 gm $31.48. Nasal ointment 2%: apply bid. 22 gm $45.68	Headache 1.7%, rash & nausea 1.1%.
Nitrofurantoin macrocrystals (Macrodantin)	100 mg q6h. Cost: 100 mg G $1.21; NB $1.86. Dose for long-term UTI suppression: 50–100 mg at bedtime	Absorption ↑ with meals. Increased activity in acid urine, much reduced at pH 8 or over. Not effective in endstage renal disease (JAC 33(Suppl A):121, 1994). Nausea and vomiting, hypersensitivity, peripheral neuropathy. Pulmonary reactions (with chronic rx): **acute ARDS type, chronic desquamative interstitial pneumonia with fibrosis.** Intrahepatic cholestasis & hepatitis similar to chronic active hepatitis. Hemolytic anemia in G6PD deficiency.
monohydrate/macrocrystals (Macrobid)	100 mg bid po. Cost: 100 mg $1.45	Contraindicated in renal failure. Should not be used in infants <1 month of age. Efficacy of Macrobid 100 mg bid = Macrodantin 50 mg qid. Adverse effects 5.6%, less nausea than with Macrodantin.
Sulfonamides [e.g., sulfisoxazole (Gantrisin), sulfamethoxazole (Gantanol)]	Sulfisoxazole (Gantrisin) peds suspension: Cost 500 mg/5 ml: 480 ml $46.02	**Short-acting are best:** high urine concentration and good solubility at acid pH. More active in alkaline urine. **Allergic reactions:** skin rash, drug fever, pruritus, photosensitization. Periarteritis nodosa & S.E. Stevens-Johnson syndrome, serum sickness syndrome, myocarditis. Neurotoxicity (psychosis, neuritis), hepatic toxicity. Blood dyscrasias, usually agranulocytosis. Crystalluria. Nausea & vomiting, headache, dizziness, lassitude, mental depression, acidosis, suppression. Hemolytic anemia in G6PD deficient & unstable hemoglobins (Hb Zurich). Do not use in newborn infants or in women near term, ↑ frequency of kernicterus (binds to albumin, blocking binding of bilirubin to albumin).
Trimethoprim (Trimpex, Proloprim, and others)	100 mg tab po q12h or 200 mg (2 tabs) po q24h. Cost: 100 mg NB $1.11, G $0.15	Rash in 3% at 100 mg bid, 6.7% at 200 mg bid. Rare reports of photosensitivity, exfoliative dermatitis, Stevens-Johnson syndrome, toxic epidermal necrolysis, and aseptic meningitis (CID 19:431, 1994). Check drug interaction with phenytoin. Increases serum K⁺ (see TMP/SMX Comments). TMP can ↑ homocysteine blood levels (J 352:1827, 1998).
Trimethoprim (TMP)/ Sulfamethoxazole (SMX) (Bactrim, Septra) Single-strength (SS) is 80 TMP/400 SMX, double-strength (DS) 160 TMP/800 SMX	**Standard po rx** (UTI, otitis media): 1 DS tablet bid, **P. carinii: see Table 13, page 96. IV rx** (base on TMP component): standard 8–10 mg/kg divided q6h, q8h, or q12h. **For shigellosis: 2.5 mg/kg IV q6h**. Cost: 160/800 po G $0.09, NB $1.02–1.72; 160/800 IV $11.21	Adverse reactions in 10% or more of pts. GI and skin. GI: nausea, vomiting, anorexia. Skin: Rash, urticaria, photosensitivity. Less often but more serious (1–10%): Stevens-Johnson syndrome and toxic epidermal necrolysis. Skin adverse reactions may represent toxic metabolites of SMX and ↓ glutathione rather than an allergy (Am J Pharm 32:361, 1998). See other sulfonamide adverse reactions above. TMP competes with creatinine for tubular secretion and serum creatinine can ↑. TMP also blocks distal renal tubule reabsorption of Na⁺ and secretion of K⁺. ↑ serum K⁺ in 21% of pts (AnIM 124:316, 1996). TMP/SMX suspected etiology of aseptic meningitis, esp. TMP component (CID 19:431, 1994). TMP/SMX contains sulfites and may trigger asthma in sulfite-sensitive pts. One of most frequent drugs to cause thrombocytopenia (AnIM 129:886, 1998).

* Cost to pharmacist according to manufacturer's listing in 2003 DRUG TOPICS RED BOOK, Medical Economics (average wholesale price).

Abbreviations: G = generic. **NB** = name brand. **MRSA** = methicillin-resistant Staph. aureus. **APAG** = antipseudomonal aminoglycoside. **NUS** = not available in the U.S.

* *NOTE: all dosage recommendations are for adults (unless otherwise indicated) and assume normal renal function.*

TABLE 10C
AMINOGLYCOSIDE ONCE-DAILY AND MULTIPLE DAILY DOSING REGIMENS
(See Table 17, page 130. If estimated creatinine clearance <90 ml/min.)

General: Dosage given as both once-daily (OD) and multiple daily dose (MDD) regimens.

Pertinent formulae:

(1) Estimated creatinine clearance (CrCl): $\dfrac{(140-age)(ideal\ body\ weight\ in\ kg)}{(72)(serum\ creatinine)}$ = CrCl for men in ml/min; multiply answer x 0.85 for CrCl of women

(2) Ideal body weight (IBW)—Females: 45.5 kg + 2.3 kg per inch over 5' = weight in kg
Males: 50.0 kg + 2.3 kg per inch over 5' = weight in kg

(3) Obesity adjustment: use if actual body weight (ABW) is ≥30% above IBW. To calculate adjusted dosing weight in kg: IBW + 0.4(ABW–IBW) = adjusted weight (CID 25:112, 1997)

DRUG	MDD AND OD IV REGIMENS/ TARGETED PEAK (P) AND TROUGH (T) SERUM LEVELS	COST Name Brand (NB), Generic (G)	COMMENTS For more data on once-daily dosing, see AJM 105:182, 1998, and Table 17, page 130
Gentamicin (Garamycin), **Tobramycin** (Nebcin)	MDD: 2 mg/kg load, then 1.7 mg/kg q8h P 4–10 μg/ml, T 1–2 μg/ml OD: 5.1 (7 if critically ill) mg/kg q24h P 16–24 μg/ml, T <1 μg/ml	Gentamicin: 80 mg NB $6.40, G $1.60 Tobramycin: 80 mg NB $6.24, G $11.96	**All aminoglycosides have potential to cause tubular necrosis and renal failure, deafness due to cochlear toxicity, vertigo due to damage to vestibular organs, and rarely neuromuscular blockade.** Risk minimal with oral or topical application due to small % absorption unless tissues altered by disease. Risk of nephrotoxicity ↑ with concomitant administration of cyclosporine, vancomycin, ampho B, radiocontrast. Risk of nephrotoxicity ↓ by concomitant AP Pen and perhaps by once-daily dosing method (especially if baseline renal function normal).
Kanamycin (Kantrex), **Amikacin** (Amikin), Streptomycin	MDD: 7.5 mg/kg q12h P 15–30 μg/ml, T 5–10 μg/ml OD: 15 mg/kg q24h P 56–64 μg/ml, T <1 μg/ml	Kanamycin: 1.0 gm $6.92–9.60 Amikacin: 500 mg NB $34.26, G $7.80 Streptomycin: 1.0 gm $6.90	In general, same factors influence risk of ototoxicity. **NOTE: There is no known method to eliminate risk of aminoglycoside nephro/ototoxicity. Proper rx attempts to ↓ the % risk.**
Netilmicin[AUS]	MDD: 2.0 mg/kg q24h P 4–10 μg/ml, T 1–2 μg/ml OD: 6.5 mg/kg q24h P 22–30 μg/ml, T <1 μg/ml		The clinical trial data of OD aminoglycosides have been reviewed extensively by meta-analysis (CID 24:816, 1997). **Serum levels:** Collect serum for 1 peak serum level (PSL) exactly 1 hr after the start of the infusion of the 3rd dose. In critically ill pts, it is reasonable to measure the PSL after the 1st dose as well as later doses as volume of distribution and renal function may change rapidly.
Isepamicin[NUS]	Only OD: Severe infections 15 mg/kg q24h, less severe 8 mg/kg q24h		
Spectinomycin (Trobicin)	2.0 gm IM x1—gonococcal infections	2 gm NB $29.76	Other dosing methods and references: For once-daily 7 mg/kg/d of gentamicin—Hartford Hospital method, see AAC 39:650, 1995.
Neomycin—oral	Prophylaxis GI surgery: 1.0 gm po x3 with erythro, see Table 15B, page 126 For hepatic coma: 4–12 gm/d, po	500 mg NB $1.24	

Tobramycin—inhaled (Tobi), See Cystic fibrosis, Table 1, page 28. Adverse effects few: transient voice alteration (13%) and transient tinnitus (3%). Cost: 300 mg $44.78

Paromomycin—oral: See Entamoeba and Cryptosporidia, Table 13, page 93. Cost: 250 mg $1.90

---

[1] Estimated CrCl invalid if serum creatinine <0.6 mg/dl. Consultation suggested

TABLE 11A: TREATMENT OF FUNGAL, ACTINOMYCOTIC, AND NOCARDIAL INFECTIONS—ANTIMICROBIAL AGENTS OF CHOICE*
(See Table 11B for Amphotericin B Preparations and Adverse Effects)

TYPE OF INFECTION/ORGANISM/ SITE OF INFECTION	ANTIMICROBIAL AGENTS OF CHOICE		COMMENTS
	PRIMARY	ALTERNATIVE	
Actinomycosis (A. israelii most common, also A. naeslundii, A. viscosus, A. odontolyticus, A. meyeri, A. gerencseriae) (CID 26:1255, 1998) Cervicofacial, pulmonary, abdominal, cerebral	**Ampicillin** 50 mg/kg/d IV x 4–6 wks, then 0.5 gm **amoxicillin** tid po x 6 mos. or **Penicillin G** 10–20 million u/d IV x 4–6 wks, then **penicillin V** 2–4 gm/d po for 6–12 mos.	**Doxycycline** or **ceftriaxone** or **clindamycin** or **erythromycin**. **Chloramphenicol** 50–60 mg/kg/d q6h IV or po has been recommended for CNS infection in pen-allergic pts.	Tuboovarian abscesses may complicate IUDs. Removal of IUD is primary rx. Prolonged abscesses or fistulae, surgery often required. While penicillin G and ampicillin IV have been effective, with home IV therapy, agents given q4, e.g., ceftriaxone, are more practical (CID 19:161, 1994). **Surgery may be superior for hemoptysis** (An Thor Surg 74:185, 2002).
Aspergillosis (A. fumigatus most common, also A. flavus and others) (CID 30:696, 2000) Allergic bronchopulmonary (Mayo Clin Proc 76:930, 2001)	**Corticosteroids**	**Itraconazole** (po) of benefit in 10/14 pts (J Am Acad Derm 23:607, 1990). Another case responded to itra 200 mg po x3 mos.	In 55 pts itra ↓ steroid reqmt., ↑ pulmonary fxn & exercise tolerance and improved chest x-ray (NEJM 342:756, 2000). Itra improved 2/3 cystic fibrosis pts with allergic bronchopulmonary aspergillosis (Allergy 57:723, 2002).
Allergic fungal sinusitis: relapsing chronic sinusitis, nasal polyps without bony invasion; asthma, eczema or allergic rhinitis. ↑ IgE levels and isolation of Aspergillus sp. (or other dematiaceous sp.) (Alternaria, Cladosporium, etc.)	**Rx controversial:** systemic corticosteroids + surgical debridement (80% respond but 2/3 recur).	**Itraconazole** (po) For failures might try **Itra** 200 mg po x12 mos (CID 31:203, 2000).	Efficacy of antimicrobial agents not proven.
Aspergilloma (fungus ball) (J Resp Dis 23:300, 2002)			Surgery if hemoptysis becomes massive (post-op complications 25%)
Invasive, pulmonary (IPA) or extrapulmonary Occurs post-transplantation and post-chemotherapy in neutropenic pts (acute leukemia). Most common pneumonia in stem cell transplant patients with graft vs host disease (CID 35:659, 2002). Usually a late (≥100 days) complication in allogeneic bone marrow & stem cell transplant recipients, but overall mortality rates vary from 78–94% (CID 28:322, 1999; CID 36:46, 2003). Typical x-ray/CT lung lesions (halo sign, cavitation, or mycotic lung sequestration) have 90% positive predictive value for invasive pulmonary aspergillosis in pts with hematologic malignancies (CID 31:859, 2000). See CID 26:781, 1998, for excellent review. Test that detects aspergillus galactomannan antigen in plasma looks hopeful (Blood 97:1604, 2001); + serum antigen predictive of IPA in neutropenic pts (J Clin Micro 42:435, 2004). Test available via MiraVista, 1-866-647-2847.	**Voriconazole** 6 mg/kg IV q12h on day 1; then either (4 mg/kg IV q12h) or (200 mg po q12h for body weight ≥40 kg, 100 mg po q12h for <40 kg) **OR** **Lipid-based ampho B** may be as effective and less nephrotoxic than standard ampho B **but much more expensive** (see footnote[3] for dosages). Some authorities now prefer lipid-based for invasive aspergillosis (CID 26:781, 1998; CID 32: 415, 2003). **OR** **Ampho B** deoxycholate (see footnote[2] page 75): Rapid increase to 1 mg/kg (1–1.25 mg/kg if neutropenic) q24h or 2.5–3.5 gm rec. by some but no data to support this practice. **OR** **Combination rx: Vori + caspo** (in above dosages) are currently preferred initial treatment in many febrile neutropenic pts, esp. in pts receiving high doses of corticosteroids. For all regimens: If response good may switch to oral **vori** after 2–3 wks.	**Itraconazole** (po) of benefit in 14–42% (CID 26:781, 1998; CID 33:358, 2001) in pulmonary aspergillosis in those pts rx ≥14 days. Dependent on underlying disease: 83% heart/kidney transplants, 54% neutropenic leukemia pts, 33% bone marrow transplant, 20% liver transplant (CID 23:608, 1996). **Ampho B** overall success rate 34–42% (CID 26:781, 1998; CID 32:358, 2001)	In 83 assessable pts, overall efficacy rate was 45% but was 56% in those receiving >7 days of caspofungin as salvage rx (ICAAC 2002, Abst. M-856). 42% with allergic or intolerant to ampho B (CID 36:1445, 2003). While new drugs may improve response & survival, IPA remains one of the most refractory fungal infections. This has led clinicians to combination therapy, albeit **to combination antifungal rx** (CID 36:1445, 2003). Case reports and small uncontrolled series reported in patients who have failed conventional ampho B: rx >100 pts have either had caspo added to ampho B-based regimen or had vori & caspo substituted for ampho B with an overall response rate of approx. 50% (ICAAC 2002, Abst. M-868, M-860, M-1238; Abst. J-1625, 2001). In an uncontrolled heart transplant pts who failed short-course ampho B, vori + caspo was superior to vori alone (L. Corey). Antagonism between the 3 classes of drugs does not seem to exist & synergism between the triazoles (vori and ampho B) and an echinocandin (caspo) (AAC 46:245, 2002; AAC 46:2564, 2002; J Infect Dis 187:1834, 2003). **No controlled clinical trials have been reported to support this approach.** Ampho B + caspo synergistic & superior to monotherapy in neutropenic animal model (AAC 46:245, 2002). Toxicity of the vori + caspo combination is acceptable but high cost is the major deterrent to combination rx.

---

1 **Oral solution preferred to tablets because of ↑ absorption** (see Table 11B, page 84).

2 **Dosages:** ABLC 5 mg/kg/d IV over 2 hrs; Ampho B cholesteryl complex 3–4 mg/kg/d IV over 2 hrs; **liposomal Ampho B** 3–5 mg/kg/d IV given over 1–2 hrs.

* From MICROMEDEX TOPICS Red Book, Medical Economics Data and Hospital Formulary Pricing Guide. **Price is average wholesale price (AWP).**

† Hydration before and after IV infusion with 500 cc saline has been shown to reduce renal toxicity.

All dosage recommendations are for adults (unless otherwise indicated) and assume normal renal function.

TABLE 11A (2)

TYPE OF INFECTION/ORGANISM/SITE OF INFECTION	ANTIMICROBIAL AGENTS OF CHOICE		COMMENTS
	PRIMARY	ALTERNATIVE	
Blastomycosis (CID 30:679, 2000) (Blastomyces dermatitidis) Cutaneous, pulmonary or extrapulmonary	Itraconazole oral solution 200–400 mg/d po for 6 mos. **or** Ampho B[2] 0.7–1 mg/kg/d to a total dose of ≥1.5 gm for very sick pts	Fluconazole 400–800 mg/d for at least 6 mos. 85%+ effective for non-life-threatening disease (CID 25:200, 1997)	Itra: in patients treated for ≥2 months, 95% cure (AJM 93:489, 1992). Ampho B successful in >90% when ≥1.5 gm total dose used (CID 22:S102, 1996). [For blood/urine antigen, call 1-866-647-2847.

Candidiasis: Candida is a major cause of nosocomial bloodstream infection, a decrease in C. albicans and increase in non-albicans species show ↓ susceptibility to antifungal agents (esp. fluconazole). These changes have predominantly affected immunocompromised pts in environments where antifungal prophylaxis (esp. fluconazole) is widely used (JAC 49:Suppl 1:3, 2002). In vitro susceptibility testing for antifungal drugs to date has not undergone rigorous in vivo validation studies, and clinical outcomes are often more dependent on host factors (Am J Med 112:380, 2002). Yet it seems prudent to use susceptibility profiles to help select empiric antifungal therapy. The following table attempts to summarize the current published reports of frequency of **(S = susceptible**, susceptible **with dose escalation (S-DD) = susceptible with dose escalation)**, may require dose escalation; **(R = resistant)**. **S-I = less active in vitro but clinically effective** interpretation as to whether a drug is clinically effective but still active in vitro but clinically effective (IDSA recommendations, 2003). In vitro testing for caspo has not standardized — only rare failures reported (Ln 359:1135, 2002).

TYPE OF INFECTION/ORGANISM/SITE OF INFECTION	% Sensitive in Vitro					Rx/% species known
	Fluconazole	Itraconazole	Voriconazole	Ampho B	Caspofungin	
	% of Candida Isolates	Risk Factors				
C. albicans — 55-65 — HIV/AIDS, surgery	97% (S)	93% (S)	99% (S)	>95% (S)	(S)	Flu,++ caspo, or ampho B
C. glabrata — 10-15 — Heme malignancies, azole prophylaxis	85-90% (S-DD)	50% (S-DD)	92% (S-I)	>95% (S-I)	(S)	Caspo, ampho B, or vori
C. parapsilosis — 15-20 — Azole prophylaxis, neonates, foreign bodies	99% (S)	4% (S-DD)	(S-DD)	>95% (S)	S-I	Flu, caspo, or ampho B
C. tropicalis — 5-10 — Neutropenia	98% (S)	58% (S)	99% (S)	>95% (S)	(S)	Flu, caspo, or ampho B
C. krusei — 2-10 — Heme malignancies, azole prophylaxis, previous ampho B	5% (R)	69% (S-DD)	99% (S)	>95% (S-I)	(S)	Caspo, ampho B, or vori
C. guilliermondi — 1	>95% (S)	?	>95% (S)	?	(S)	Flu, caspo, or ampho B
C. lusitaniae — 1 — Previous ampho B rx	>95% (S)	?	>95% (S)	(R)	(S)	Flu, caspo, or vori

++ If patient had prior heavy basal exposure.

TYPE OF INFECTION	Risk Factors	PRIMARY / ALTERNATIVE	COMMENTS
Bloodstream: clinically stable with or without venous catheter • Appropriate blood cultures require therapy • Remove & replace venous catheter ("not over a wire") if possible (CID 34:591 & 600, 2002), esp. in non-neutropenic; mortality vs 4%, catheter not removed. Other studies support (CID 36:1221, 2003). • Observe for metastatic lesions, esp. endophthalmitis, ophthalmologic exam recommended for all pts with candidemia. • Treat for 2 wks after last pos. blood culture & resolution of signs & symptoms of infection.	Use ampho B or caspo (CID 35:1073, 2002; 36:1497, 2003)	**Fluconazole** ≥6 mg/kg/d or 400 mg IV or po x1 d, then po for 14 d. after last + blood culture **or** **Caspofungin** 70 mg IV on day 1 followed by 50 mg IV qd (reduce to 35 mg IV qd with moderate hepatic insufficiency). Would use in place of flu in those heavily pretreated with azoles (CID 26:1221, 2003) **or** **Ampho B** 0.6 mg/kg/d IV, total dose 5–7 mg/kg/d — In pts who fail to respond or deteriorate, higher doses of either drug may be used (**ampho B** 0.6–1 mg/kg/d) or **fluconazole 800 mg/d IV** (re po) CID 25:43, 1997). Be sure catheter is removed. **or** **Voriconazole**[NFDA-L] 6 mg/kg q12h x1 d, IV, then maintenance dose 3 mg/kg q12h IV for serious candida infections.	In a multicenter trial fluconazole = ampho B but less toxicity (NEJM 331:1325, 1994; AAM 7:155-2429, 1995), microbiologic failure 10-14% in both. Similar results found in cancer pts (AJM 101:170, 1996). Observational studies suggest flu & ampho B are similarly effective in neutropenic pts (IDSA Guidelines, 2003). A randomized study (224 pts, 10% were neutropenic) found caspofungin equivalent to ampho B (0.6-1 mg/kg/d) for invasive candidiasis. For candidemia 71.7% rx with caspo vs 62.8% with ampho B had successful outcomes but caspo had significantly less toxicity (NEJM 347:2020, 2002).

---

[1] Oral solution preferred to tablets because of ↑ **absorption** (see Table 11B, page 84).

[2] Hydration before and after infusion with 500 cc saline has been shown to reduce renal toxicity.

[3] ABLC or liposomal ampho B recommended for pts intolerant of or refractory to ampho B, i.e., failure of 500 mg ampho B, initial renal insufficiency (creatinine >2.5 mg/dl or CrCl <25 ml/min), a sig. ↑ in serum Cr (to >2.5 mg/dl for adults or 1.5 mg/dl for children) or severe acute administration-related toxicity (CID 26:1383, 1998). Since efficacy similar and toxicity less, some now recommend lipid-based ampho B for all (unless cost a major issue) (CID 37:415, 2003).

* From 2003 Drug Topics RED Book, Medical Economics Data and Hospital Formulary Pricing Guide. Price is average wholesale price (AWP).

All dosage recommendations are for adults (unless otherwise indicated) and assume normal renal function

TABLE 11A (3)

TYPE OF INFECTION/ORGANISM/ SITE OF INFECTION	ANTIMICROBIAL AGENTS OF CHOICE		COMMENTS
	PRIMARY	**ALTERNATIVE**	
Candidiasis (continued) **Bloodstream: unstable, deteriorating** (pulmonary, eye, hepatosplenic) ± **neutropenia** *For endoph/thalmitis, see below*	**Ampho B** 0.8–1 mg/kg/d IV **± 5FC** 37.5[1] mg/kg q6h or (**lipid-based ampho B (ABLC), 5 mg/kg/d** or **Fluconazole** 400–800 mg po IV. If start ampho B, switch to flucon 400 mg po qd x14 d. after 1st positive blood culture, resolution of neutropenia & disappearance of signs/ symptoms of candidal infection or **Combination of fluconazole** 800 mg/d **+ ampho B** 0.7 mg/kg/d for first 5–6 days, then switch to flu 800 mg/d	**Voriconazole loading dose 6 mg/kg q12h x1 d. IV, then maintenance dose 3 mg/kg q12h IV** for serious candida infections or **Caspofungin** 70 mg IV on day 1 followed by 50 mg IV qd (reduce to 35 mg IV qd with moderate hepatic insufficiency)	In a randomized study of 219 pts with non-neutropenic candidemia, fluconazole (800 mg/d) + ampho B (0.7 mg/kg/d for the 1st 5 days) was slightly better than flu alone. Primary analysis, success on day 36 was 69% vs 57%; overall success rate 69% vs 56% (p= .043) and clearance of fungemia 94% vs 83% (p= .02). The flu alone group was slightly sicker (APACHE II 16.9 vs 16.8, p= .039) and renal toxicity in combination group (23% vs 3%, p <.001) (CID 36: 1221, 2003). Given difficulty with interpretation of this study, the editors would reserve combination of flu + ampho B for only the sickest candidemic patient. Voriconazole may have a role in this clinical setting (Euro Con Clin Micro & Inf Dis 2002, Abst. 237 (IDSA 2000, Abst. 352). Only open labeled & observational studies available for ampho B (AJM 108:88, 1988; Cancer 76:2357, 1995), lipid-associated ampho B (AAC 43:1944, 1995) & fluconazole (AJM 91:137, 142, 1991). Caspofungin successful in a single case report (CID 31:1155, 2002).
Chronic disseminated candidiasis (hepatosplenic candidiasis)	**Ampho B** 0.6–0.7 mg/kg/d or a lipid-based ampho 3–5 mg/kg/d in acutely ill or pt with refractory disease for 1–2 weeks then flucon-azole 400 mg po qd or longer OR **Fluconazole** 6 mg/kg/d (400 mg po qd) in stable patient	**Fluctyosine + ampho B** for refractory disease	Respond to ampho B but relapse is usual. Flucon used and may be less toxic, but experience limited.
Chronic mucocutaneous	**Ketoconazole** 400 mg po (as single day dose with food) for 3–8 months	Usually children: Peds dose of **fluconazole** 3–6 mg/kg/d as single daily dose	
Cutaneous *(including paronychia, Table 1, page 18)*	Apply topically **ampho B, clotrimazole, econazole, miconazole or nystatin** 3–4x daily **Ciclopirox olamine** 1% cream/lotion. Apply topically bid x7–14 d		Cost (30 gm tube cream): AAC $29, Clo $19, MIC $21, Nys $3.58. Cic $18.26
Endocarditis • Both native & prosthetic valve replacement should be surgical replacement of infected valve • Causes of fungal endocarditis: C. albicans 24%, non-albicans Candida sp. 24%, Aspergillus sp. 24%, others 27% (CID 32:50, 2001)	**Ampho B** 0.6 mg/kg/d IV or 7 days, then **ampho B or lipid-based ampho B** 3–5 mg/kg/d. Continue 6–8 weeks after surgery + **Fluctyosine** 25–37.5 mg/kg/d	**Fluconazole** 200–400 mg/d for chronic suppression; may be of value when valve cannot be replaced (CID 7:22:302, 2002)	Candida cidal vs candistat & may be of value; no data. Candida endocarditis has propensity to relapse; requires careful follow-up for at least a year (Chest 99:1531, 1991)
Endophthalmitis (IDSA Guidelines, 2003) • Complication of hematologenous candidemia, thus ophthalmological consult recommended for all pts with candidemia (Med 53:47, 1974) • Typically occurs unilateral, white exudates on retinal exam and/or solation of fungus Ophthalmic • Long-term therapy of 6–12 weeks typically required for complete resolution or stabilization of disease	**Ampho B or lipid-based ampho B** (ABLC 4.5 mg/kg/d) **± 5FC** or **Fluconazole** 400 mg IV or po either as initial rx or follow-up after ampho B Role of intravitreal ampho B not well defined but commonly used in pts with substantial vision loss (CID 27:1130, 1998)		Treatment results mixed in comparison of intraocular fluconazole (CID 20:657, 1995), ABLC (CID 27:1130, 1998)
Oral (thrush)—not AIDS patient (See next page for vaginitis)	**Fluconazole** 200 mg single dose or 100 mg/d for 5–14 days, OR **itraconazole** oral solution 200 mg (20 ml) qd without food x7 days	**Nystatin pastilles** (200,000 u) lozenge qid, 500,000 u (swish & swallow) qid or **Nystatin** (100,000 u/ml) suspension 400,000–600,000 u (swish & swallow) 5x/d qid x14 d or **Clotrimazole** 1 troche (10 mg) 5x/d x14 d	**Fluconazole:** Single dose 100 mg; 16/16 clinical cure. 75% mycologic at 2 weeks (AAC 34:2267, 1990). Maintenance rx required in HIV/AIDS pts. Usually improves in 3–4 days, longer rx & relapse. C. krusei fungemia reported in flucon-rx pts (NEJM 325:1315, 1991).

[1] Some experts reduce dose of 5FC to 25 mg/kg q6h

* From 2003 Drug Topics Red Book, Medical Economics Data and Hospital Formulary Pricing Guide. **Price is average wholesale price (AWP).**
† All dosage recommendations are for adults (unless otherwise indicated) and assume normal renal function

TABLE 11A (4)

TYPE OF INFECTION/ORGANISM/ SITE OF INFECTION	ANTIMICROBIAL AGENTS OF CHOICE		COMMENTS
	PRIMARY	ALTERNATIVE	
Candidiasis/Oral (thrush) (continued)			
AIDS patients **Stomatitis, esophagitis, vaginitis** • Oral colonization with candida correlates with HIV RNA levels in plasma, unless so with CD4 counts (<50 with HIV infection) (JID 180:534, 1999). Since protease inhibitors & recurrent oral candidiasis decreased vs rx with (other antiretroviral agents p < .001) (JAIDS 21:20, 1999). May be due to direct effect on candida aspartic protease (J AIDS 22:106, 1999). **Post-treatment chronic suppression** (secondary prophylaxis) for disabling recurrent oral, esophageal vaginitis infection (AIDS Res Hum Retroviruses 10:1619, 1999). However, some use **fluconazole 100 mg po once/wk.**	**Fluconazole 200 mg po 1st day** then 100 mg po qd x14 d. (21 d. or 2 wks following resolution of symptoms for esophagitis) or **Itraconazole oral solution 200 mg po qd** 100 mg po bid x14 d. Some recommend anti-topical agents[1] for oral with esophageal involvement when CD4 <50 & receiving (or will receive) HAART. **Current recommendation is to avoid chronic suppressive rx & only rx acute episode** (AIDS Res Hum Retroviruses 10:1619, 1999). However, some use **fluconazole 100 mg po 150 mg qd** following HAART.	**For fluconazole-refractory disease:** Options include: 1. **Fluconazole** 400–800 mg po qd or bid or 2. **Itraconazole solution** 100 mg po qd or bid or 3. **Ampho B** 0.3–0.5 mg/kg IV qd or 4. **Voriconazole** (see Table 11B, page 84 for dose) or 5. **Caspofungin** 50 mg IV qd If fluconazole-refractory esophagitis, failed fluconazole suppression, may be forced to rx with **ampho B** (0.3 mg/kg IV qd or 1 mg/kg IV q week)	**Fluconazole-refractory disease remains low** (4% in ACTG 816) & is seen in pts with low CD4 counts (<50/mm³). **Flu** superior to oral suspension of nystatin (CID 24:1204, 1997). In pts with oral thrush, but not if achieved oral candidiasis (41/74 (55%) pts unresponsive to flu (AIDS Res Hum Retrovir 15:1413, 1999). **Ampho B oral suspension** gave 42.6% response rate in 54 pts refractory to flu, but 70% of those relapsed (AIDS 14:845, 2000). For esophagitis, **caspofungin** as effective as **ampho B IV** but less toxic (CID 33:1529, 2001; AAC 45:451, 2002; AJ AIDS 31:183, 2002). **Voriconazole** as effective as **fluconazole** for esophagitis (CID 33:1447, 2001). Fluconazole 200 mg qd doses reduce risk of candida esophagitis & cryptococcosis (NEJM 332:700, 1995). Disadvantages: Concern of enhanced risk of emergence of fluconazole (azole)-resistant Candida species.
Peritonitis (Chronic Ambulatory Peritoneal Dialysis) Based on Peritoneal Dialysis International 20:396, 2000. See Table 19, page 135	**Ampho B.** continuous IP dosing at 1.5 mg/L of dialysis fluid x4–6 wks	**Ampho B.** 0.5 mg/kg IV x7–14 d.	Remove cath immediately or if no clinical improvement in 4–7 d.
Urinary • Risk factors urinary tract instrumentation, recent antibiotic rx & advanced age • Usually represents colonization of urinary catheter, a benign event • Rarely may be the source of dissemination if pt has symptoms of UTI, neutropenic, low birth-weight infant, has renal allograft or is undergoing urologic manipulation. Then: • Persistent candiduria in immunocompromised pt warrants ultrasound or CT of kidneys	**Remove urinary catheter or stent;** 40% will clear but only 20% if replaced (CID 30:14, 2000) Antifungal rx not indicated unless pt has symptoms of UTI, neutropenic, low birth-weight infant, has renal allograft or is undergoing urologic manipulation. Then: **fluconazole 200 mg/d po or IV x7–14 d.**	**Ampho B** 0.5 mg/kg/d IV x7–14 d.	Fluconazole alone is successful in presence of bezoar (Ped Nephrol 17:550, 2002). In a placebo-controlled trial, candiduria was cleared more rapidly in pts treated with flucon 200 mg/d x14 d. 2 weeks after completion was not different than placebo group; 60% for catheterized pts & 73% for non-cath pts cleared pts (CID 30:19, 2000). Bladder washout with ampho B not recommended: will not treat upper tract infection. 5FC may be of value in non-albicans UTI but resistance develops rapidly. Caspofungin was effective in clearing candiduria in 12 pts (most with candidemia) but urine levels low (IDSA 2003, Abst. 135). **NOTE:** Vori not in urine in active form.
Vaginitis—Non-AIDS patients Review article JAMA 51(RR-6), 2002 (Candida vaginitis in AIDS patients: see above) (See Table 1, page 17)	Oral: **Fluconazole** 150 mg po x1 or **Itraconazole** 200 mg po bid x1 d.	Intravaginal: Multiple **imidazoles** with 85–95% cure rates. See doses in footnote[2] below, various over-the-counter preparations, see below in footnote[2]	**In general, oral and vaginal rx are similarly effective.** Rx aided by avoiding tight clothing, e.g., pantyhose. Oral drugs + rectal candida and may ↓ relapses. Comparable cure rate reported in both HIV+ and HIV– pts (CID 22:726, 1996) found incidence of flu refractory disease remains low (CID 26:557, 1998). Boric acid solution intravaginally has also been used (CID 24:649, 1997).
"Candida syndrome"[17]	In a double-blind study, **nystatin did not reduce systemic or psychological symptoms** vs placebo (NEJM 323:1717, 1990).		

[1] Oral agents: Nystatin, clotrimazole troche 10 mg 5x/d

[2] **Butoconazole** 2% cream (5 gm) qhs x3 d; **clotrimazole** 100 mg vaginal tabs (2 qd hs x3 d), or 1% cream (5 gm) qhs x7-14 d, or 100 mg vaginal tab (1 qd hs x7 d) or 100 mg vaginal tab (1 qd hs x3 d**) or **miconazole** 100 mg vaginal suppos. (1 qd hs x7 d), or 2% cream (5 gm) qhs x7 d or 0.8% cream (5 gm) qhs x7 d or **tioconazole** 6.5% vag. ointment x1 dose** or 200 mg vaginal suppos. (1 qd hs x3 d) or 5 gm intravaginal qd x3 d or **terconazole** 80 mg vaginal tab (1 qd hs x3 d), or 0.4% cream (5 gm) qd hs x7 d or 0.8% cream 5 gm intravaginal qd x3 d or **tioconazole** 6.5% vag. ointment x1 dose** ** = over-the-counter product

From 2003 Drug TOPICS RED Book, Medical Economics Data and Hospital Formulary Pricing Guide. **Price is average wholesale price (AWP).**

All dosage recommendations are for adults (unless otherwise indicated) and assume normal renal function

TABLE 11A (5)

TYPE OF INFECTION/ORGANISM/ SITE OF INFECTION	ANTIMICROBIAL AGENTS OF CHOICE		COMMENTS
	PRIMARY	ALTERNATIVE	
Chromomycosis (J Am Acad Derm 44:585, 2001) (Cladosporium or Fonsecaea); Cutaneous (usually feet, legs)	If lesions small and few, **surgical excision** with **cryosurgery with liquid nitrogen**. If lesions chronic, extensive, burrowing: **Itraconazole**	**Itraconazole** 100 mg po qd x18 months (or until response) Fluconazole experience disappointing	2 relapses (18, 24 mos.) **Terbinafine**[NUS] impressive in small number of pts (A/TMH 55:45, 1996; Cutis 66:45, 2000)
Coccidioidomycosis mmitis) (see AnIM 130:293, 1999; IDCP 8:21, 1999; IDCP 8:21, 1999) (San Joaquin or Valley			**13/13 patients rx Itra responded** (CID 15:553, 1992)
Primary pulmonary (San Joaquin or Valley Fever)			
Uncomplicated pulmonary in normal host. Influenza-like illness of 1-2 wks duration	**Antifungal rx not generally recommended** but pt should be monitored periodically and rx if fever, wt loss and/or fatigue do not resolve within several wks to 2 months (see below)		**Cure rate (ampho B) 50-70%. Responses are similar.** Itra may have slight advantage esp. in soft tissue infection. Relapse rates after rx 40%; coccidioidin skin test (RR = 4.8) (CID 25:1205, 1997). Following CF titers after completion of rx important.
Primary pulmonary in pts with ↑ risk for complications or dissemination. Rx indicated: • Immunosuppressive disease (AIDS), post-transplantation, or therapies (steroids) • Pregnancy in 3rd trimester • Diabetes • ↑ Complement fixation antibody titer >1:16 • pulmonary infiltrates • Documented extrapulmonary involvement—dissemination (identification of schedules or culture of organism from ulcer, joint effusion, pus from abscess or bone lux, etc.)	**Mild to moderate severity:** **Itraconazole** solution 200 mg po or IV bid OR **Fluconazole** 400 mg po qd for 3-12 months **Locally severe or extensive disease:** **Ampho B** 0.6-1 mg/kg/d x7 d, then 0.8 mg/kg/good. Total dose 2.5 gm or more. **Consultation with specialist recommended:** surgery may be required.	**Ampho B** (IV as for pulmonary (above) /AnIM 119:28, 1993); 0.1-0.3 mg daily intrathecal (intraventricular) via reservoir device.	Important and rising titers should probably warrant readministration of rx (CID 25:1211, 1997). In a randomized double-blind study of 198 pts with progressive non-meningeal cocci, 57% responded to flu vs 72% to itra (p=0.05) by 12 mos. (AnIM 133:676, 2000). Those with skeletal infections responded twice as frequently to itra than flu. Relapse seen in 18% after itra. Lifetime suppression in HIV+ patients: flu 200 mg po qd or Itra 200 mg po bid (Mycosis 46:42, 2003). Targeted fluconazole prophylaxis post rx of pt with rx of cocci or sero-pos. may reduce reactivation post-transplant (Transpl Inf Dis 5:3, 2003).
Meningitis occurs in 1/3 to 1/2 of pts with disseminated coccidioidomycosis			
Adult	**Fluconazole** 400-800 mg po indefinitely		**37/47 patients responded to flucon** (3 yrs) /AnIM 119:28, 1993). 14/18 pts rx with azoles relapsed when drug discontinued, therefore recommended that **fluconazole be continued indefinitely** (AnIM 124:305, 1996). One study also found itra 400-800 mg po to be effective (AnIM 112:108, 1990). Voriconazole successful in high doses (6 mg/kg q12h IV) followed by oral suppression (400 mg q12h) in a pt who failed flucon (CID 36:1619, 2003).
Child	**Fluconazole** (po) (Pediatric dose not established, 6 mg/kg qd used)		
Cryptococcosis (CID 30:710, 2000)			
Non-meningeal (non-AIDS) Risk 57% in organ transplant (Transpl Inf Dis 4:183, 2002)	**Fluconazole** 400 mg/d IV or po for 8 wks to 6 mos **For more severe disease:** **Ampho B** 0.5-0.8 mg/kg/d IV till response then change to **Fluconazole** 400 mg/d po for 8-10 week course	**Itraconazole** 200-400 mg po solution qd for 6-12 mos OR **Ampho B** 0.5-1 mg/kg/d IV + **flucytosine** 37.5 mg/kg qd x6 wks.	Adjust flucyt dose and interval to produce serum levels of peak 70-80 mg/L, trough 30-40 mg/L. **Flucon alone 90% effective for meningeal and non-meningeal forms** (74% on steroid rx). French study suggests fluconazole equally effective as ampho B (CID 22:S154, 1996) and was 92% effective in cancer pts (CID 32:E145, 2001).
Meningitis (non-AIDS)	**Fluconazole** 37.5 mg/kg) IV + **flucytosine** 37.5 mg/kg) qd'h po until pt afebrile and cultures negative (NEJM 301:126, 1979) then stop ampho B/flucyt, start **fluconazole** 200 mg po qd x8-10 wks (NEJM 113:183, 1979) OR **Ampho B** 0.5-0.8 mg/kg/d IV (for less severe disease), recommend continuing flu for 2 yrs to reduce relapse rate (no controlled data available) (CID 28:291, 1999).		**Flucytosine levels must be measured**; adjust dose and interval to give serum level peak 70-80 mg/L, trough 30-40 mg/L. **Fluconazole alone has been used successfully** (CID 28:629, 1999) but poor response if pts in coma (CID 37:673, 2003). Hydrocephalus may be successfully rx with VP or VA[2] shunting (CID 28:629, 1999) but poor response if pts in coma (CID 37:673, 2003).

[1] Some experts would reduce to 25 mg/kg q6h

VP = ventriculoperitoneal. **VA** = ventriculoatrial

* From 2003 DRUG TOPICS RED BOOK, Medical Economics Data and Hospital Formulary Pricing Guide. **Price is average wholesale price (AWP).**

All dosage recommendations are for adults (unless otherwise indicated) and assume normal renal function

TABLE 11A (6)

TYPE OF INFECTION/ORGANISM/ SITE OF INFECTION	ANTIMICROBIAL AGENTS OF CHOICE		COMMENTS
	PRIMARY	ALTERNATIVE	

Cryptococcosis (continued)

HIV+/AIDS: Cryptococcemia and/or Meningitis
↓ in era of HAART (see CID 30:710, 2000).

Treatment (see Comments) (see Neurol 56:257, 2001; CID 36:789, 2003).

Cryptococci in blood may be manifest by positive blood culture or positive serum for cryptococcal antigen

With HAART, symptoms of acute meningitis may return; immune reconstitution (AIDS 12:1491, 1999). If failure to respond to initial rx, think dual infection with tbc, neurosyphilis, toxo, etc. (Neurol 51:1213, 1998).

Ampho B 0.7–1 **mg/d. IV + flucytosine[1]** 25 **mg/kg po q6h x 2 wks** or until clinically stable **followed by flu 400 mg/d.** for **minimum of 10 wks**, then switch to 200 mg (suppression) (see below). Ampho B alone: 0.7–1.0 mg/kg/d IV x2 wks or until afebrile, headache, nausea and vomiting gone. Then dc ampho B, start **flucon 400 mg po** qd to complete 8–10 week course. Then maintain on flucon 200 mg po qd. Start Highly Active Antiretroviral Therapy (HAART) if possible.	**Fluconazole** 400 mg po qd x6–10 wks. then suppressive rx (see Comments) or **Fluconazole** 400 mg po qd + **flucytosine[1]** 37.5 mg/kg po q6h x10 wks (↑ toxicity) or **Liposomal amphotericin** 5 mg/kg qd x2 wks followed by fluconazole as above (Mycosis 46:24, 2003) or **Ampho B lipid complex** IV 5 mg/kg/d (MAOM) IV 1x/week or **Itraconazole** 200 mg po bid if flu intolerant or failure	If normal mental status, >20 cells/mm³ CSF, and CSF crypto anti-gen <1:1024, flucon alone is reasonable (CID 22:322, 1996); no help in monitoring therapy. Serum cryptococcal antigen useful in dx (95% sens.), no help in monitoring therapy. Improved survival if ↑ intracranial pressure lower with CSF removal. No data on steroids. Must monitor 5-FC levels: peak 70–80 mg/l, trough 30–40 mg/l. Higher levels assoc. with bone marrow toxicity. Itraconazole does not penetrate CSF. (CID 22:329, 1996). Even with rx (ampho B + 5FC regimen) 29/236 pts died within 1st 2 wks & 62 (26%) by 10 wks; only 129 (55%) were alive & culture-neg. at 10 wks (CID 28:82, 1999). In 163 pts (15 on HAART) survival was 85%, 6 months after discharge from hospital & receiving flucon suppression in Uganda (IDSA 2003, Abst 630). Itraconazole not as effective as fluconazole. "Not recommended", 13/57 (23%) pts relapsed vs 2/51 (4%) receiving fluconazole (p = 0.006) (CID 36:1329, 2003). Recurrences of crypto meningitis in 22 pts who dc flu sup-pression with >100 CD4 & undetectable VL x3 mos. in Thailand (CID 36:1329, 2003).

Suppression

Fluconazole 200 mg po qd. (If CD4 count rises to >100/mm³ with effective antiretroviral rx, some authorities now recommend dc of suppressive rx. See www.hivatis.org. Authors would only dc if CSF culture negative.)		

Dermatophytosis

Erythrasma (Corynebacterium minutissimum)

Erythromycin 250 mg qid po for 14 days	{2% aqueous clindamycin topically}	Diff. dx with Tinea versicolor, Tinea cruris. Erythrasma gives coral red fluorescence with Woods light.

Onychomycosis (Tinea unguium)
(See CID 23:305, 1994; JAm Acad Med Assn 39:127, 2001; Brit J Derm 148:402, 2003). A topical nail lacquer (ciclopirox) has been approved but resulted in cure in only 5-8% after 48 wks (Med Lett 42:51, 2000). But ↑ to 50% cure in another study (J Am Acad Derm 44:479, 2001). Terbinafine[2] ↑ cure rate & ↓ relapse vs itra at 5 yrs (AcDerm 138:353, 2002) & ↑ cure rate after 1 yr vs flu. (Brit J Derm 142:97, 2000); appears to be most cost-effective (see Table 11B, page 84).

Fingernail Rx Options: **Terbinafine[2]** 250 mg po qd (children <20 kg: 67.5 mg/d, 20–40 kg: 125 mg/d, >40 kg: 250 mg/d) x12 wks (70-81% effective)[3] or **Itraconazole[2]** 200 mg po bid x6 wks (79% effective)[3] or **Fluconazole** 150–300 mg po x1 wk/mo. x2 mos.[NFDA1]	**Toenail Rx Options:** **Terbinafine[2]** 250 mg/kg/d for 30 d.[NFDA1] or **Itraconazole[2]** 200 mg po qd x3 mos.[NFDA1] or **Fluconazole** 150–300 mg po x1 wk/mo. x3–4 mos.[NFDA1]

NOTE: For safe effective, see footnotes 2 & 3

Tinea capitis ("Ringworm") (Trichophyton tonsurans, Microsporum canis, N. America; other sp. elsewhere) (PIDJ 18:191, 1999)

Terbinafine 250 mg po qd x4 wks for ↓ T. ton-surans, 6-8 wks for Microsporum canis[NFDA1]. Children 125 mg qd.	**Itraconazole[2]** 3–5 mg/kg/d for 30 d[NFDA1] or **Fluconazole** 8 mg/kg qwk x8-12 wks. or **Griseofulvin** adults 500 mg po x4–6 wks, children 10–20 mg/kg/d until hair regrows, usually 6-9 wks	All agents with similar cure rates (60-100%) in clinical studies (Ped Derm 17:304, 2000). Griseofulvin considered drug of choice by some although concerns for resistance and toxicities. Addition of topical ketoconazole or selenium sulfate shampoo reduces transmissibility (IJ Derm 39:261, 2000).

---

[1] Flucytosine = 5-FC.

[2] **Serious but rare cases of hepatic failure** have been reported in pts receiving terbinafine & should not be used in pts with chronic or active liver disease. (See Table 11B, page 84). Suggest checking ALT & AST before prescribing (Arch J Health Sys Pharm 58:1076, 2001).

[3] Use of itraconazole has been associated with myocardial dysfunction and with onset of congestive heart failure (see Ln 357:1766, 2001).

From 2003 **DRUG TOPICS RED BOOK**, Medical Economics Data and Hospital Formulary Pricing Guide. **Price is average wholesale price (AWP)**.

All dosage recommendations are for adults (unless otherwise indicated) and assume normal renal function

TABLE 11A (7)

TYPE OF INFECTION/ORGANISM/ SITE OF INFECTION	ANTIMICROBIAL AGENTS OF CHOICE		COMMENTS
	PRIMARY	**ALTERNATIVE**	
Dermatophytosis (continued)			
Tinea corporis, cruris, or pedis (Trichophyton rubrum, T. mentagrophytes, Epidermophyton floccosum) "Athlete's foot, jock itch," and ringworm	**Topical rx:** Generally applied 2x/d. Available as creams, ointments, sprays, lotions, solutions & "over the counter". Apply 2x/d for 2-3 wks. See footnote[1] for names and prices. Recommend: butenafine (Lotrimin Ultra or Lamisil AT; contain butenafine & terbinafine—both are fungicidal & effective)[SEPDA]	**Terbinafine** 250 mg po x2 wks[SEPDA] OR **itraconazole** 200 mg po x2 x4 wks OR **fluconazole** 150 mg po 1x/wk for 2-4 wks[SEPDA] **Griseofulvin:** adults 500 mg po q4-14 wks, children 10-20 mg/kg/d. Duration: 2-4 wks for corporis, 4-8 wks for pedis	Keto po often effective in severe recalcitrant infection. Follow for hepatotoxicity. Terbinafine: 87% achieved mycological cure in double-blind study (32 pts) (J Med Assoc Thai 76:388, 1993; Brit J Derm 130(543):22, 1994) and fluconazole 78% (J Am Acad Derm 40:531, 1999).
Tinea versicolor (Malassezia furfur or Pityrosporum orbiculare)	**Ketoconazole** (400 mg po single dose or 200 mg po x7 days) or (2% cream applied 1x q/d 2 wks)	**Fluconazole** 400 mg po single dose or **itraconazole** 400 mg po qd x3-7 days	Keto (po) x1 97% effective in 1 study. Another alternative Selenium sulfide (Selsun), 2.5% lotion, apply as lather, leave on 10 min then wash off, 1x/d x7 d or x3-6wk/wk x2-4 weeks
Fusariosis Causes infection in eye, skin, sinus and disseminated diseases—increased in transplant patients (CID 34:909, 2002)	**Voriconazole** 6 mg/kg IV q12h x2 then 4 mg/kg IV q12h] or (200 mg po q12h for body weight ≥40 kg, but 100 mg po q12h for body weight <40 kg)	**Ampho B** 1–1.2 mg/kg po or lipid-associated ampho B	Voriconazole successful in 9/21, 4 eye, 2 bloodstream, 2 sinus & 1 skin (CID 35:909, 2002; 36:1122, 2003; 37:311, 2003)
Histoplasmosis (Histoplasma capsulatum): See CID 30:688, 2000; ID Clin N A 17:1, 2003. Best diagnostic test is urinary antigen (ELISA) (CID 22:S102, 1996; MiraVista Diagnostics (1-866-647-2847).			
Immunocompetent patient:	**Minimal disease: No rx**		**With ≥2 months itra rx, 86% success in chronic pulmon-ary & extrapulmonary disease** in 81 patients with ≥ diseas palatal, neph-rotoxicity (mostly v 37%). No difference in mortality after 10 additional weeks of itra in both arms (AnIM 137:105, 2002).
Pulmonary, localized, disseminated	**Moderate: Itraconazole** 200 mg/d solution po for 9 months. If life-threatening 200 mg po 1d x3, then 200 mg po bid until response, then low doses followed by 200 mg bid x4 wks[8] (see 1:89-5, 1989) [Panel: CID 24:1195, 1997]		
	Severe, including meningitis: Ampho B 0.5-1 mg/kg IV x7 d, followed by 0.8 mg/kg qod IV. **Itra not recommended for meningitis** (South Med J 96:410, 2003)		
		For less severe disease: **Itraconazole** (300 mg bid po x3 d, then 200 mg bid x2 wks) or (400 mg qd x12 wks (85–90% response) then 200 mg qd (see footnote 3 page 79). **Not recommended for meningitis.** IV if unable to take po.	Liposomal Ampho B superior at 2 wks vs Ampho B (88% vs 64%) clinical success) in 81 patients with a diseas palatal, neph-rotoxicity (mostly v 37%). No difference in mortality after 10 additional weeks of itra in both arms (AnIM 137:105, 2002). **Itra (ACTG 120) 50/59 (85%) pts responded,** cleared fungemia with only 5% toxicity. Avoid concomitant rifampin, which reduces itra serum concentration (A/M 98:336, 1995). **Itra best drug for suppression at 200 mg qd x7 d/wk** had probable hepatic toxicity (A/DS & Human Retro 16:100, 1997. Flu less effective than itra & induces flu resistance (CID 33:1910, 2001).
Immunocompromised patient (AIDS) (CID 24:1195, 1997, & 32:1215, 2001) Recently reported following antitumor necrosis factor-α rx, infliximab (A/RCCM 167:1279, 2003)	**Lipid-based and Ampho B: Liposomal Ampho B** 3 mg/kg IV x14 d, then suppressive therapy with **itraconazole** 200 mg po qd (AnIM 137:435, 2002) **Ampho B** 0.5-1 mg/kg/d IV x7 d, followed by 0.8 mg/kg qod or (3x/wk) to total dose of 10-15 mg/kg, then suppressive therapy as above		Voriconazole IV superior of choice in Mexico, usually N. asteroides.
Madura foot (See Comments) (See Nocardia, Pseudallescheria boydii, below)	None, unless Nocardia (see below)	In U.S., usually Pseudallescheria boydii (Scedosporium apiosp.), usually Nocardia brasiliensis, in Japan, N. asteroides.	
Mucormycosis (Zygomycosis) = Rhizopus, Rhizomucor, Absidia	**Ampho B** Increase rapidly to 0.8–1.5 mg/kg IV, when improving, then qod. Total dose usually 2.5–3 gm	Treatment requires control of underlying condition, esp. diabetic ketoacidosis, neutropenia. Surgical debridement usually required and discontinue deferoxamine if applicable. Deferoxamine rx (risk of mucormycosis), use hydroxypyridinone chelators.	
Rhinocerebral, pulmonary (AnIM 159:1301, 1999)	**Lipid-based Ampho B.** **Azoles and caspofungin usually inactive**	[Ref:] AJRCCM 167:1279, 2003. Liposomal Ampho B 5mg/kg/d IV x for 5 days, then every 3-3.5 mg/kg/d x5-9 days Abelcet (ABLC) 5 mg/kg/d lipo-somal amphotericin successful in 2 cases (J Int 41:265, 2000). Itra which fallen under development (CID 36:1488,2003)	

[1] Drug name (trade name) & wholesale price for 15 gm. All are applied to affected area bid. **Prescription drugs:** butenafine (Mentax) $27, ciclopirox (Loprox) $14, clotrimazole (Lotrimin) $13, Mycelex $10), econazole (Spectazole) $13, ketoconazole (Nizoral) $18, miconazole (Monistat, Micatin) $13 (Micatin-S1), naftifine (Naftin) $17, oxiconazole (Oxistat) $14, sulconazole (Exelderm) $10, terconazole (Terazol) $9. **Non-prescription (over-the-counter):** clotrimazole (Lotrimin $5, Tinactin $5), miconazole (Micatin $5), tolnaftate (Tinactin $5, Ting or Tolnate $2), undecylenic acid (Cruex $5, Desenex $5), Lotrimin AT 1%, 12 gm $6.17, Lamisil AT 1%, 12 gm $6.79.

[2] **Oral solution preferred to tablets because of ↑ absorption** (see Table 11B, page 84).

From 2004 DRUG TOPICS RED BOOK. Medical Economics Data and Hospital Formulary Pricing Guide. **Price is average wholesale price (AWP).**

All dosage recommendations are for adults (unless otherwise indicated) and assume normal renal function

TABLE 11A (8)

TYPE OF INFECTION/ORGANISM/ SITE OF INFECTION	ANTIMICROBIAL AGENTS OF CHOICE		COMMENTS
	PRIMARY	ALTERNATIVE	
Nocardiosis (N. asteroides & N. brasiliensis). Culture & sensitivities may be valuable in refractory cases. Reference Labs, R.J. Wallace (903) 877-7660 or CDC (404) 639-3158 *JIDCP 8:27, 1999)*			
Cutaneous and lymphocutaneous (sporotrichoid)	TMP/SMX 5–10 mg/kg/d of TMP & 25–50 mg/kg/d of SMX IV, q.4 div. doses/d, po or IV	Sulfisoxazole 2 gm po q4 or Minocycline 100–200 mg po bid, successful in 6/6 cases	877-7660 or CDC (404) 639-3158 *JIDCP 8:27, 1999)*
Pulmonary, disseminated, brain abscess (Brain abscess: 3 mos for immuno-competent host (38%) & 6 mos. for immuno-compromised (62% organ transplant, malignancy, chronic lung disease, diabetes, ETOH use, steroid Rx, & AIDS).	TMP/SMX: Initially 15 mg/kg/d of TMP & 75 mg/kg/d of SMX IV or po, div. in 2–4 doses. After 3–4 wks. ↓ dose to 10 mg/kg/d of TMP in 2–4 doses po. Do serum levels per Comment	TMP/SMX: Initially 15 mg/kg/d of TMP & 75 mg/kg/d of SMX IV or po + amikacin 7.5 mg/kg IV q12h) x3–4 wks & then po regimen	Measure sulfonamide blood levels with sulfa-containing regimen used *(Medicine 88:38, 1999).* Survival may be improved when sulfa-containing regimen used *(Medicine 88:38, 1999).* Measure sulfonamide blood levels early to ensure absorption of po rx. Desire peak level of 100–150 µg/ml 2 hrs post-po dose.
Paracoccidioidomycosis (South American blastomycosis)/P. brasiliensis	Itraconazole 200 mg/d po x 6 months or Ketoconazole 400 mg/d po for 6–18 months	Ampho B 0.4–0.5 mg/kg/d IV to total dose of 1.5–2.5 gm or sulfonamides (dose: see Comment)	Improvement in >90% pts on itra or keto.NF94 Sulfa: 4–6 gm/d for several weeks, then 500 mg/d for 3–5 yrs also used *(CID 14(Supp):S68, 1992).* Low-dose itra (50–100 mg/d), keto (200–400 mg/d), & sulfadiazine (up to 6 mg/d) showed similar clinical responses in 4–6 mos. in a randomized study, 14/14, 14/14, 13/14 respectively *(Med Mycol 40:411, 2002).* HIV+1, TMP/SMX suppressive rx indefinitely *(CID 21:1275, 1995).* Terbinafine has good in vitro activity *(JCM 40:2828, 2002).*
Lobomycosis (keloidal blastomycosis)/ P. loboi	Surgical excision. clofazimine or ampho B		
Penicilliosis (Penicillium marneffei). Common disseminated fungal infection in AIDS pts in SE Asia *(resp. Thailand & Vietnam)* *(CID 24:1080, 1997; Int J Inf Dis 3:48, 1998)*	Ampho B 0.5–1 mg/kg/d x2 wks followed by Itraconazole 400 mg/d for 10 wks followed by 200 mg/d po indefinitely for HIV-infected pts *(CID 26:1107, 1998).* See Comment	Itra 200 mg po tid x3 d, then 200 mg po bid x12 wks, then 200 mg po qd. (IV if unable to take po)	3rd most common OI in AIDS pts following TBc and cryptococcal meningitis. Skin lesions resemble molluscum or TBc *(CID 23:125, 1996).* Rare reports without disseminated systemic cryptococcal infection or molluscum contagiosum). In AIDS pts long-term suppression with itra was effective in preventing relapses in 36/36 pts, whereas 20/35 pts receiving placebo relapsed within 6 mos. *(NEJM 339:1739, 1998).*
Phaeohyphomycosis (black molds) dematiaceous fungi) *(see CID 34:467, 2002)* Species. Scedosporium prolificans. Bipolaris, Wangiella, Exophiala, Exophiala, Phialemonium, Scytalidium, Alternaria, & others)	Surgery + itraconazole 400 mg po, duration not defined, probably 6 monthsNF94+	Voriconazole has some in vitro activity, but clinical experience limited to date vs S. prolificans *(AAC 45:2151, 2001).*	Notoriously resistant to antifungal drugs including amphotericin. In vitro voriconazole more active than itra *(J Clin Micro 39:954, 2001).* Case reports of successful rx of disseminated and CNS disease with voriconazole *(CID 31:1499 & 673, 2000; Clin Microbiol Inf 9:750, 2003; Eur J Clin Micro Inf Dis 20:107, 2001).*
		Itraconazole + terbinafine synergistic against S. prolificans *(AAC 44:470, 2000).* No clinical data but combination could show ↑ toxicity *(see Table 11B, page 84).*	
Pseudallescheria boydii (Scedosporium apiospermum) (not considered a true dematiaceous fungi) *(Med 81:333, 2002)* Skin, subcutaneous (Madura foot), brain abscess, recurrent meningitis	Voriconazole 200 mg po *(see Table 11B, page 84).* Surgery + itraconazole 200 mg IV q12h for 7 days then either (4 mg/kg IV q12h) or (200 mg po q12h for body weight ≥40 kg, but 100 mg po q12h for body weight <40 kg) *(PIDJ 21:240, 2002)*	Surgery + itraconazole 200 mg po bid until clinically well.NF94 (Many species now resistant or refractory to itra) or MiconazoleNF94 600 mg IV q8h	
Sporotrichosis *(CID 29:231, 1999; CID 30:684, 2000; CID 36:34, 2003; ID Clin N.A. 17:59, 2003)*			
Cutaneous/Lymphonodular	Itraconazole 100–200 mg/d solution po 3–6 mos. (then 200 mg po bid long-term for HIV-infected pts*)	Fluconazole 400 mg po qd x6 mos or Sat. soln. potassium iodide (SSKI). Start with 5–10 drops tid (in 5–10 drops (in H₂O). Start with 5–10 drops tid, gradually ↑ to 40–50 drops tid for 3–6 mos. Take after meals.	Ref. cit. *CID 17:210, 1993.* Some authorities use ampho B as primary. Mexican resistant strains reported *(AJM 95:279, 1993).* Itra rx for up to 24 months effective in multifocal osteoarticular infection *(CID 23: 394, 1996).* SSKI side-effects: nausea, rash, fever, metallic taste, salivary gland swelling.

† **Oral solution preferred to tablets because of ↑ absorption** *(see Table 11B, page 84).*

* From 2003 DRUG TOPICS RED BOOK, Medical Economics Data and Hospital Formulary Pricing Guide. **Price is average wholesale price (AWP).**

All dosage recommendations are for adults *(unless otherwise indicated) and assume normal renal function*

TABLE 11A (9)
ANTIMICROBIAL AGENTS OF CHOICE

TYPE OF INFECTION/ORGANISM/ SITE OF INFECTION	PRIMARY	ALTERNATIVE	COMMENTS
Sporotrichosis *(continued)*			
Osteoarticular, pulmonary, meningeal	**Osteoarticular, pulmonary: Itraconazole** 300 mg PO bid x6-12 mos. Then 200 mg po bid (long-term for HIV-infected pts) [IV if unable to take po]	**Disseminated, meningeal: Ampho B** 0.5 mg/kg/d to total of 1–2 gm, followed by **Itra** 200 mg bid or **flu** 800 mg qd	
Extracutaneous. Osteoarticular, pulmonary, disseminated, meningeal			

Abbreviations: **AM/CL** = amoxicillin clavulanate, **Ampho B** = amphotericin B. **Clot** = clotrimazole, **de** = discontinue, **Flu** = fluconazole, **Flucyt** = flucytosine, **G** = generic; **Griseo** = griseofulvin; **I** = investigational; **IMP** = imipenem; **IT** = intrathecal or intraventricular, **Itra** = itraconazole, **IUD** = intrauterine device, **IV** = intravenous, **keto** = ketoconazole, **NB** = name brand; **NFDA-I** = not FDA-approved indication; **NUS** = not available in the U.S.; **PSL** = peak serum level; **R/O** = rule out; **TMP/SMX** = trimethoprim/sulfamethoxazole, **vag. oint.** = vaginal ointment

TABLE 11B: ANTIFUNGAL DRUGS: ADVERSE EFFECTS, COMMENTS, COST

DRUG NAME, GENERIC (TRADE)/ USUAL DOSAGE/COST*	ADVERSE EFFECTS/ADVERSE EFFECTS, COMMENTS, COST
Non-lipid amphotericin B deoxycholate (Fungizone) 0.3–1 mg/kg/d as single infusion 50 mg $10 to 25	**Non-lipid amphotericin B (Fungizone)** **Admin.:** Commercial ampho B is a colloidal suspension that must be prepared in electrolyte-free D5W at 0.1 mg/ml to avoid precipitation. No need to protect drug suspensions from light. Ampho B infusions often cause chills/fever, myalgia, anorexia, nausea, rarely hypotension. Postulated due to release of proinflammatory cytokines but does not appear to be histamine release (*Pharmaco 23:966, 2003*). Manufacturer recommends a test dose of 1 mg, but often not done (1° have the 1st dose is a test dose). Duration of infusion usually 4 or more hrs. No difference found in 1- vs. 4-hr infusions (*AAC 34:1402, 1992; AJM 93:123, 1992*) except chills/fever occurred sooner with 1-hr infusion. Frequency and severity of febrile reactions decrease with repeated infusions (*CID 33:75, 2001*). Rare premedication reactions (severe dyspnea and rapid infiltrates suggesting pulmonary edema) appear to be associated with rapid infusion (*CID 33:75, 2001*).

Severe rigors respond to meperidine (25–50 mg IV). Premedication with acetaminophen, diphenhydramine, hydrocortisone (25–50 mg) and heparin (1000 units) had no influence on rigors/fevers (*CID 10:755, 1995*). If cytokine postulate correct, NSAIDs or high-dose steroids may prove efficacious but their use may risk worsening infection under iv or increase iv risk of nephrotoxicity (i.e., NSAIDs). Clinical side effects ↓ with ↑ age (*CID 26:334, 1998*).

Toxicity: Major concern is nephrotoxicity. Initially (1st day) by kaliuresis and hypokalemia, then fall in serum bicarbonate (may proceed to renal tubular acidosis), ↓ in renal erythropoietin and anemia, and rising BUN/serum creatinine. Hypomagnesemia may occur.

Can reduce risk of renal injury by **(a) pre- and post-infusion hydration with 500 ml saline (if clinical status will allow salt load)**, (b) avoidance of other nephrotoxins, e.g., radiocontrast, aminoglycosides, cis-platinum, (c) perhaps use of lipid prep of ampho B. Use of low-dose dopamine did not significantly reduce renal toxicity (*AAC 47:3139, 1998*). In a single randomized controlled trial of 80 neutropenic pts with refractory fever & suspected or proven invasive fungal infections, 24-hr **continuous infusion** compared to the classical dosing **rapid infusion** of 0.95 mg/kg/d over 4 hrs (p <0.02-0.0003) & appeared as effective as rapid infusion but in very few proven fungal infections (7 & 3, respectively) (*BMJ 322:1, 2001*). Continuous infusion also allows a dramatic ↑ in administered dosage without sig. toxicity [26% ↓ in max. serum Cr (p=0.0005) ↑↑ renal tolerance]. This is disturbing that this exciting observations have not led to controlled trials examining effectiveness at rapid infusion in rx of life-threatening fungal infections (*CID 36:952, 2003*). Await trials of efficacy in larger number of proven infections! |
Mixing ampho B with lipid emulsion results in precipitation and is discouraged (*Am. J. Health Pharm 52:1463, 1995*).	
Lipid-based ampho B products:[1]	**Ampho B lipid complex (ABLC) (Abelcet):** **Admin.:** Indicated for rx of invasive fungal infections in pts refractory or intolerant to non-lipid ampho B. Consists of ampho B complexed with 2 lipid bilayer ribbons. Compared to standard ampho B, larger volume of distribution, rapid blood clearance and high tissue concentrations (liver, spleen, lung). Dosage: **5** mg/kg/d as single infusion 2.5 mg/kg/hr; adult and ped. dose the same. Do NOT use an in-line filter. Do not dilute with saline solution or mix with other **drugs or electrolytes** (*CID 41:1297, 1997*).
Amphotericin B lipid complex (ABLC) (Abelcet): 5 mg/kg/d as single infusion 100 mg IV $206 ($575/350 mg)	
Lipid-based ampho B products *(con't)*:	**Toxicity:** Fever and chills in 14–18%; nausea 9%, vomiting 8%; serum creatinine ↑ in 11%; renal failure 5%, anemia 4%; ↓ K 5%; rash 4%

[1] Published data from patients intolerant of or refractory to conventional ampho B (Amp B d). **None of the lipid ampho B preps has shown superior efficacy compared to ampho B in prospective trials (except liposomal ampho B).** Liposomal ampho B was **more effective** than ampho B in rx of disseminated histoplasmosis at 2 wks (*AnIM 137:105, 2002; CID 37:415, 2003*). **Dosage equivalency has not been established** (*CID 36:1500, 2003*). Nephrotoxicity less with all lipid ampho B preps (*IDCP 7:516, 1998; CID 27:603, 1998; CID 26:1383, 1998*).

[2] Cost is >10-fold higher than standard ampho B. Differences in nephrotoxic side effects are of uncertain clinical significance. In one study, nephrotoxicity (↑ serum creatinine ≥2.0x) in some (59% vs 38%, p=0.05). Mild elevations in serum creatinine were observed in 1/3 of both (*BJ Hemat 103:198, 1998; Focus on Fungal Infect 9:20, 1999; Bone Marrow Tx 20:39, 1997; CID 26:1383, 1998*).

* From 2003 Drug Topics Red Book, Medical Economics Data and Hospital Formulary Pricing Guide. **Price is average wholesale price (AWP).**
All dosage recommendations are for adults (unless otherwise indicated) and assume normal renal function

TABLE 11B (2)

DRUG NAME, GENERIC (TRADE)/ USUAL DOSAGE/COST*	ADVERSE EFFECTS/COMMENTS
Liposomal amphotericin B (L-AmB, AmBisome): 1–5 mg/kg/d as single infusion 50 mg $196 ($1372/250 mg)	**Liposomal amphotericin B (AmBisome):** **Admin.:** Approved for empirical rx for presumed fungal infections in febrile neutropenic pts; rx of pts with aspergillus, candida and/or cryptococcus infections refractory to conventional ampho B, or in pts where renal impairment or unacceptable toxicity precludes the use of conventional ampho B; rx of visceral leishmaniasis; treatment of pts with aspergillosis, candidiasis and/or cryptococcosis who are intolerant to conventional ampho B. Dosage: **3–5 mg/kg** IV as single dose infused over a period of approx. 120 min. Infusion time can be reduced to 60 min.[1] 1 mg/kg was as effective as 4 mg/kg/d (6 mos. survival rates 43% vs 37%, respectively) in pts with invasive aspergillosis complicating bone marrow tx and/or neutropenia from malignancy (CID 27:1406, 1998). **Major toxicity:** Generally less than ampho B. Nephrotoxicity 18.7% vs 33.7% for ampho B, chills 47% vs 75%, nausea 39.7% vs 38.7%, vomiting 31.8% vs 43.9%, hypokalemia 20.4% vs 25.6%, ↑ K 20.4% vs 25.6%, ↓ Mg 20.4% vs 25.6%. Acute infusion-related reactions are common with liposomal ampho B: 20–40%. 86% occurred within 5 min. of infusion, including chest pain, dyspnea & hypoxia or severe abdominal, flank or leg pain; 14% developed flushing & urticaria near the end of 4-hr infusion. Reactions may be due to complement activation by the liposome (CID 36:1213, 2003).
Amphotericin B cholesteryl complex (amphotericin B colloidal dispersion, ABCD, Amphotec): 3–4 mg/kg/d as single infusion. 100 mg $160	**Ampho B cholesteryl complex (Amphotec):** **Admin.:** Approved for rx of aspergillosis in pts who either failed or were intolerant to standard ampho B. Consists of ampho B deoxycholate stabilized with cholesteryl sulfate resulting in a disc-shaped colloidal complex. Compared to standard ampho B, larger volume of distribution, rapid blood clearance, high tissue concentrations. Dosage: Initial dose for adults & children: **3–4 mg/kg/day.** If necessary, can ↑ to 6 mg/kg/day. Dilute in D5W & infuse at 1 mg/kg/hr. Do NOT use in-line filter. **Toxicity:** Chills 50%, fever 33%, ↑ serum creatinine 12–28%, ↓ Ca 6%, ↓ K 17%.
Caspofungin (Cancidas) 70 mg IV once, followed by 50 mg IV qd (reduce to 35 mg IV qd with moderate hepatic insufficiency) 70 mg $500, 50 mg $388 Ref.: In 362:1142, 2003	An echinocandin which inhibits synthesis of β-(1,3)-D-glucan, a critical component of fungal cell walls. Fungicidal against candida (MIC <2 μg/ml) including most resistant to other antifungals & active against aspergillus. Approved for rx of candidemia & other candida infections (peritonitis, intra-abdominal abscess, esophageal candidiasis, pleural space infection) & refractory aspergillosis & 48.9% successful in 57 pts with invasive aspergillosis infections in severely impaired hosts who had failed other antifungals. **Toxicity** remarkably non-toxic with no nephrotoxicity reported. Only 2% of 263 pts in double-blind trial discontinued drug due to drug-related adverse event (Transpl Inf Dis 1:25, 2002). 14% had ↑ transaminases (similar to triazoles). Most common adverse effect: pruritus at infusion site & headache, fever, chills, vomiting, & diarrhea in approx. 10% of pts. Class C for pregnancy (embryotoxic in rats & rabbits), so only of potential benefits outweigh risks. See Table 22, page 141 for drug-drug interactions, esp. cyclosporine (hepatic toxicity) & tacrolimus (drug level monitoring recommended) (Curr Med Res Opin 19:263, 2003; JAC 49:889, 2002).
Fluconazole (Diflucan) 100 mg tabs $8.54 150 mg tabs $13.60 200 mg tabs $13.98 400 mg IV $147.58 Oral suspension: 40 mg/ml, $126.98/35 ml bottle	IV → oral bease of excellent bioavailability. **Pharmacology:** absorbed po, water solubility enables IV. Peak serum levels (see Table 9, page 61). T½ 30 hrs (range 20–50 hrs). 12% protein bound. **CSF levels 50–90% of serum in normals.**[1] in meningitis. No effect on mammalian steroid metabolism. **Drug-drug interactions common, see Table 22.** Side-effects overall 16% (incidence common in HIV+ pts [21%]). Nausea 3.7%, skin rash 1.8%, lab abnormalities: ↑ SGOT 5%, ↑ SGPT 5%, vomiting 1.7%, abdominal pain 1.7%, diarrhea 1.5%. Rare: severe hepatotoxicity, exfoliative dermatitis. Anaphylaxis (CID 13:81, 1993), thrombocytopenia, leucopenia. Good reference: NEJM 330:263, 1994
Flucytosine (Ancobon) 500 mg (oral) tab $3.59	AEs: Overall 30%. GI 6% (diarrhea, anorexia, nausea, vomiting); hematologic: 22% [leucopenia, thrombocytopenia, when serum level > 100 μg/ml (esp. in azotemic pts)]; hepatotoxic [asymptomatic ↑ SGOT, reversible); skin rash 7%; aplastic anemia (rare–2 or 3 cases). False ↑ in serum creatinine on EKTACHEM analyzer (JAC 26:177, 1990).
Griseofulvin (Fulvicin, Grifulvin, Grisactin) 500 mg G $1.56, susp 125 mg/ml: 120 ml $6	Photosensitivity, urticaria, GI upset, fatigue, leucopenia (rare). Interferes with warfarin anticoagulation. Increases blood and urine porphyrins, should not be used in patients with porphyria. Minor disulfiram-like reactions. Exacerbation of systemic lupus erythematosus.
Imidazoles, topical For vaginal and/or skin use	Not recommended in 1st trimester of pregnancy. Local reactions: 0.5–1.5%: dyspareunia, mild vaginal or vulvar erythema, burning, pruritus, urticaria, rash. Rarely similar symptoms in sexual partner. Cost of treating vaginitis: miconazole x3 d $13, clotrimazole x7 d $12, miconazole x3 d $30, terconazole x3 d $34, tioconazole x1 dose $24. Oral agents preferred because of convenience, compliance, and cost. Fluconazole 150 mg po x1 dose $12

*From 2003 Drug Topics Red Book, Medical Economics Data and Hospital Formulary Pricing Guide. **Price is average wholesale price (AWP).**
All dosage recommendations are for adults (unless otherwise indicated) and assume normal renal/renal function

TABLE 11B (3)

DRUG NAME, GENERIC (TRADE)/ USUAL DOSAGE/COST*	ADVERSE EFFECTS/COMMENTS
Itraconazole (Sporanox) 100 mg cap $8.16 10 mg/ml oral solution (fasting state) (150 ml: $139) (AAC 42:1862, 1998) IV usual dose 200 mg bid x 4 doses then 200 mg qd for a maximum of 14 days ($21.19/250 mg)	**Itraconazole tablet and solution forms are not interchangeable, solution preferred.** Many authorities recommend measuring drug serum concentration after 2 wks on prolonged rx to ensured satisfactory absorption. To obtain the highest plasma concentration, the tablet is given with food and acidic drinks (e.g., Coca-Cola) while the solution is taken in the fasted state; under these conditions, the peak conc. of the capsule is approx. 3 μg/ml and of the solution 5.4 μg/ml. Peak levels are reached faster (2.2 vs 5 hrs) with the solution. **Peak plasma concentrations after IV injection (200 mg) compared to oral capsule (200 mg): 2.8 μg/ml (on day 7 of rx) vs 2 μg/ml (on day 36 of rx).** Protein-binding for both preparations is over 99%, which explains the virtual absence of penetration into the CSF. **Peak plasma concentrations after IV injection (200 mg) compared to oral capsule (200 mg):** Most common adverse effects are drug-related nausea 10%, diarrhea 8%, vomiting 6%, and abdominal discomfort 5.7%. Allergic rash 8.6%, ↑ bilirubin 6%, edema 3.5%, and hepatitis 2.7% reported. ↑ doses may produce hypokalemia 8% and ↑ blood pressure. Other concern, as with fluconazole and ketoconazole, is **drug-drug interactions; see Table 22.** Some interactions can be life-threatening. **Delirium reported** (Psychosomatics 44:260, 2003). **Reported to produce impairment in cardiac function** (see footnote 3 page 79)
Ketoconazole (Nizoral) 200 mg tab $4.00	Gastric acid required for absorption—cimetidine, omeprazole, antacids block absorption. In achlorhydia, dissolve tablet in 4 ml 0.2N HCl, drink with a straw. Coca-Cola ↑ absorption by 65% (AAC 39:1671, 1995). CSF levels "none." **Drug-drug interactions important, see Table 22. Some interactions can be life-threatening. Dose-dependent nausea and vomiting.** Rare hepatic toxicity (reversible) reported in about 1:10,000 exposed pts—usually after several days to weeks of exposure. Liver toxicity of hepatocellular type reported in about 1:10,000 exposed pts—usually after several days to weeks of exposure. At doses of ≥800 mg/d seen ↓ testosterone and plasma cortisol levels fall. With high doses, adrenal (Addisonian) crisis reported
Miconazole (Monistat IV) 200 mg IV vial—not available in U.S.	IV miconazole indicated in patient critically ill with Pseudallescheria boydii. Used in some centers as prophylaxis or in ↑ initial rx regimens in febrile neutropenic pts (AJM 86:81103, 1987; J Clin Onc 8:280, 1990). Very toxic due to vehicle needed to get drug into solution.
Nystatin (Mycostatin) 30 gm cream $28.52 500,000 u oral tab $0.36	Topical: virtually no adverse effects. Less effective than imidazoles and triazoles. PO: large doses give occasional GI distress and diarrhea.
Terbinafine (Lamisil) 250 mg tab $9.88	Rare cases (8) of idiosyncratic & symptomatic hepatic injury and more rarely liver failure leading to death or liver transplantation reported in pts receiving terbinafine for onychomycosis. Therefore, the rx is **not recommended** for pts with **chronic or active liver disease** although in patients with hepatotoxicity may occur in pts with or without pre-existing disease. Pretreatment screening of serum transaminase (ALT & AST) is advised & alternate rx used for those with abnormal levels. Pts started on terbinafine should be warned about symptoms suggesting liver dysfunction (persistent nausea, anorexia, fatigue, vomiting, RUQ pain jaundice, dark urine or pale stools). If symptoms develop, drug should be discontinued & liver function immediately evaluated. In controlled trials, changes in ocular lens and retina reported—clinical significance unknown. Major drug-drug interaction is 100% ↑ in rate of clearance by rifampin. AEs: usually mild; transient and rarely caused discontinuation of rx. % with AE: headache 2.7, rash 5.6 vs 2.2; taste abnormality 2.8 vs 0.7. Inhibits CYP2D6 enzymes (see Table 22).
Voriconazole (Vfend) IV: **Loading dose 6 mg/kg q12h x1** and IV, then **Maintenance dose 4 mg/kg q12h IV** for invasive aspergillus & serious mold infections; **3 mg/kg q12h IV** for less severe infections Oral: **>40 kg body weight:** 400 mg po q12h x1 d, then 200 mg po q12h **<40 kg body weight:** 200 mg po q12h x1 d, then 100 mg po q12h **Take oral dose 1 hour before or 1 hour after eating.** Reduce to ½ maintenance dose for moderate hepatic insufficiency. 50 mg tab $7.81; 200 mg tab $31.25, 200 mg IV $106.25	A unique triazole with enhanced activity against Aspergillus sp. (MIC 90 = 0.25–2 μg/ml), including Ampho resistant strains (A. terreus) (JCM 37:2343, 1999). Candida sp. (MIC 0.03–2 μg/ml but may be higher for some resistant sp.). Fusarium sp. (MIC 0.25–8) & various molds. Steady state serum levels reach 2.5–4 μg/ml. Effective in infections caused by slow including C. krusei & in ≥50% of invasive aspergillosis infections (N Engl J Med 347:408, 2002). Toxicity similar to other azole/triazoles requiring uncommon serious hepatic toxicity (hepatitis, cholestasis & fulminant hepatic failure, 4 cases after first dose), & possibly related to voriconazole concentration & liver enzyme tests (AST, ALT, alk phos, total bili) should be monitored during rx & drug dc'd if abnormalities develop. Rash reported in up to 20%, occ. photosensitivity & rare Stevens-Johnson, hallucinations, & anaphylactoid infusion reactions with fever and hypertension (Clin Eur Dermatol 26:648, 2001). **Approx. 30% experience a transient visual disturbance** following IV or po ("altered/enhanced visual perception", blurred or colored visual change or photophobia) within 30–60 minutes. These changes resolve within 30–60 min in patients with repeated doses (do not drive at night for outpatient rx). No persistence of effect reported. Cause unknown. In patients with CrCl <50, the intravenous vehicle (SBECD-sulfobutyl-ether-β cyclodextrin) may accumulate. Potential for drug-drug interactions high—see Table 22 (CID 36:630, 1087, 1122, 2003). **NOTE:** Not in urine in active form.

TABLE 12A: TREATMENT OF MYCOBACTERIAL INFECTIONS*

Tuberculin skin test (TST). Same as PPD *(MMWR 52/RR-2):15, 2003]*

Criteria for positive TST after 5 tuberculin units (intermediate PPD) read at 48–72 hours:

≥5 mm induration: + HIV, immunosuppressed, recent close contact
≥10 mm induration: < 15 mg prednisone/day, healing TBc on chest x-ray, recent close contact of potentially infectious cases, low income, IVDUsers, NH residents, chronic illness, silicosis
≥15 mm induration: countries with high prevalence; low income; otherwise healthy

Two-stage to detect sluggish positivity: if "+" PPD pos. but < 10 mm, repeat intermediate PPD in 1 week. Response to 2° PPD can also happen if pt received BCG in childhood.

BCG vaccine as child: if ≥10 mm induration, & from country with TBc, should be attributed to M. tuberculosis.
Routine anergy testing no longer recommended in HIV+ or HIV-negative patients *(JAMA 283:2003, 2000).*

CAUSATIVE AGENT/DISEASE	MODIFYING CIRCUMSTANCES	SUGGESTED REGIMENS	
		INITIAL THERAPY	CONTINUATION PHASE OF THERAPY
Mycobacterium tuberculosis tuberculosis exposure but TST negative (household members & other close contacts of potentially infectious cases)	Neonate—Rx essential	INH (10 mg/kg/day for 3 months)	Repeat tuberculin skin test (TST) in 3 mos. If mother's smear negative & infant's TST negative & chest x-ray (CXR) normal, stop INH. In UK, BCG is then given *(Ln 2:1479, 1990),* unless mother HIV+. If infant's repeat TST positive &/or CXR abnormal (hilar adenopathy &/or infiltrate), INH + RIF (10–20 mg/day) (or SM). Total rx 6 months. If mother is being rx because of possible exposure, 2nd PPD not indicated.
	Children <5 years of age—Rx indicated	As for neonate for 1st 3 months	If repeat TST at 3 months is negative, stop, if repeat TST positive, continue INH for total of 9 months. If INH not given initially, repeat TST at 3 mos. If positive rx with INH for 9 mos. *(see Category II below).*
	Older children & adults—Risk 2–4% 1st year	No rx	

CAUSATIVE AGENT/DISEASE	MODIFYING CIRCUMSTANCES	SUGGESTED REGIMENS	
		INITIAL THERAPY	ALTERNATIVE
II. Treatment of latent infection with M. tuberculosis (formerly known as "prophylaxis") *(AJRCCM 161:S221, 2000; NEJM 347:1860, 2002).*	(1) + tuberculin reactor & HIV + (risk of active disease 10%/yr, AIDS 170x.)	INH (5 mg/kg/day; maximum 300 mg) for adults. 10 mg/kg/day for children. May use twice-weekly INH with DOT *(MMWR 52:735, 2003).* If HIV+ & CD4 < 200 or if oral candidiasis includes children, HIV–, HIV+, older, fibrotic lesions on chest x-ray. In some cases, 6 mos. may be given for cost-effectiveness *(AJRCCM 161:S221, 2000).* Do not use 6 mo. regimen in HIV+ persons <18 yrs old, or those with fibrotic lesions on chest film *(NEJM 345:189, 2001).*	If compliance problem: **INH by DOT 15 mg/kg 2x/wk x9 mos.** 2-month **RIF + PZA** regimen effective in HIV– and HIV+ *(AJRCCM 161:S221, 2000; JAMA 283:1445, 2000).* **However, there are recent descriptions of severe & fatal hepatitis in pts on RIF + PZA** *(MMWR 52:735, 2003).* Therefore, this regimen is no longer recommended for LTBI *(MMWR 52:735, 2003).*
A. INH indicated due to high-risk Assumes INH susceptibility likely highly effective in preventing active TB for ≥20 years.	(2) Newly infected persons (TST conversion within 2 yrs) (3) Past tuberculosis, not rx with adequate chemotherapy (INH, RIF, or alternatives) (4) + tuberculin reactors with CXR consistent with non-progressive tuberculous disease (risk 0.5–5.0%/yr)		RIF 600 mg/d po for 4 mos. (HIV– and HIV+).
	(5) + tuberculin reactors with other specified predisposing conditions: illicit injection drug use *(MMWR 38:236, 1989),* silicosis, diabetes mellitus, prolonged adrenocorticoid rx (>15 mg prednisone/day), immunosuppressive rx, hematologic diseases (Hodgkin's, leukemia), end-stage renal disease, clinical condition with substantial rapid weight loss or chronic under-nutrition, previous gastrectomy *(AARD 134: 355, 1986).*		
* NOTE: For HIV, see SANFORD GUIDE TO HIV/AIDS THERAPY and/or MMWR 48:RR-10, 1999			

CAUSATIVE AGENT/DISEASE	MODIFYING CIRCUMSTANCES	SUGGESTED REGIMENS		
		INITIAL THERAPY	ALTERNATIVE	COMMENTS
B. TST (reactor (organisms likely to be INH-susceptible)	Age no longer considered modifying factor (see Comments)	**INH** 5 mg/kg/day, max. 300 mg/d for adults; 10 mg/kg/day for children. Results with 6 mos. rx not quite as effective as 12 mos. (65% vs 0.14 reduction in disease); 9 mos. is current recommendation. See II.A above for details and alternate rx.		Reanalysis of earlier studies favors **INH** prophylaxis (if INH related, hepatitis case fatality rate <1% and TB case fatality ≤8.7%, which appears to be the case) *(AJM 152:2517, 1990).* Recent data suggest nausea benefit too. Cost-effectiveness also favors **INH** prophylaxis *(AJM 127: 1051, 1997).* Overall risk of hepatotoxicity 0.1–0.15% *(JAMA 281:1014, 1999).*

See pages 90 & 92 for all footnotes and abbreviations

* Dosages are for adults (unless otherwise indicated) and assume normal renal/renal function

* See pages 90, 91 and 92 for footnotes and abbreviations

DOT = directly observed therapy

TABLE 12A (2)

II. Treatment of latent infection with M. tuberculosis ("prophylaxis") TST positive (organisms likely to be susceptible) (continued)

CAUSATIVE AGENT/DISEASE	MODIFYING CIRCUMSTANCES	SUGGESTED REGIMENS — INITIAL THERAPY	ALTERNATIVE	COMMENTS
	Pregnancy—Any risk factors (II.A above)	Treat with INH as above. For women who are HIV+ or who have been recently infected, rx should not be delayed even during the first trimester.		Risk of INH hepatitis may be ↑: those who are HIV+ or who [AJRCCM 149:1359, 1994; 161:199, 1995].
	Pregnancy—No risk factors	No initial rx (see Comment)		Delay rx until after delivery [AJRCCM 161:1359, 1996]. IDSA guideline lists rifabutin at 300 mg/d dose as another alternative; however, current recommended max. dose of rifabutin is 300 mg/d.
C. TST positive & drug resistance likely (For data on worldwide prevalence of drug resistance, see NEJM 344:1294, 2001; JID 185:1197, 2002)	INH-resistant (or adverse reaction to INH), RIF-sensitive organisms likely	RIF 600 mg/d po for 4 mos. (HIV+ or HIV−)		Estimate that rifabutin alone has protective effect of 56%; 26% of pts reported adverse effects (only 2/157 did not complete 6 mos. rx) [AJRCCM 155:1735, 1997].
	INH- and RIF-resistant organisms likely	Efficacy of all regimens unproven [PZA 25-30 mg/kg/d to max. of 2 gm/d + ETB 15-25 mg/kg/d po) x6–12 mos.	[(PZA 25-30 mg/kg/d to max. of 2.0 gm/d) + (levofloxacin 500 mg/d or oflox 500 mg/d or oflox 400 mg)] all po, x6–12 mos.	PZA + oflox has been associated with asymptomatic hepatitis [CID 24:1264, 1997].

SUGGESTED REGIMENS

SEE COMMENTS FOR DOSAGE AND DIRECTLY OBSERVED THERAPY (DOT) REGIMENS (in vitro susceptibility known)

CAUSATIVE AGENT/DISEASE	MODIFYING CIRCUM-STANCES	INITIAL PHASE[a] — Regimen[1]	Drugs	Interval/doses[2,3] (min. duration)	CONTINUATION PHASE OF THERAPY[b] — Regimen[1]	Drugs	Interval/Doses[2,3] (min. duration)	Range of Total Doses (min. duration)
III. Mycobacterium tuberculosis — A. Pulmonary TB (General reference on rx in adults & children: Ln 362:887-899; MMWR 52(RR-11):1, 2003) Isolation essential: Pts with active TB should be isolated in single rooms, not cohorted. Older observations on infectivity of susceptible & resistant M. tbc before and after rx [ARRD 85:511, 1962] the HIV+ individual. Extended isolation may be appropriate. DOT regimens recommended if possible [JAMA 279:943, 1998] (continued on next page)	Rate of INH resistance known to be <4% (drug-susceptible organisms) [Modified from MMWR 52(RR-11):1, 2001]	1	INH RIF PZA ETB	7 d/wk x56 doses (8 wk) or 5 d/wk x40 doses (8 wk)*	1a	INH/RIF	7 d/wk x126 doses (18 wk) or 5 d/wk x90 doses (18 wk)*	182-130 doses (26 wk)
					1b	INH/RIF	2x/wk x36 doses (18 wk)	92-76 [26 wk]
					1c*	INH/RIF	1x/wk x18 doses (18 wk)	74-58 [26 wk]
					1c*	INH/RFP	1x/wk x18 doses (18 wk)	62-58 [26 wk]
		2	INH RIF PZA ETB	7 d/wk x14 doses (2 wk), then 2x/wk x12 doses (6 wk) or 5 d/wk x10 doses (2 wk) then 2x/wk x12 doses (6 wk)*	2a	INH/RIF	2x/wk x36 doses (18 wk)	62-58 [26 wk]
					2b*	INH/RFP	1x/wk x18 doses (18 wk)	44-40 [26 wk]
		3	INH RIF PZA ETB	3x/wk x24 doses (8 wk)	3a	INH/RIF	3x/wk x54 doses (18 wk)	78 [26 wk]
		4	INH RIF ETB	7 d/wk x56 doses (8 wk) or 5 d/wk x40 doses (8 wk)*	4a	INH/RIF	7 d/wk x217 doses (31 wk) or 5 d/wk x155 doses (31 wk)*	273-195 [39 wk]
					4b	INH/RIF	2x/wk x62 doses (31 wk)	118-102 [39 wk]

COMMENTS

Regimen[c]	Dose in mg/kg (max. daily dose)					
	INH	RIF	PZA	ETB	SM	RFB
Daily: Child	10-20 (300)	10-20 (600)	15-30 (2000)	15-25	20-40 (1000)	10-20 (300)
Adult	5 (300)	10 (600)	15-30 (2000)	15-25	15 (1000)	5 (300)
2x/wk (DOT): Child	20-40 (900)	10-20 (600)	50-70 (4000)	50	25-30 (1500)	—
Adult	15 (900)	10 (600)	50-70 (4000)	50	25-30 (1500)	NA
3x/wk (DOT): Child	20-40 (900)	10-20 (600)	50-70 (3000)	25-30	25-30 (1500)	NA
Adult	15 (900)	10 (600)	50-70 (3000)	25-30	25-30 (1500)	NA

Second-line anti-TB agents can be dosed as follows to facilitate DOT: Cycloserine 500-750 mg qd (5x/wk) po; Ethionamide 500-750 mg qd (5x/wk) po; Kanamycin or capreomycin 15 mg/kg qd (3-5x/wk) IM/IV; Ciprofloxacin 750 mg qd (5x/wk) po; Ofloxacin 600-800 mg qd (5x/wk) po; Levofloxacin 750 mg qd (5x/wk) po [CID 21:1245, 1995].

Risk factors for drug-resistant TB: Recent immigration from Latin America or Asia or living in area of >4% 1° resistance (>4%) or previous rx without RIF: exposure to known MDR TB. Incidence of MDR TB in U.S. appears to have stabilized and may be slightly decreasing [NEJM 338:1641, 1998]; however, primary drug resistance is particularly high (>25%) in parts of the former Soviet Union, Russia, Estonia & Latvia [NEJM 344:1294, 2001; NEJM 347:1850, 2002].

(continued on next page)

* Dosages are for adults (unless otherwise indicated) and assume normal renal/renal function   † DOT = directly observed therapy

See pages 90 & 92 for all footnotes and abbreviations

TABLE 12A (3)

CAUSATIVE AGENT/DISEASE	MODIFYING CIRCUM-STANCES	SUGGESTED REGIMEN*	DURATION OF TREATMENT (mo.)*	SPECIFIC COMMENTS*	COMMENTS
III. Mycobacterium tuberculosis A. Pulmonary TB (continued from previous page) REFERENCE: CID 22:683, 1996	INH (± SM) resistance	RIF, PZA, ETB (an FQ may strengthen the regimen for pts with extensive disease). Emergence of FQ resistance is a concern (LnID 3:432, 2003)	6	In British Medical Research Council trials, 6-mo. regimens have yielded >95% success rates despite resistance to INH if 4 drugs were used in the initial phase & INH + ETB or SM was used throughout the 6 mos. (ARRD 136:1339, 1987). FQs were not employed in BMRC studies, but may strengthen the regimen for pts with more extensive disease. INH should be stopped in cases of INH resistance [see AnIM 52:1781, 1/1/11, 2003]	(continued from previous page) For MDR TB, consider rifabutin (~30% RIF-resistant strains are rifabutin-susceptible). Note that CIP not as effective as INH or RIF in one TB regimen for susceptible TB (CID 22:287, 1996). Gatifloxacin and levofloxacin have enhanced activity compared with CIP against M. tuberculosis (AAC 46:1022, 2002). Linezolid has excellent in vitro activity, including MDR strains (AAC 47:416, 2003). Mortality reviewed: Ln 349:71, 1997. Rapid (24-hr) diagnostic tests for M. tuberculosis: (1) The Amplified Mycobacterium tuberculosis Direct Test amplifies and detects M. tuberculosis ribosomal RNA; (2) The AMPLICOR Mycobacterium tuberculosis Test amplifies and detects DNA. Both tests have sensitivities and specificities >95% in sputum samples that are AFB-positive. In negative smears, specifically AFB-positive, sensitivity remains >95% but sensitivity is 40–77% (Am J Crit Care Med 155:1497, 1997). Note that MDR may grow out on standard blood agar plates in 1–2 wks (JClin 41:1710, 2003).
Multidrug-Resistant Tuberculosis (MDR TB): Defined as resistant to at least 2 drugs. Pt clusters with high mortality (AnIM 118:17, 1993).	Resistance to INH & RIF (± SM)	FQ, PZA, ETB, ± alternative agent*	18–24	In such cases, extended tx is needed to ↓ the risk of relapse. In cases with extensive disease, the use of an additional agent (alternative agents) may be prudent to ↓ the risk of failure & additional acquired drug resistance. Resectional surgery may be appropriate. Use the first-line agents to which the organism is susceptible. Add 2 or more alternative agents in case of extensive disease. Surgery should be considered.	
	Resistance to INH, RIF (± SM), & ETB or PZA	FQ, ETB or PZA (if active), IA, & 2 alternative agents*	24		
	Resistance to RIF	INH, ETB, FQ, supplemented with PZA for the first 2 mos. (an IA may be included for pts with extensive disease)	12–16	Daily & 3x/wk regimens of INH, PZA, & SM given for 9 mos. were effective in a BMRC trial (ARRD 115:727, 1977). However, extended use of an IA may not be feasible. It is not known if ETB would be as effective as SM in this regimen. An isoniazid regimen x12–18 mos. should be effective. But for more extensive disease &/or to shorten duration (e.g. 9–12 mos.), an IA may be added in the initial 2 mos. of rx.	

CAUSATIVE AGENT/DISEASE; MODIFYING CIRCUMSTANCES	SUGGESTED REGIMENS		COMMENTS
	INITIAL THERAPY	CONTINUATION PHASE OF THERAPY (in vitro susceptibility known)	
B. Extrapulmonary TB	INH + RIF (or RFB) + PZA daily x2 weeks Authors add pyridoxine 25–50 mg po daily to regimens that include INH.	INH + ETB when susceptibility to INH and RIF established. See Table 9C, page 61, for CSF drug penetration.	6-month regimens probably effective. Most experience with 9–12 month regimens. Am Acad Ped (1994) recommends 6 mos. rx for pulmonary tuberculosis. IDSA recommends 6 mos. for meningitis, miliary, bone/joint. DOT useful here as well as for pulmonary tuberculosis. Pediatric & disseminated disease, genitourinary may require 9–12 mos. rx, 6–9 mos. for lymph node, pleural, pericardial, peritoneal TBc. Bone & joint, CNS (including brain) TBc. Corticosteroids "strongly recommended" only for pericarditis & meningeal TBc (MMWR 52:RR-11/1, 2003).
C. Tuberculous meningitis For critical appraisal of adjunctive steroids: CID 25:872, 1997	INH + RIF + PZA ETB + PZA	INH + RIF + ETB for 9 months	3 drugs often recommended for initial rx. May substitute ethionamide (Pediatrics 99:226, 1997). Dexamethasone (for 1st month) has been shown to ↓ complications & diagnostic sensitivity and provides rapid dx (Neuro M3:2228, 1995; Arch Neurol 53:771, 1996).
D. Tuberculosis during pregnancy	INH + RIF + ETB		PZA not recommended (teratogenicity data inadequate. Because of potential ototoxicity to fetus throughout gestation (16%), SM should not be used unless other drugs contraindicated. Add pyridoxine 25 mg/kg/d for pregnant women on INH. Breast-feeding safe (MMWR 52:RR-11/1, 2003).
E. Treatment failure or relapse: Usually due to poor compliance or resistant organisms (AJM 102:164, 1997).	Directly observed therapy (DOT). Check susceptibilities. (See section III.A, page 86, above.)		Patient's whose sputum has not converted after 5–6 mos. = treatment failures. Failures may be due to non-compliance or resistant organisms. Check susceptibilities on current isolates. Non-compliance common, therefore institute DOT. If isolates show resistance, modify regimen to include at least 2 effective agents, preferably ones which patient has not received. Surgery may be necessary. In HIV+ pts, reinfection is a possible explanation for "failure"

See pages 90 & 92 for all footnotes and abbreviations   * Dosages are for adults (unless otherwise indicated) and assume normal renal function   **DOT = directly observed therapy

TABLE 12A (4)

CAUSATIVE AGENT/DISEASE	MODIFYING CIRCUMSTANCES	SUGGESTED REGIMENS		COMMENTS
		PRIMARY	ALTERNATIVE	

III. Mycobacterial tuberculosis (continued)

CAUSATIVE AGENT/DISEASE	MODIFYING CIRCUMSTANCES	SUGGESTED REGIMENS PRIMARY/ALTERNATIVE	COMMENTS
F. HIV infection or AIDS—pulmonary or extrapulmonary (NOTE: 60–70% of HIV+ pts have extrapulmonary TB)		**INH + RIF** (or **RFB**) daily x4 months (total 6 mos). May treat up to 9 mos. in pts with delayed response. (Authors add **pyridoxine** 25–50 mg daily to regimens that include INH)	1. Because of the possibility of developing resistance to RIF in pts with low CD4 cell counts who receive weekly or biweekly doses of RFB, it is recomm. that such pts receive daily (or minimally 3x/ weekly) doses of RFB for initiation & continuation phase of rx (MMWR 51:214, 2002). 2. Clinical and microbiologic response same as in HIV-negative patient although there is considerable overlap in outcomes among currently available studies (CID 32:623, 2001). 3. Post-treatment suppression not necessary among patients with durable response. 4. Rate of INH resistance known to be <4% for [1] rates of resistance see Section III.A. 5. For more information, see MMWR 47(RR-20):1, 1998; CID 28:139, 1999; MMWR 52(RR-11):1, 2003 6. May use partially intermittent therapy: 1 dose/day for 2 weeks, then 2-3 doses/week for 24 weeks (MMWR 47(RR-20):1, 1998)
Concomitant protease inhibitor (PI) therapy (Modified from MMWR 49:185, 2000)		**Initial & cont. therapy:** Use **(nelfinavir** 1250 mg bid) or (**indinavir** 800 mg q8h) as the PI component of antiretroviral rx. **INH + SM + PZA** x2 mos., then **INH + SM** q wk for 7 mos. **INH + rifabutin** 150 mg + **PZA** mg/kg + **ETB** 15 (mg/kg) all po daily for 2 mos., then **INH + rifabutin** for 4–7 mos.	**Comments:** Rifamycins induce cytochrome CYP450 enzymes (RIF> RFB > RFP) & reduce serum levels of concomitantly administered PIs. Conversely, PIs (ritonavir > amprenavir > indinavir = nelfinavir > saquinavir) inhibit CYP450 & cause ↑ serum levels of RIF, RFP & RFB. If dose of RFB is not reduced, toxicity ↑. **Do not use RIF + PI.** RIF/PI combinations are therapeutically effective but PI blood levels may be high & unpredictable. If RFB is reduced to 150 mg q24h or 300 mg 2–3 times/wk, there is no effect on nelfinavir levels at dose of 1250 mg/day (Can J ID 10:21B, 1999). **Alternative regimen:** (See ATS Consensus: AJRCCM 152:51, 1997; IDC No. Amer., March 2002; CMR 15:716, 2002)

IV. Other Mycobacterial Disease ("Atypical") (See ATS Consensus: AJRCCM 152:51, 1997; IDC No. Amer., March 2002; CMR 15:716, 2002)

CAUSATIVE AGENT/DISEASE	MODIFYING CIRCUMSTANCES	SUGGESTED REGIMENS PRIMARY	ALTERNATIVE	COMMENTS
A. M. bovis	Only fever (>38.5°C) for 12–24 hrs. Systemic illness or sepsis	**INH + RIF + ETB**		Infection includes M. bovis. All isolates resistant to PZA. 9–12 months of rx used by some authorities. Isolation not required.
B. Bacillus Calmette-Guerin (BCG) (derived from M. bovis)		**INH** 300 mg x6 months		Intravesical BCG effective in superficial bladder tumors and carcinoma in situ. Adverse effects: fever 2.9%, granulomatosis, pneumonitis, hepatitis 0.7%, sepsis 0.4% (J Urol 147:596, 1992). With sepsis, consider brief adjunctive prednisolone. Resistant to PZA.
C. M. avium-intra-cellulare complex (MAC, MAI or Battey bacillus) disseminated disease (subcutaneous, pulmonary, bone) *Excellent rev.: AJM 102 (5C):1, 1997* ATS Consensus Statement: AJRCCM 156:51, 1997 *Clin Chest Med 23:633, 2002*	**Immunocompetent patients** with chronic pulmonary disseminated disease (subcutaneous, bone)	**(INH** 300 mg) + (RIF 600 mg) + **ETB** x6 mos. **Clarithro** 500 mg po bid or **azithro** 500 mg mg po qd x2 mos., then 15 mg/kg. Add **SM** or **AMK** mg po qd or bid. Then 250 mg po qd x3 mos. or 1200 mg po as effective. May also qd or 500 mg po qd (until clar. then 250 mg po qd x3 mos. resist. improv.). Rx until culture neg. x1 yr. Alternative: **Clarithro** 500 mg po qd + **ETB** 15–25 (mg/kg) qd + **RFB** 300 mg po qd for up to 24 mos. (Curr Int Dis Repts 2:193, 2000; CID 32:1547, 2001).		"Classic" pulmonary MAC: Men 50–75, smokers, COPD. May be associated with hot tub use (Clin Chest Med 23:675, 2002). "New" pulmonary MAC: Women 50–70, scoliosis, mitral valve prolapse, pectus excavatum ("Lady Windermere syndrome"). MAC can be associated with interferon gamma deficiency (NEJM 335:1956, 1941; 335:1956, 1992). Susceptibility testing of MAC not recommended except clarithro testing of isolates from pts who have failed prior clarithro. Clarithro + RFB shown effective for cervical adenitis in children (J Peds 128:383, 1996). 3x/wk azithro (600 mg po), ETB (25 mg/kg po), RFB (300 mg po), & rifab 2x/wk SM may be as effective as 5x/wk regimen (patients >1.2 × 10⁵ CD4/mm³) (CID 37:1234, 2003). Late relapses" (following completion of therapy) after treatment with clarithro or azithro in pts with nodular bronchiectasis usually represent reinfection, not failure of rx (CID 186:266, 2002). Combination of clarithro + ETB + RFB effective in mouse model (AID 187:1977, 2003).
	Immunocompromised **Primary prophylaxis**—Pt's CD4 count <50–100/mm³. Discontinue when CD4 count increases to >100/mm³ in response to HAART (CID 34: 662, 2002). Guideline: AnIM 137-435, 2002	**PRIMARY** **Azithro** 1200 mg po weekly OR **Clarithro** 500 mg po bid	**ALTERNATIVE** **RFB** 300 mg po qd OR **Azithro** 1200 mg po weekly + **RIF** 300 mg po qd	RFB reduces MAC infection rate by 55% (no survival benefit); Azithro by 69% (30% survival benefit). RFB + RFB more effective than either alone but not as well tolerated (NEJM 335:392, 1996). Azithro + RFB more effective than either alone but not as well tolerated (NEJM 335:392, 1996). Many drug–drug interactions (see Table 22, pages 143, 144, 145. RFB ↑ metabolism of ZDV with 32% ↓ in AUC. Clarithro ↑ blood levels of non-sedating antihistamines with attendant risk of arrhythmias. Drug-drug interactions of rifamycins & important in whom HAART used (CID 28:419, 1999). Need to be sure no active M. tbc (NEJM 335:384 & 428, 1996). Clarithro prophylaxis & in 11% of pts on azithro but has not been observed with RFB prophylaxis (CID 27:807, 1998). Clarithro resistance may promote selection of rifamycin-resistant M. tbc

See pages 90 & 92 for all footnotes and abbreviations

Dosages are for adults (unless otherwise indicated) and assume normal renal function   †DOT = directly observed therapy

TABLE 12A (5)

CAUSATIVE AGENT/DISEASE; MODIFYING CIRCUMSTANCES	SUGGESTED REGIMENS PRIMARY	ALTERNATIVE	COMMENTS
IV. Other Mycobacterial Disease ("Atypical") *(continued)*			
C. M. avium-intracellulare complex *(continued)*			
Immunocompromised pts *(continued)*	**(**Claritthro 500 mg* po bid or azithro 600 mg po qd) **+** ETB 15–25 mg/kg **+** RFB 300 mg po qd	**(**Clarithro 500 mg* po bid or azithro 600 mg po qd) **+** ETB + RFB + one or more (Cipro 750 mg po bid or Oflox 400 mg po qd or Amikacin 7.5–15 mg/kg IV q24h)	Median time to neg. blood culture: clarithro + ETB 4.4 wks vs azithro + ETB >16 wks. At 16 wks, clearance of bacteremia seen in 37.5% of azithro- & 85.7% of clarithro-treated pts (*CID 27:1278, 1998*). More effective with ETB (*CID 31:1245, 2000*). Addition of clarithro (56%) at 24 wks when combined with ETB (*CID 31:1245, 2000*). Addition of RFB to clarithro + ETB → emergence of resistance to clari but has no effect on rate of survival (*CID 28:1080, 1999*). Data on clofazimine difficult to assess; Earlier study suggested ↓ survival (*CID 25:1063, 1996*).
Treatment presumptive dx or after positive blood, marrow, or other usually sterile body fluids, e.g., -- liver	**Higher doses of clari (1000 mg po bid) may be associated with ↑ mortality** (*CID 29:125, 1999*).		Combination of clari + azithro not recommended. Ref: *AnIM 121:905, 1994*. To avoid RFB toxicity, reduce RFB to 300 mg. Recurrences almost universal without chronic suppression. However, in patients on HAART with robust CD4 cell increase, may be possible to discontinue chronic suppression (*JID 178:1446, 1998; NEJM 340:1205, 1999*).
Chronic post-treatment suppression—secondary prophylaxis	**Always necessary.** (Clarithro or azithro) + ETB (lower dose to RFB 15 mg/kg/d (dosage above)	Clarithro or azithro or RFB (dosage above)	Isolated from pulmonary lesions and blood in pts with pulm. disease. Rx similar to RIF (and MAC). Susceptibilities similar to MAC, but highly resistant to RIF (*CID 24:140, 1997*).
D. Mycobacterium celatum	Regimen(s) not defined	May be susceptible to clarithro, FQ (*Clin Microbiol H 3:582, 1997*). Resistant to RIF (*AnIM 38:175, 1994*). Most reported cases resistant to RIF (*CID 24:144, 1997*). Easily confused with *M. tuberculosis* & may be highly resistant to RIF (*CID 24:140, 1997*).	
E. Mycobacterium chelonae/abscessus **Mycobacterium chelonae ssp. chelonae**	Treatment: Surgical excision may facilitate clarithro rx in subcutaneous abscess and is important adjunct to rx (*CID 24:1147, 1997*).	Clarithro 500 mg po bid x6 mos. (*AnIM 119:482, 1993; CID 24:1147, 1997; E.CMID 19:43, 2000*). Amik may also be effective. For serious disseminated infections add tobramycin + IMP for 1* 2–6 wks (*CMR 15:716, 2002*).	*M. abscessus* susceptible to AMK (70%), cefoxitin (95%), clarithro (95%). Single isolates of *M. abscessus* often not associated with disease. Clarithro-resistant strains now described (*JCCM 39:2745, 2001*). *M. chelonae* sensitive to tobramycin (100%), clarithro (100%), IMP (60%), gatifloxacin (90%), moxifloxacin (90%). Resistant to cefoxitin, FQ (*AAC 46:3283, 2002; AJRCCM 156:S1, 1997*).
F. Mycobacterium fortuitum	Treatment: optimal regimen not defined. Surgical excision of infected areas.	**AMK + cefoxitin + probenecid** 2–6 weeks, then (po TMP/SMX or doxycycline 2–6 mos. (*JID 152:50, 1985*). Usually responds to 6–12 mos. of oral rx with 2 drugs to which is susceptible (*AJRCCM 156:S1, 1997*).	**Resistant to all standard anti-TBc drugs.** Sensitive in vitro to doxycycline, minocycline, cefoxitin, IMP, AMK, TMP/SMX, CIP, ofloxz, azithro, clarithro, gatifloxacin (AAC 46:3283, 2002), linezolid (AAC 47:1736, 2003), with neomacrolides (clarithro, azithro) moxifloxacin (AAC 36:180, 1992), but may be resistant to azithromycin, rifabutin (AAC 39:567, 1997).
G. Mycobacterium haemophilum	Regimen(s) not defined in animal model, **clarithro + rifabutin** effective (*AAC 39:2316, 1995*). Combination of CIP + RFB + clarithro reported effective but clinical experience limited (*CMR 9:435, 1996*). Surgical debridement may be necessary (*CID 26:505, 1998*).		Clinical: Ulcerating skin lesions, synovitis, osteomyelitis. Lab: Requires supplemented media to isolate. Sensitive in vitro to: CIP, cycloserine, rifabutin. Over ½ resistant to: INH, ETB, PZA (*AnIM 120:118, 1994*).
H. Mycobacterium genavense	Regimens used include 2 or more of: **RIF, RFB, ETB, clofazimine, clarithro & amikacin.** Either RIF + RFB & RFB (& to reduce Lab) shown effective in reducing bacterial counts; CIP not effective (*JAC 42:483, 1998*).		Clinical: Dissem. MAC-like illness. Risk factor: CD4 <50. Symptoms of fever, weight loss, diarrhea. Lab: Subcultures grow only on Middlebrook 7H11 agar containing 2 μg/ml mycobactin J—growth still insufficient in 1 month with ≥2 drugs (*Arch Int Med 155:400, 1995*). Growth in BACTEC vials slow (mean 42 days). Survival ↑ from 81 to 263 days in pts tx for at least 1 month with ≥2 drugs (*CMR 15:716, 2002*).
I. Mycobacterium gordonae	Regimen(s) not defined, but consider **RIF + ETB + KM + CIP** (*CID 14:1229, 1992*). Surgical excision.		In vitro: sensitive to ETB, RIF, AMK, CIP, clarithro, linezolid (*AAC 47:1736, 2003*). Resistant to INH (*JCM 29:1667, 1994*).

See pages 90 & 92 for all footnotes and abbreviations

* Dosages are for adults (unless otherwise indicated) and assume normal renal function
RIF = rifampin, RFB = rifabutin, INH = isoniazid, ETB = ethambutol, PZA = pyrazinamide, CIP = ciprofloxacin, FQ = fluoroquinolone, AMK = amikacin, KM = kanamycin, TMP/SMX = trimethoprim/sulfamethoxazole, CLO = clofazimine, DOT = directly observed therapy

TABLE 12A (6)

CAUSATIVE AGENT/DISEASE; MODIFYING CIRCUMSTANCES	SUGGESTED REGIMENS		COMMENTS
	PRIMARY	ALTERNATIVE	
IV. Other Mycobacterial Disease			
J. Mycobacterium kansasii	"Atypical" (continued) Daily po: **INH** (300 mg) + **RIF** (600 mg) + **ETB** (15 mg/kg/d) x2 mos, then 15 mg/kg/d for 18 mos. Rx until culture-neg. sputum x12 mos; 15 mos. if HIV+ pt.) (See Comment)	If RIF-resistant: daily po: **INH** (900 mg) + **sulfamethoxazole** (1.0 gm three times/day) + **ETB** (50 mg/kg/d three times/wk) + **sulfamethoxazole** (3.0 gm three times/wk)	Susceptibility testing: Test only RIF. Testing INH and streptomycin give misleading results. All isolates are resistant to PZA. Rifapentine, azithro, ETB shown effective alone or in combination with RIF (AAC 42:2794, 1998). INH-resistance does not affect outcome (Chest 123:2003). If HIV+ pt taking protease inhibitor, substitute either clarithro (500 mg bid) or RFB (150 mg/d) for RIF (A/RCCM 156:S1, 1997). Because of variable susceptibility to INH, some would substitute clarithro 500–750 mg daily for INH. However, resistance to clarithro has been reported (DMID 31:360, 1998).
K. Mycobacterium marinum	(**Clarithro** 500 mg bid) or (**doxy-cycline** 100–200 mg po bid) or **ETB** for 3 mos. (A/RCCM 156:S1, 1997).	(**Clarithro** 500 mg bid) or (**minocycline** 100–200 mg po bid) or **TMP/SMX** 160/800 mg po bid, or (**RIF** + **ETB**) for 3 mos. Surgical excision.	Resistant to INH & PZA (A/RCCM 156:S1, 1997). Also susceptible in vitro to linezolid (AAC 47:1736, 2003). CIP, gatifloxacin, moxifloxacin also show moderate in vitro activity (AAC 46:1114, 2002).
L. Mycobacterium scrofulaceum	Surgical excision. Chemotherapy seldom indicated. Although regimens not defined, clarithro + CLO with or without ETB have also been used.		In vitro resistant to INH, RIF, ETB, PZA, AMK, CIP (CID 20:549, 1995). Susceptible to clarithro, strep, erythromycin.
M. Mycobacterium simiae	Regimen(s) not defined. Start 4 drugs as for disseminated MAI.		Most isolates resistant to all 1st-line and tbc drugs. Isolates often not clinically significant (CID 26, 625, 1998).
N. Mycobacterium ulcerans (Buruli ulcer)	**RIF** + **AMK** (7.5 mg/kg IM bid) or [**ETB** + **TMP/SMX** (160/800 mg po bid)] for 4–6 weeks. Surgical excision.	Some recommend **RIF** + **SM** (A/RCCM 156:S1, 1997).	Treatment generally disappointing—see review, Ln 354:1013, 1999. RIF + dapsone only slightly better (80% improved than placebo (75%) in small study (LID 6:560, 2002).
O. Mycobacterium xenopi	Regimen(s) not defined (CID 24:226 & 233, 1997). Some recommend **macrolide** + (**RIF** or **rifabutin**) + **ETB** + **SM** (A/RCCM 156:S1, 1997) or **RIF** + **INH** + **ETB** (Resp Med 97:439, 2003).		In vitro sensitive to clarithro, strep, RIF, ETB, INH (AAC 45:3229, 2001) and many standard antimycobacterial drugs. Clarithro-containing regimens effective in mice (AAC 45:3229, 2001). FQs, linezolid also active in vitro.
Mycobacterium leprae (leprosy) Paucibacillary (tuberculoid or indeterminate) Multibacillary (lepromatous or borderline) See Comment for erythema nodosum leprosum	**Dapsone** 100 mg daily unsupervised + **RIF** 600 mg po 1x/month supervised for 6 months. **Dapsone** 100 mg daily + **CLO** 50 mg daily (unsupervised) + (**RIF** 600 mg + **CLO** 300 mg 1x/month supervised) for 24 months (WHO Tech Rpt 874, 1998). Newer data suggest 12 mos. is effective (Ln 353:655, 1999).	**Ethionamide** (250 mg) or **prothi-onamide** (375 mg daily) may be substituted for CLO	Side-effects overall 0.4%. Single lesion paucibacillary disease may be treated with single-dose rx (RIF 600 mg + oflox 400 mg + minocycline 100 mg) (Ln 353:655, 1999). Side-effects overall 5.1%. For erythema nodosum leprosum: prednisone 60–80 mg/d or thalidomide 300 mg/d (BMJ 144:775, 1998; AJM 100:487, 2000). CLO available from Novartis. Pefloxacin 800 mg and ofloxacin 400 mg po on a daily basis, not bactericidal effect with a 1 g + minocycline clinically effective with a 1 g + minocycline in small trials (Int J Leprosy 58:281, 1990; AAC 38:662, 1994). Clarithro also rapidly bactericidal (AAC 38:565, 1994). Dapsone as effective as combination rx for multibacillary leprosy (AAC 38:2249, 1994). Regimens incorporating clarithro, minocycline, RIF (AAC 41:1618, 1997). High relapse rate in pts treated with daily RIF + oflox for 4 wks of leprosy not found (AAC 41:1953, 1997). Resistance to dapsone, RIF, ofloxacin reported (Ln 349:103, 1997). See also IJCP 11:32, 2002. DOT = directly observed therapy

Abbreviations: AMK = amikacin; **ATS** = American Thoracic Society. **Azithro** = azithromycin. **BL/BLI** = β-lactam/β-lactamase inhibitors; **CIP** = ciprofloxacin. **CLO** = clofazi-mine; **CXR** = chest x-ray; **ddC** = discontinue; **ddC** = zalcitabine; **DOT** = directly observed therapy; **ETB** = ethambutol; **FQ** = fluoroquinolones; **IA** = Injectable agent; may include aminoglycosides (strep-tomycin, amikacin, or kanamycin) or the polypeptide capreomycin; **IDSA** = Infectious Diseases Society of America. **IMP** = imipenem cilastatin; **INH** = isoniazid; **INH-CR** = complete INH resistance. **KM** = kanamycin. **Neomacrolides** (new acrolides) = azithromycin or clarithromycin; **NUS** = not available in the US. **PAS** = para-aminosalicylic acid; **PZA** = pyrazinamide; **RFB** = rifabutin; **RFP** = rifapentine; **RIF** = rifampin; **rx** = treatment; **sens** = sensitive; **SM** = streptomycin; **TBc** = tuberculosis; **TMP/SMX** = trimethoprim/sulfamethoxazole

FOOTNOTES: [1] In order of preference. [2] When DOT is used, drugs may be given 5 d/wk & the necessary number of doses adjusted accordingly. Although there are no rx studies that compare 5 with 7 daily doses, extensive experience indicates this would be an effective practice. [3] Patients with cavitation on initial chest x-ray & positive cultures at completion of 2 months of rx should receive a 7-month (31 wk; either 31 doses [daily] or 62 doses [2x/wk] continuation phase. [4] 5-day a wk administration is always given by DOT. [5] Not recommended for HIV-infected pts with CD4 cell counts <100 cells/µL [6] Options 4, 5, 6 should be used only in the case of drug intolerance. If options 4, 5, or 6 are used, the total duration of therapy would increase and would be based on bacteriologic response. [7] Not recommended. [8] Options 1–3 cannot be given. [9] Alternative agents — found to have a pos. culture from the 2-month specimen, should have rx extended an extra 3 months. [10] DOT is not necessary during the continuation phase if doses are given daily. [11] Alternative agents = ethionamide, cycloserine, p-aminosalicylic acid, clarithromycin, AMK, linezolid. * Dosages are for adults (unless otherwise indicated) and assume normal renal function.

See pages 90 & 92 for all footnotes and abbreviations

TABLE 12B: DOSAGE, PRICE AND SELECTED ADVERSE EFFECTS OF ANTIMYCOBACTERIAL DRUGS[1]

AGENT (TRADE NAME)	USUAL DOSAGE	ROUTE[1]/ DRUG RESISTANCE (RES) US/COST	SIDE-EFFECTS, TOXICITY AND PRECAUTIONS	SURVEILLANCE
FIRST LINE DRUGS				
Ethambutol (Myambutol)	25 mg/kg/d for 2 months & then 15 mg/kg/d as 1 dose [Bacteriostatic to both extracellular & intracellular organisms] (<10% protein binding)	po RES± 0.3% (0–0.7%) 400 mg tab $2.00	**Optic neuritis** with: decreased visual acuity, central scotomata, and loss of green and red perception; peripheral neuropathy and headache (−1%), rashes (rare), arthralgia (rare), hyperuricemia (rare). Anaphylactoid reaction (rare). *Comment:* Primarily used to inhibit resistance. Disrupts outer cell membrane in M. avium w/↑ activity to other drugs.	Monthly visual acuity & red/green with dose >15 mg/kg/day ≥10% loss considered significant. Usually reversible if drug discontinued.
Isoniazid (INH) (Nydrazid, Laniazid, Teebaconin)	Daily dose: 5–10 mg/kg up to 300 mg (max) as 1 dose. Intermittent dosing: 15 mg/kg (900 mg maximum dose) [Bacteriocidal to both extracellular and intracellular organisms] (<10% protein binding) Add pyridoxine in alcoholic, pregnant, or malnourished pts.	po RES: 4.1% (2.6–8.9%) 300 mg tab $0.02 IM (IV route not FDA-approved but has been used, esp. in AIDS) 100 mg/ml in 10 ml vials (IM) $16.64	Overall: −1%. **Hepatitis** (children 10%, mild ↑ SGOT, normalizes with continued rx, −20% with chronic therapy ranges 1.2%, <50 years 2.3%) (also ↑ with daily alcohol & previous exposure to hepatitis C). Usually asymptomatic—*CID* 36:293, 2003). May be fatal. With prodromal sx, dark urine do LFTs; discontinue if SGOT >3-5x normal. **Peripheral neuropathy** (17% on 6 mg/kg, less on 300 mg, incidence ↑ in slow acetylators); **pyridoxine** 10 mg daily will ↓ incidence; other neurologic sequelae: convulsions, optic neuritis, toxic encephalopathy, psychosis, muscle twitching, dizziness, coma (all rare); allergic skin rashes, fever, minor disulfiram-like reaction, flushing after Swiss cheese. Drug-induced lupus (20%). **Drug-drug interactions common, see Table 22**	Pre-rx liver functions. Repeat if symptoms (fatigue, weakness, malaise, anorexia, nausea & vomiting) >5 days (*AJRCCM* 152:1705, 1995). Some recommend SGOT at 2, 4, 6 months esp. if age >50 years. Clinical evaluation every month.
Pyrazinamide	25 mg/kg (maximum 2.5 gm/d) po as 1 dose [Bacteriocidal for intra-cellular organisms]	po 500 mg tab $1.04	**Arthralgia; hyperuricemia** (with or without symptoms); hepatitis (not over 2% if recommended dose not exceeded); gastric irritation, photosensitivity (rare)	Pre-rx liver functions. Monthly SGOT, uric acid. Measure serum uric acid if symptomatic gouty attack occurs.
Rifamate[®]— combination tablet	2 tablets single dose qd	po 1 tablet contains 150 mg INH, 300 mg RIF		As with individual drugs.
Rifampin (Rifadin, Rimactane, Rofact)	10.0 mg/kg/day up to 600 mg/day as 1 dose [Bacteriocidal to all populations of organisms]	po RES: 0.25% (0–0.3%) 300 mg cap $1.90 (IV available, Merrell-Dow. Cost 600 mg $90.28)	INH/RIF dr/d in −3% for toxicity, gastrointestinal irritation, antibiotic-associated pseudomembranous colitis, allergic skin rash (1%), anaphylactoid reactions (rare). In HIV+ pts, rashes (rash), thrombocytopenia (1%), leukopenia, hemolytic anemia, transient **abnormalities in liver function**. **"Flu syndrome"** (fever, chills, headache, bone pain, shortness of breath) seen if RIF taken irregularly or if daily dose restarted after an interval of no rx. **Discolors urine, sweat, tears, & contact lens an orange-brownish color.** May cause drug-induced lupus erythematosus (*Ln* 349:1521, 1977).	Pre-rx liver function. Repeat if symptoms. **Multiple significant drug-drug interactions, see Table 22.**
Rifater[®]— combination tablet (See Side-Effects)	Wt ≥55 kg, 6 tablets single dose qd	po (1 h before meal) $1.91	1 tablet contains 50 mg INH, 120 mg RIF, 300 mg PZA. Used in 1st 2 months of rx (PZA 25 mg/kg). Purpose is convenience in dosing, ↑ compliance (*AnIM* 122: 951, 1995) but cost 1.58 more. Side-effects = individual drugs.	As with individual drugs; PZA 25 mg/kg
Streptomycin	15 mg/kg IM qd, 0.75–1.0 gm/day initially for 60–90 days, then 1.0 gm 2–3 times/week (15 mg/kg maximum) IM qd as 1 dose	IM (or IV) RES: 3.9% (2.7–7.6%) 1.0 gm $6.45	Overall 8%. **Ototoxicity**: vestibular dysfunction (vertigo), paresthesias: dizziness & nausea (all less in pts receiving <1.0 gm/day), tinnitus and high frequency loss (2.4%), peripheral neuropathy (rare); allergic skin rashes (4–5%), drug fever. Available from X-Gen Pharmaceuticals, 607-732-4411. Reference re: IV: *CID* 21:1150, 1994.	Monthly audiogram. In older pts, serum creatinine or BUN at start of rx and weekly if pt stable
SECOND LINE DRUGS (more difficult to use and/or less effective than first line drugs)				
Amikacin (Amikin)	7.5–10.0 mg/kg qd	IV or IM RES (est. 0.1%) 500 mg NB $33, G $18.70	See Table 10, pages 63 & 73	Monthly audiogram. Serum creatinine or BUN weekly if pt stable

Note: Malabsorption of antimycobacterial drugs may occur in patients with AIDS enteropathy. For review of adverse effects, see *AJRCCM* 167:1472, 2003.
[2] **% resistance** of M. tuberculosis
See pages 90 & 92 for all footnotes and abbreviations

* Dosages are for adults (unless otherwise indicated) and assume normal renal function   [1] **DOT** = directly observed therapy

TABLE 12B (2)

SECOND LINE DRUGS (more difficult to use and/or less effective than first line drugs) *(continued)*

Drug	IM or IV	po	Adverse Effects / Comment	Monitoring
Capreomycin sulfate (Capastat sulfate)	1 gm/day (15 mg/kg/day) qd as 1 dose — RES: 0.1% (0-0.9%) 1 gm $25.54		Nephrotoxicity (36%), ototoxicity (auditory 11%), eosinophilia, leucopenia, skin rash, fever, hypokalemia, neuromuscular blockade.	Monthly audiogram, biweekly serum creatinine or BUN
Ciprofloxacin (Cipro)	po. IV 750 mg bid $4.80	750 mg/day	TB not an FDA-approved indication for CIP. Desired CIP serum levels 4-6 µg/ml. (*Ln* 345:1148, 1995). Discontinuation rates 6-7%. CIP well tolerated (*AJRCCM* 151:2006, 1995). CIP-resistant M. Tb identified in New York (*Ln* 345:1148, 1995). See Table 10, pages 65 & 70 for adverse effects	None
Clofazimine (Lamprene)	po with meals 50 mg $0.13	50 mg/d (unsupervised) + 300 mg 1x/month supervised or 100 mg/d	Skin: pigmentation (**pink-brownish black**) 75-100%, dryness 20%, pruritus 5%. GI: abdominal pain 50% (rarely severe leading to exploratory laparoscopy), splenic infarction (VR), bowel obstruction (VR), GI bleeding (VR). Eye: conjunctival irritation, retinal crystal deposits.	None
Cycloserine (Seromycin)	RES: 0.1% (0-0.3%)	po 250 mg cap $4.00 — 750-1000 mg/day (15 mg/kg/day) 2-4 doses/day [Bacteriostatic for both extracellular & intracellular organisms]	Convulsions, **psychoses** (5-10% of those receiving 1.0 gm/day), headache, somnolence; hyperreflexia; increased CSF protein and pressure, **peripheral neuropathy**. 100 mg pyridoxine (or more) daily should be given concomitantly. Contraindicated in epileptics	None
Dapsone		po 100 mg $0.20 — 100 mg/day	Blood: ↓ hemoglobin (1-2 gm) & ↑ retics (2-12%), in most pts. Hemolysis in G6PD deficiency. **Methemoglobinemia** (rare). CNS: peripheral neuropathy (rare). GI: nausea, vomiting. Renal: albuminuria, nephrotic syndrome. Erythema nodosum leprosum in pts rx for leprosy (½ pts 1st year).	None
Ethionamide (Trecator-SC)	RES: 0.8% (0-1.5%) 250 mg tab $2.19 [Bacteriostatic for extracellular organisms only]	po 500-1000 mg/day (10-15 mg/kg/day) 1 doses/day	**Gastrointestinal irritation** (up to 50% on large dose); goiter; hepatitis; peripheral neuropathy (rare); convulsions (rare); changes in affect (rare); difficulty in diabetes control; rashes; hepatitis; purpura; stomatitis; gynecomastia; menstrual irregularity. Give drug with meals or antacids; 50-100 mg pyridoxine per day concomitantly; SGOT monthly. Possibly teratogenic.	Liver functions monthly
Ofloxacin (Floxin)	po. IV 400 mg bid — 400 mg (po) $5.44		Not an FDA-approved indication. Overall adverse effects 11%, 4% discontinued due to side-effects. GI: nausea 3%, diarrhea 1%. **CNS** insomnia 3%, headache 1%, dizziness 1%.	None
Para-aminosalicylic acid (PAS, Paser) (Na+ or K+ salt)	RES: 0.8% (0-1.5%) 450 mg tab $0.08 (see Comment)	4-6 gm bid (200 mg/kg/day) [Bacteriostatic for extracellular organisms only]	**Gastrointestinal irritation** (10-15%); goitrogenic action (rare); depressed prothrombin activity (rare); G6PD-deficiency hemolytic anemia (rare); drug fever; rashes; hepatitis; myalgia; arthralgia. Retards hepatic enzyme induction; may ↓ INH hepatotoxicity. Available from CDC, (404) 639-3670; Jacobus Pharm. Co. (609) 921-7447.	None
Rifabutin (Mycobutin)	po 150 mg $4.54	300 mg/day (prophylaxis or treatment)	Polymyalgia, polyarthralgia, leucopenia, granulocytopenia. Anterior uveitis when given with concomitant clarithromycin; avoid 600 mg dose (*NEJM* 330:438, 1994). Uveitis reported with 300 mg/day (*NEJM* 12:510, 1994). Reddish urine, orange skin (pseudojaundice).	None
Rifapentine (Priftin)	po 150 mg $2.91	600 mg twice weekly for 1st 2 mos., then 600 mg q week	Similar to other rifabutins. (See *RIF, RFB.*) Hyperuricemia seen in 21%. Causes red-orange discoloration of body fluids. Note ↑ prevalence of RIF resistance in pts on weekly rx (*Ln* 353:1843, 1999).	None
Thalidomide (Thalomid)	po 50 mg $11.35	100-300 mg po qd (may use up to 400 mg po qd for severe erythema nodosum leprosum)	**Contraindicated in pregnancy. Causes severe life-threatening birth defects. Use in females requires concomitant use of two reliable contraceptive methods (Pregnancy Category X). Frequently causes drowsiness or somnolence. May cause peripheral neuropathy.** (*AJM* 108:487, 2000)	Available only through pharmacists participating in System for Thalidomide Education and Prescribing Safety (S.T.E.P.S.)

* Adult dosage only; **Mean (higher in Hispanics, Asians, and patients < 10 years old); ** Average wholesale price according to 2003 DRUG TOPICS RED BOOK, Medical Economics
Abbreviations: VR = very rare, **esp.** = especially, **dc** = discontinue, **RES** = % resistance to M. tuberculosis

* Dosages are for adults (unless otherwise indicated) and assume normal renal function • † **DOT** = directly observed therapy

See pages 90 & 92 for all footnotes and abbreviations

TABLE 13A: TREATMENT OF PARASITIC INFECTIONS

Many of the drugs suggested are not licensed in the United States. The following are helpful resources available through the Center for Disease Control and Prevention (CDC) in Atlanta. Website is www.cdc.gov. General advice for care of parasitic diseases other than malaria: (770) 488-7760 or (770) 488-7775.
For CDC Drug Service[1] 8:00 a.m.–4:30 p.m. EST: (404) 639-3670 (or -2888); emergency after hours: (404) 639-2888; fax. (404) 639-3717.
For malaria: Prophylaxis advice (770) 488-7788 or (877) 394-8747; treatment (770) 488-7788; website: www.cdc.gov/travel; fax (888) 232-3299
NOTE: All dosage regimens are for adults with normal renal function unless otherwise indicated.
For licensed drugs, suggest checking package inserts to verify dosage and side-effects. Occasionally, post-licensure data may alter dosages as compared to package inserts.
For abbreviations of journal titles, see Table 7 page 45. **Reference with pediatric dosages: Medical Letter on-line version: www.medletter.com (April 2002)**

INFECTING ORGANISM	SUGGESTED REGIMENS		COMMENTS
	PRIMARY	**ALTERNATIVE**	
PROTOZOA—INTESTINAL (non-pathogenic): E. hartmanni, E. dispar, E. coli, Iodamoeba butschlii, Endolimax nana, Chilomastix mesnili)			
Balantidium coli	**Tetracycline** 500 mg po qid x10 d.	**Metronidazole** 750 mg po tid x5 d.	See Table 10B for side-effects.
Blastocystis hominis	Role as pathogen supported random. trial: metro vs placebo	**Metronidazole** 750 mg po tid x10 d. **High dose** increases risk of adverse effects. **Alternative: Iodoquinol** 650 mg po x20 d. Metro resist. reported (Trop Med Int Health 4:274, 1999)	
Cryptosporidium parvum Treatment is unsatisfactory Ref.: NEJM 346:1723, 2002	**Immunocompetent pt:** No specific therapy. Hydration only. **Pts with AIDS:** Restore immune function with active antiretroviral therapy. If anti-HIV fails, then try antidiarrheal; if anti-HIV fails or **nitazoxanide** or (**paromomycin** + **azithro**)—see Alternative Regimens	**If HAART fails:** (1) **Nitazoxanide (Alinia)** 0.5–1.0 gm po bid (x14 d if HIV +). Peds dose: 100–200 mg po bid x3 d. **OR** (2) **Paromomycin** 1.0 gm po 2v/d. + **azithro** 600 mg po x4 wks	**Nitazoxanide:** Approved in liquid formulation for rx of children; tabs for adults pending at FDA. 50% effective children with crypto. **NO benefit in children if HIV+.** 60% cure in adults with HIV. Refs.: Med Lett 45:29, 2003; Tr RSTMH 92:663, 1998). Active vs giardia plus other parasites (Trends in Parasit 18:36, 2002).
Cyclospora cayetanensis	Immunocompetent pts. **TMP/SMX-DS** tab 1 po qid x10 d. then po bid x7 d.	AIDS Pts. **TMP/SMX-DS** tab 1 po qid x10 d. then tab 1 bid 3x/wk.	Ref.: CID 23:429, 1996. If sulfa-allergic: **CIP** 500 mg po bid x7 d. & then 1 tab po 3x/wk x2 wks.
Dientamoeba fragilis	**Iodoquinol** 650 mg po tid x20 d.	**Tetracycline** 500 mg po qid x10 d. **OR Metronidazole** 500–750 mg po tid x10 d.	Other alternatives: doxy 100 mg po bid x10 d; paromomycin 500–750 mg po tid x10 d.
Entamoeba histolytica; amebiasis Reviews: Ln 351:1025, 2003; NEJM 348:1563, 2003.			
Asymptomatic cyst passer	**Paromomycin** (aminosidine in U.K.) 500 mg po tid x7 d. OR **Iodoquinol** 650 mg po tid x20 d.	**Diloxanide furoate**[AUS] (Furamide) 500 mg po tid x10 d. Manufacturer: Boots, United Kingdom	Metronidazole not effective vs cysts.
Pt with diarrhea/dysentery; mild/moderate disease. Oral rx possible	**Metronidazole** 500–750 mg po tid x10 d. Either [**paromomycin** 500 mg po tid x7 d.] or [**iodoquinol** 500 mg po tid x20 d.]	**Tinidazole**[AUS] 1.0 (kids 50 mg/kg) po q12h x3 d.) or (**ornidazole**[AUS] 500 mg po q12h x5 d.) followed by:	Drug side-effects in Table 10B. Colitis can mimic ulcerative colitis, amebooma can mimic adenocarcinoma of colon. **Dx:** antigen detection & PCR better than O&P (Clin Micro Rev 16:713, 2003). Watch out for non-pathogenic E. dispar (J 351:1672, 1998).
Severe or extraintestinal infection. e.g., hepatic abscess	**Metronidazole** 750 mg **iv** or **po** tid x10 d. followed by **paromomycin** 500 mg po tid x7 d. Outside U.S. may substitute **tinidazole** (600 mg bid or 800 mg tid x5 d.) for metro.	(**Tinidazole**[AUS] 2.0 gm po x1) OR (**quinacrine**[AUS] 100 mg po tid after meals x5 d.)[6] See Comment.	**Serology positive (antibody present) with extraintestinal disease.**
Giardia lamblia; giardiasis Ref.: MMWR 49:S5–7, 2000	**Metronidazole** (250, not 500 mg) po tid x5 d. OR **furazolidone** 100 mg qid x7–10 d.	**Paromomycin** 500 mg 4x/d. x7 d. Rx if pregnant.	**Refractory pts:** (metro **750 mg po + quinacrine 100 mg**)—both 3x/d. x14 d. Ref: CID 33:22, 2001. Another option for AIDS pts: **Nitazoxanide** 1.5 gm po bid x3 d. (AJM 132:885, 2000).
Isospora belli	**TMP/SMX-DS** tab 1 po bid x10 d.. If AIDS pt.: TMP/SMX-DS qid x10 d. & then bid x3 wks.	**Pyrimethamine** 75 mg/d po + **folinic acid** 10 mg/d po) once/d po bid x7—87% response (AHM 132:885, 2000)	Chronic suppression in AIDS pts, either 1 TMP/SMX-DS tab po bid or (pyrimethamine 25 mg/d po + folinic acid 5 mg/d po)

---

[1] **Drugs available from CDC Drug Service: 404-639-2888 or -3670; Bithionol, dehydroemetine, diethylcarbamazine (DEC), melarsoprol, nifurtimox, stibogluconate (Pentostam), suramin.**

[2] Both quinacrine and tinidazole available from Panorama Compounding Pharmacy (818) 247-9767; (818) 988-7979.

* All doses are for adults (unless otherwise indicated) and assume normal renal function. See page 103 for abbreviations.

TABLE 13A (2)

INFECTING ORGANISM	SUGGESTED REGIMENS		COMMENTS
	PRIMARY	ALTERNATIVE	
PROTOZOA—INTESTINAL (continued)			
Microsporidiosis (Ref: CID 27:1, 1998)			
Ocular Encephalitozoon hellem (Nosema corneae, Vittaforma corneae (Nosema sp.)	**Albendazole** 400 mg po bid x3 weeks	In HIV+ pts, reports of response of E. hellum to **fumagillin** eyedrops (see Comment). For V. corneae, may need keratoplasty.	To obtain fumagillin: 1-800-547-1392. Neutropenia & thrombocytopenia serious adverse events. Dx: Most labs use modified trichrome stain. Need electron micrographs for species identification. FA and PCR methods in development.
Intestinal (diarrhea): Enterocytozoon bieneusi, Encephalitozoon (Septata) intestinalis	**Albendazole** 400 mg po bid x3 weeks	Oral **fumagillin 20 mg po tid** reported effective for E. bieneusi (NEJM 346:1963, 2002)—see Comment	
Disseminated: E. hellum cuniculi or intestinalis; Pleistophora sp.	**Albendazole** 400 mg po bid x3 weeks	No established rx for Pleistophora sp.	Other species reported pathogenic: Trachipleistophora sp., Brachiola vesiculorum.
PROTOZOA—EXTRAINTESTINAL			
Amebic meningoencephalitis			
Acanthamoeba sp.— no proven rx Rev.: Clin Micro Rev 16:273, 2003	Success with IV **pentamidine**, topical **chlorhexidine & 2% ketoconazole** cream & then po **itra** (NEJM 331:85, 1994). 2 children responded to rx: TMP/SMX + **rifampin + itra** (PIDJ 20:623, 2001).		For treatment of keratitis, see Table 1, page 9
Balamuthia mandrillaris	**Pentamidine** amebastatic in vitro		A cause of chronic granulomatous meningitis
Naegleria fowleri: >95% mortality. Sappinia diploidea	**Ampho B** 1 mg/kg/d IV + 0.1–1.0 mg/d into lateral ventricle via an Omaya reservoir. Duration?	One pt responded to clarithro + **fluconazole** + sulfadiazine + **fluconazole**	Case report: Ampho, miconazole, & RIF (NEJM 306:346, 1982).
Babesia microti; babesiosis (CID 22:1117, 2001)	**Atovaquone** 750 mg bid po x7–10 d. + **azithro** 500 mg (day 1) then 250 mg/d. x7 d. (NEJM 343:1454, 2000)	**Clinda** (600 mg po tid) + (**quinine** 650 mg po tid) x7 d. For adults, can give **clinda** IV as 1.2 gm bid.	Can cause overwhelming infection in asplenic patients.
Ehrlichiosis—See Table 1, pages 38–39			
Leishmaniasis—See Table 1. NOTE: Responses of various species differ—see references.			
Visceral—Kala-azar L. donovani: India/Africa, L. infantum: Mediterranean, L. chagasi: New World **WARNING: Avoid combined antimony & ampho B** (Ln 351:1928, 1998)	**Antimony** (see Astra Medica, Glenview) dx of infusion. **Adults:** 2.5 mg/kg/d, po either qd once or twice daily x28 d. **Children** (<12 yrs old): 2.5 mg/kg/d, in 3 div. doses after meals x28 d. Refs: NEJM 347:1737, 1739, & 1794, 2002; PIDJ 22:434, 2003.	**Lipid formulations of ampho B** effective in short-course regimens but impractical due to expense. **Children** Liposomal ampho B 10 mg/kg/d x2 d → 98% success (CID 36:560, 2003). **Adults:** 3 mg/kg/d on days 1–5, 14, & 21.	Antimony resistance is a problem in India (JID 180:564, 1999). **Antimony (stibogluconate** or **meglumine antimoniate)** 20 mg/kg/d of antimony (Sb) (in 2 div. doses) IM or IV x28 d. Not marketed in U.S. Contact CDC Drug Service: (404) 639-3670.
Miltefosine Effective vs L. major (NEJM 346:891, 2002)	**Fluconazole** 200 mg po once daily x6 wks Antimony as for Visceral	**AmB** 1 mg/kg IV qod x20–30 doses	Approx. cure rates: antimony 60%, AmB >75%
Mucosal—L. braziliensis			
Cutaneous: **Most resolve spontaneously; Rx goal: ↓ time to cure** L. mexicana and L. braziliensis in New World L. tropica and L. major in Old World	Antimony as for Visceral	**Miltefosine** approx. 2.25 mg/kg once daily po x3–4 wks. Cure in 94% (CID 33:e57, 2001). Contact Astra Medica or Zentaris. GI¹ unease in 40% of pts.	Other options all IV: **Antimony** as for visceral, or **Pentamidine** 2–4 mg/kg qd or q2 days IV x15 doses

NOTE: All dosage recommendations are for adults (unless otherwise indicated) and assume normal renal/renal function. See page 103 for abbreviations.

TABLE 13A (3)

INFECTING ORGANISM	SUGGESTED REGIMENS		COMMENTS
	PRIMARY	**ALTERNATIVE**	

PROTOZOA—EXTRAINTESTINAL *(continued)*

Malaria (Plasmodium species)—NOTE: CDC Malaria info—prophylaxis (877) 394-8747; treatment (770) 488-7788. Websites: www.cdc.gov/ncidod/dpd/parasites/malaria/default.htm; www.who.int/health-topics/malaria.htm.

Prophylaxis—Drugs plus personal protection: screens, nets, 30–35% DEET skin repellent (avoid 95% products in children), permethrin spray on clothing and nets

For areas free of chloroquine (CQ)-resistant P. falciparum: Haiti, Dominican Republic, Central America west and north of the Panama Canal, and parts of the Middle East	**CQ** 500 mg (300 mg base) po per week starting 1–2 wks before travel, during travel, & 4 wks post-travel.		The areas free of CQ-resistant falciparum malaria continue to shrink: Central America north of Panama Canal, Haiti, and parts of Middle East. CQ-resistant falciparum malaria reported from Saudi Arabia, Yemen. *(Antim 128:931, 1998)*
For areas free of CQ-resistant P. falciparum	**Atovaquone 250 mg—proguanil 100 mg (Malarone):** comb. tablet, 1 tab q24h with food 1–2 d. prior to, during, & 7 d. post-travel. Peds dose in footnote[2]. Cost/2 wks: $125.	**Doxycycline** 100 mg po daily for adults & children >8 yrs. Start 1–2 days before travel, daily during travel, and for 4 wks after travel. Cost/2 wks: $80	**MQ current best option.** Insufficient data with prolonged exposure during pregnancy. **Primaquine:** Used only if prolonged exposure to endemic area (e.g., Peace Corps). **Can cause hemolytic anemia if G6PD deficiency present.**
	Mefloquine (MQ) 250 mg (228 mg base) po per week, 1 wk. before, during, & for 4 wks after travel. Peds dose in footnote[2]		Malarone: **Avoid doxycycline and primaquine.** MO not recommended if cardiac conduction abnormalities, seizures, or psychiatric disorders, e.g., depression, psychosis. MO outside U.S. 275 mg tab, contains 250 mg of base.
	Another option for adults: **primaquine (PQ)** 30.0 mg base po daily in non-pregnant G6PD-neg. travelers (85% protective vs P. falciparum & >92% vs P. vivax *(CID 33:1990, 2001).*		*Malarone* resistance: *CID 37:450, 2003*

Treatment *(NEJM 335:800, 1996)* **(P. falciparum, P. vivax, P. malariae, P. ovale)**

Blood smear consistent with P. vivax &/or P. ovale	**For chloroquine (CQ)-sensitive malaria: CQ** (1.0 gm (=600 mg base) po, 0.5 gm in 6 hrs, then 0.5 gm daily x2 d)	Tylenol prolonged time to clear parasitemia *(Ln 350:704, 1997)* As CQ-resistant P. falciparum. Rx as CQ-resistant P. falciparum: see below.	CQ-resistant P. vivax reported from Oceania and South America. Rx as CQ-resistant P. falciparum. **Pregnancy** CQ safe all trimesters. No PQ in pregnancy or to newborns—risk of hemolysis. For PQ use 0.3 mg base per kg po, then 5 mg/kg/d (15 mg base) daily x14 d.
CDC: Malaria treatment— (770) 488-7788 or website: www.cdc.gov	**Primaquine (PQ)** 26.3 mg (15 mg base) po daily x14 d. OR 79 mg (45 mg base) po per week x8 wks. Check for G6PD deficiency before Rx.	After CQ (as for matrices, give PQ 26.3 mg (15 mg base)) po daily x14 d. screen for G6PD def. to avoid severe hemolysis.	For prevention of relapse (P. ovale or P. vivax) use 0.3 mg base/kg/d x14 d.

Blood smear consistent with P. falciparum or P. malariae	**Chloroquine (CQ)** 325 mg (=250 mg base). Given as above (CQ for CQ-sensitive P. vivax above). Don't have PO therapy possible.	**Quinine sulfate (QS)** 650 mg po 3x/d (1+ **doxycycline** 100 mg po 2x/d)—both x7 d. **Peds QS** 25 mg/kg/d in 3 div. doses x 3–7 d + **Fansidar** x1 dose on last d.	Assumes CQ-sensitive (Central America west of Panama Canal), Haiti, and most of Middle East. **Other rx alternatives:** (1) **quinine** 650 mg q8h x3–7 d, then 500 mg q12h 12 hrs later *(JID 180:2077, 1999)*. (2) **Halofantrine** 500 mg q6h x3 doses. Repeat regimen in 1 wk. **Pregnancy** High morbidity/mortality. Despite concerns of potential
Blood smear shows P. falciparum assumed CQ-resistant	**Quinine sulfate (QS)** 650 mg po 3x/d x3–7 d + (**doxycycline** 100 mg po 2x/d x7 d)	or **Atovaquone/proguanil** 250/100 mg, 4 adult tabs po 1x/d x3 days	fetal toxicity, use **quinine** or IV **quinidine** followed by **Fansidar** (sulfadoxine-pyrimethamine) 3 tablets (each tab 25/500 mg) or 1500 mg **sulfadoxine** + 75 mg **pyrimethamine** x1 dose. Alternatives:
Rx same for CQ-resistant P. vivax	or **Atovaquone/proguanil 1 gm/400 mg (4 adult tabs) po 1x/day for 3 days**, with food. Peds dose in footnote[3]	**Mefloquine (MQ)** 750 mg po then 500 mg 12 hrs later. Peds: **Artesunate** *(Ref.: CID 37:1340, 2003)* 4 mg/kg/d po q8h x3 days + (**doxycycline** 2 mg/kg/d up to 100 mg po q24h x3 d.) or a single po dose of quinine. **Atovaquone/proguanil** single daily dose by weight: 11–20 kg, 1 adult tab; 21–30 kg,	[Quinine + doxycycline (despite fetal concerns)] OR [quinine + clindamycin *(AAC 46:2315, 2002)*]
			2 adult tabs; 31–40 kg, 3 adult tabs; >40 kg, 4 adult tabs. **Mefloquine** <45 kg, 15 mg/kg, then 10 mg/kg 8–12 hrs later. **Halofantrine** <40 kg, 8 mg/kg q6h x3, repeat in 1 week.	

Footnotes:

[1] **CQ** = chloroquine phosphate, **MQ** = mefloquine, **PQ** = primaquine, **QS** = quinine sulfate

[2] **Peds prophylaxis dose by weight** *(Ref.: CID 34:493, 2002)*: Mefloquine weekly dose by **weight in kg**: <15 = 5 mg/kg; 15–19 = ¼ adult dose; 20–30 = ½; 31–45 = ¾; >45 = adult dose. **Atovaquone/proguanil by weight in kg**, single daily dose: 11–20 kg, 62.5/25 mg; 21–30 kg, 125/50 mg; 31–40 kg, 187.5/75 mg; >40 kg, 250/100 mg. **Doxycycline** 2 mg/kg/d up to 100 mg po daily—both x7 d.

[3] **Pediatric treatment dosage** *(Ref.: CID 37:1340, 2003)*: CQ 25 mg/kg/d (max. 2 gm/d) po div. q8h x2 d. + a single po dose of quinine. Fansidar single dose by age (yr) of pt: <1 = ¼ tab, 1–3 = ½, 4–8 yrs = 1 tab, 9–14 = 2 tabs, >14 = 3 tabs. **Atovaquone/proguanil** single daily dose by weight in kg: 11–20 kg, 500/200 mg; 31–40 mg, 750/300 mg. >40 kg, 1 gm/400 mg, po x 3 days. **Mefloquine** <45 kg, 15 mg/kg, then 10 mg/kg 8–12 hrs later. **Halofantrine** <40 kg, 8 mg/kg q6h x3, repeat in 1 week.

NOTE: All dosage recommendations are for adults (unless otherwise indicated) and assume normal renal function. See page 103 for abbreviations.

TABLE 13A (4)

INFECTING ORGANISM	SUGGESTED REGIMENS		COMMENTS
	PRIMARY	**ALTERNATIVE**	
PROTOZOA—EXTRAINTESTINAL/Malaria Treatment *(continued)*			
Blood smear consistent with P. falciparum **Pt too ill for initial po therapy** **NOTE:** Steroids are harmful in cerebral malaria. Drug resistance ref. *Ln Inf Dis 2:209, 2002*	In U.S. **Quinidine gluconate** in normal saline (10 mg/kg IV over 1 hr, then 0.02 mg/kg/min. (monitor EKG) x72 hrs] OR [15 mg/kg IV over 4 hrs, then 7.5 mg/kg IV over 4 hrs q8h x72 hrs] Until patient can take po meds. **NOTE:** No loading dose if meflo-	Outside U.S. **Quinine dihydrochloride**[AS](1) [15 mg/kg IV loading dose over 4 hrs, then 10 mg/kg over 2-8 hrs q8h x72 hrs] OR **Artemether**[AS](1) 3.2 mg/kg IM, then 1.6 mg/kg IM, daily. For each, switch to po regimen when possible to	May be manifest as cerebral malaria, renal failure, or ARDS. Monitor parasitemia: if rx effective, expect ≥75% ↓ parasite count after 48 hrs of rx. If parasitemia exceeds 15%, consider **exchange transfusion** (CID 34:1192, 2002). CDC: Malaria info (770) 488-7788
	quine or quinine in past 24 hrs.	finish 7 days of rx.	**Pregnancy:** See Comment, po therapy, bottom of page 95
Microsporidia—systemic—see page 91			
Pneumocystis carinii Pneumonia (PCP). Official new name is **Pneumocystis jiroveci** (yee-row-vet-zee) *EID 8:891, 2002.* Resistance to TMP/SMX and atovaquone may emerge (JAMA 286:2450, 2001)			
Not acutely ill, able to take po meds. PaO₂ >70 mmHg	**TMP/SMX-DS,** 2 tabs po q8h x21 d.) OR [**Dapsone** 100 mg po qd + **trimethoprim** 5 mg/kg po tid x21 d.]	**[Clindamycin** 300-450 mg po q6h + **primaquine** 15 mg (base po qd) x21 d.] OR **Atovaquone** suspension 750 mg po bid with food x21 d.	
	NOTE: Concomitant use of corticosteroids usually reserved for sicker pts with PaO₂ <70 (see below)		
Acutely ill, po rx not possible. PaO₂ <70 mmHg	**Prednisone** (15-30 min before TMP/SMX) 40 mg po bid x5 d, then 40 mg po qd x5 d, then 20 mg po qd x11 d.) + **TMP/SMX** [15 mg of TMP component/kg/d] IV div q6-8h x21 d.)	**Prednisone** as in primary rx **PLUS [Clinda** 600 mg IV q8h + **(primaquine** 30 mg base po qd) x21 d.] OR **Pentamidine** 4 mg/kg IV x21 d.	**After 21 days, chronic suppression in AIDS pts (see below).** **PCP** can occur in absence of HIV infection and steroids (CID 23:215 & 219, 1997).
	Can substitute IV prednisolone for prednisone		
Primary prophylaxis and post-treatment suppression Refs. MMWR 51(RR-8), 6/14/2002; AnIM 137:435, 2002	**(TMP/SMX-DS** or **-SS,** 1 tab po qd or 1 DS 3x/wk) OR **(dapsone** 100 mg po qd). DC rx if CD4 >200 x3 mos. (NEJM 344:159, 2001).	**[Pentamidine** 300 mg IV & mist. water by aerosol (q4 wks) OR **(dapsone** 200 mg po + **pyrimethamine** 75 mg po + **folinic acid** 25 mg po—**all once a week**)] OR **atovaquone** 1500 mg po qd with food.	**TMP/SMX-DS** regimen provides cross-protection vs toxo and other bacterial infections. Dapsone + pyrimethamine protects vs toxo. Atovaquone suspension 1500 mg once daily as effective as daily dapsone (NEJM 339:1889, 1998) & inhaled pentamidine (JID 180:369, 1999).
Toxoplasma gondii (Reference: Remington and McLeod in INFECTIOUS DISEASES, Gorbach et al., Eds., 2nd Ed., 1997, pp 1620-40)			
Immunologically normal patients (For pediatric doses, see reference)	Treat as for active chorioretinitis		
Active chorioretinitis Acquired w/lymphadenopathy (No accident)	**Pyrimethamine** (pyr) 50-100 mg po load [then 25 mg qd] + **[leucovorin (folinic acid)** 10 mg or more/day]—**see Comment** + **sulfadiazine** (see Comment) 1-1.5 gm po qid + **[leucovorin (folinic acid)** 10 mg or more/day]—**see Comment**	(No accident) Treat only if symptoms severe/persistent symptoms or evidence of vital organ damage	For active chorioretinitis
Acquired w/transfusion or IV (accident) lowered resistance due to steroids or cytotoxic drugs	pyr 1-2 wks beyond resolution of signs/symptoms; continue leucovorin 1 wk after stopping pyri.		
Pregnancy—1st to 18 weeks of gestation, or to term if fetus not infected	**Spiramycin** [From FDA, call (301) 827-2335] 1.0 gm po q8h x3-4 wks. **NOTE:** Use caution in interpretation of commercial tests for toxoplasma IgM antibody, for help, call (650) 853-4828 FDA Advisory (301) 594-3060 or Toxoplasma Serology Lab of Palo Alto Med. Found (650) 853-4828		For congenital toxo, toxo meningitis in adults, and chorio-retinitis, **add prednisone 1 mg/kg/d in 2 divs. doses** until CSF protein conc. falls or vision-threatening inflammation has subsided. Adjust folinic acid dose by following CBC results. IgG avidity test of help in 1ˢᵗ trimester (JID 183:1248, 2001).

---

(1) Sulfonamides for toxo. Sulfadiazine now commercially available. Sulfisoxazole much less effective.
NOTE: All dosage recommendations are for adults (unless otherwise indicated) and assume normal renal function. See page 103 for abbreviations.

TABLE 13A (5)

INFECTING ORGANISM	SUGGESTED REGIMENS		COMMENTS
	PRIMARY	ALTERNATIVE	
PROTOZOA—EXTRAINTESTINAL/Toxoplasma gondii (continued)			
Acquired immunodeficiency syndrome (AIDS)			
Cerebral toxoplasmosis Ref. See *Remington & McLeod* ref., above	[Pyrimethamine (pyri) 200 mg x1 po, then 75–100 mg/d po) + **(sulfadiazine** 1–1.5 gm po q6h)] + **(folinic acid** 10–15 mg/d po) x3–6 wks and then suppressive rx (see below) OR (4) **TMP/SMX** 10/50 mg/kg/d po or IV div q12h x30 d (*AAC* 42:1346, 1998)	[**Pyri** + **folinic acid** (as in primary regimen)] + 1 of the following: (1) **Clinda** 600 mg po/IV q6h or (2) **clarithro** 1.0 gm po bid or (3) **azithro** 1.2–1.5 gm po qd or (4) **dapsone** 100 mg po qd: Treat 3–6 wks, then suppression.	Use alternative regimen for pts with severe sulfa allergy. If multiple ring-enhancing brain lesions (CT or MRI), ~85% of pts respond to 7–10 days of empiric rx. If no response, suggest brain biopsy.
Primary prophylaxis, AIDS pts—IgG toxo antibody + CD4 count <100/µl.	(**TMP/SMX-DS**, 1 tab po qd) or (**TMP/SMX SS**, 1 tab po qd)	[**Dapsone** 50 mg po qd) + (**pyri** 50 mg po q week) + **folinic acid** 25 mg po q week)] OR **atovaquone** 1500 mg po qd	Prophylaxis for pneumocystis also effective vs toxo. Refs.: *MMWR* 51 (RR-8), 6/14/2002; *AnIM* 137:435, 2002 (pyri + sulfa) prevents PCP and toxo. (clinda + pyri) prevents toxo only.
Suppression after rx of cerebral toxo	Sulfadiazine 500–1000 mg po qid + (**pyri** 25–50 mg po qd) + (**folinic acid** 10–25 mg po qd). SC if CD4 count <200 x3 months.	[(**Clinda** 300–450 mg po q6–8h) **(pyri** 25–50 mg po qd) + **folinic acid** 10–25 mg po qd)] OR **atovaquone** 750 mg po q6–12h	
Trichomonas vaginalis	See *Vaginitis, Table 1, page 17*		
Trypanosomiasis Refs.: *LnID* 2:437, 2002; *Ln* 362:1469, 2003			
T. brucei gambiense or T. brucei rhodesiense: African sleeping sickness			
Early infection without CNS symptoms or abnormal CSF	Pentamidine isethionate 4 mg/kg IM daily x10 days	[**Suramin**[CDC] test dose of 0.2 gm IV, then 20 mg/kg, up to max. of 1.0 gm, IV on days 1, 3, 7, 14 & 21. Children: 20 mg/kg on same schedule]	CSF abnormal if 5 cells/µl or ↑ protein concentration. Melarsoprol-induced encephalopathy in 10% of pts. NOTE: T. brucei rhodesiense are resistant to nifurtimox and eflornithine.
Late infection with CNS symptoms and abnormal CSF	Melarsoprol[CDC] 2.2–3.6 mg/kg/d IV x3 doses, repeat after 1 week and again after 10–21 days (active vs rhodesiense)	Eflornithine 100 mg/kg q6h IV x14 d. and then 75 mg/kg po for 21–30 d. **for gambiense but not rhodesiense**	Under study as facial cream (Vaniqa) to remove unwanted hair.
↓Prednisone 1 mg/kg/d po may be used in encephalopathy (see Comment)	Prednisone 1 mg/kg/d po may be used in encephalopathy (see Comment). See *Peds ref.* in *Table 13B, page 102*	Peds. dose of eflornithine, 100 mg/kg IV q6h x4 wks.	
T. brucei gambiense relapse post-rx with melarsoprol	Eflornithine 100 mg/kg q6h IV x14 d., then 75 mg/kg po for 21–30 d.		
T. brucei gambiense prophylaxis	Pentamidine isethionate 3 mg/kg IM q 6 months	[Not for casual visitor.]	Risk to tourists low. Not effective for T. brucei rhodesiense.
T. cruzi—Chagas disease or acute American trypanosomiasis Ref.: *Ln* 357:797, 2001	Nifurtimox[CDC] 8–10 mg/kg/d po div. 4x/d. after meals x120 d. Ages 11–16 yrs: 12.5–15 mg/kg/d div. qid po x90 d. Children <11: 15–20 mg/kg/d div. qid po x90 d.	Benznidazole[AG] 5–7 mg/kg/d po div. 2x/d x30–90 d. (*AJTMH* 63:111, 2000). NOTE: Avoid tetracycline and steroids	Treatment 70–95% effective. Nifurtimox reported 70–95% effective. Immunosuppression for heart transplant can reactivate chronic Chagas disease.
NEMATODES—INTESTINAL (Roundworms)			
Angiostrongylus cantonensis For significance of eosinophilia, see *CID* 34:407, 2002	Mebendazole 100 mg bid x5 d.	Anthelminthic therapy may worsen meningitis (*NEJM* 346:668, 2002)	For eosinophilic meningitis, corticosteroids of benefit (*CID* 31:660, 2000).
Angiostrongylus costaricensis (*AJM* 111:109, 2001)	Mebendazole 200–400 mg tid x10 d.	Thiabendazole 75 mg/kg/d in 3 div. doses (max. 3 gm/d)	Can cause inflammatory mass that mimics appendicitis.

[1] **CDC** = available from CDC Drug Service

[2] **Melarsoprol** 2.2 mg/kg IV x10 d. as effective as standard regimen (*Ln* 355:1419, 2000).

NOTE: All dosage recommendations are for adults (unless otherwise indicated) and assume normal renal function. See page 103 for abbreviations.

TABLE 13A (6)

INFECTING ORGANISM	SUGGESTED REGIMENS		COMMENTS
	PRIMARY	ALTERNATIVE	
NEMATODES—INTESTINAL (Roundworms) *(continued)*			
Ascaris lumbricoides (**ascariasis**)	Albendazole 400 mg po x1 dose or mebendazole 100 mg po bid x3 d. or 500 mg po x1 dose	Pyrantel pamoate 11 mg/kg po x1 dose (max. 1.0 gm)	Can present with intestinal obstruction.
Capillaria philippinensis (**capillariasis**)	Mebendazole 200 mg po bid x20 d.	Albendazole 200 mg po bid x10 d.	
Enterobius vermicularis (**pinworm**)	Albendazole 400 mg po x1, repeat in 2 wks OR mebendazole 100 mg po x1, repeat in 2 wks	Pyrantel pamoate 11 mg/kg (to max. dose of 1.0 gm) po x1 dose; repeat every 2 wks x2	Side-effects in Table 13B, pages 101, 103
Hookworm (Necator americanus and Ancylostoma duodenale)	Albendazole 400 mg po x1 or mebendazole 100 mg po bid x3 d.	Pyrantel pamoate 11 mg/kg to max. dose of 1.0 gm) po daily x3	NOTE: Ivermectin not effective. Eosinophilia may be present but eggs detectable in stool.
Strongyloides stercoralis (**strongyloidiasis**)	Ivermectin 200 µg/kg po x1-2 d.	Thiabendazole 25 mg/kg po bid (max. 3 gm/d) x2 d (7-10 d for disseminated hyperinfection syndrome)	Case report of ivermectin failure in pt with hypogammaglobulinemia (J Med Sci 311:178, 1996).
Trichostrongylus orientalis	Albendazole 400 mg po x1 dose	Pyrantel pamoate 11 mg/kg po bid x3 d.	Mebendazole 100 mg po bid x3 d.
Trichuris trichiura (**whipworm**)	Albendazole 400 mg po once daily x3 days	Mebendazole 100 mg po bid x3 d.	May need repeat tx if heavily infected.
NEMATODES—EXTRAINTESTINAL (Roundworms)			
Anisakis simplex (**anisakiasis**)	Physical removal: endoscope or surgery	Questionable response to albendazole (Ln 360:54, 2002)	Anisakiasis acquired by eating raw fish: herring, salmon, mackerel, cod, squid. Similar illness due to Pseudoterranova species acquired from cod, halibut, red snapper
Ancylostoma braziliense, causes **cutaneous larva migrans**	Ivermectin 200 µg/kg po x1 dose/d. x1-2 d	Albendazole 200 mg po bid x3 d.	Also called "creeping eruption," dog and cat hookworm. Ivermectin cure rate 77% (1 dose) to 97% (2-3 doses) (CID 31:493, 2000).
Dracunculus medinensis: **Guinea worm**	Surgical removal pre-emergent worm	Metronidazole 250 mg po bid x10 d. used to ↓ inflammatory response and facilitate removal. Immersion in warm water promotes worm emergence. Mebendazole 400-800 mg/d. x6 d. may kill worm.	
Filariasis			
Lymphatic (**Elephantiasis**): Wuchereria bancrofti or Brugia malayi or B. timori	Ivermectin[1] (see Comment) 100-440 µg/kg x1 dose OR (for children) ivermectin 200-400 µg/kg and albendazole 400 mg, one dose of each (Ln 350:480, 1997).	Diethylcarbamazine[3] (DEC)[1,4] po over 14 days. Day 1, 50 mg; day 2, 50 mg tid; day 3, 100 mg tid; days 4-14, 2 mg/kg tid. (See Comment)	Ivermectin kills microfilaria but not adult worms. Diethylcarbamazine: If no microfilariae in blood, can give full doses from day 1.
Cutaneous			
Loiasis: **Loa loa, eyeworm disease**[2]	Diethylcarbamazine (DEC)[1,4] ...dose as for Wuchereria, except use 3 mg/kg tid days 4-14.		DEC 300 mg/wk po effective prophylaxis
Onchocerca volvulus[3] (**onchocerciasis—river blindness**) (Ln 360:203, 2002)	Ivermectin 150 µg/kg po x1 dose; repeat q6 months to suppress dermal and ocular microfilariae. If eye involved, start prednisone 1 mg/kg/d po several days before ivermectin. NOTE: Worm survival requires symbiotic bacteria Wolbachia (Science 295:1365, 2002)		Ivermectin ↓ number of microfilariae in skin and impairs female worm fertility; does not kill adult worms (nothing does). Ivermectin OK in pregnancy.
Body cavity			
Mansonella perstans (**dipetalonemiasis**)	Mebendazole[1] 100 mg po bid x30 d. or albendazole 400 mg po bid x10 d.	Diethylcarbamazine[1] as above for Wuchereria	Usually asymptomatic. Articular pain, pruritus, lymphadenopathy reported. May have allergic reaction from dying organisms.
Mansonella streptocerca	Diethylcarbamazine[1] as above for Wuchereria OR Ivermectin 150 µg/kg x1		Chronic pruritic hypopigmented lesions that may be confused with leprosy. Can be asymptomatic.
Mansonella ozzardi	Ivermectin 200 µg/kg x1 dose may be effective		Usually asymptomatic + eosinophilus. Ivermectin has no activity against this species.

[1] May need antihistamine or corticosteroid for allergic reaction from disintegrating organisms

[2] Diethylcarbamazine available from Wyeth-Ayerst (610) 971-5509

[3] Occasional serious reactions reported in pts with both loiasis and onchocerciasis given ivermectin (Ln 350:18, 1997)

NOTE: *All dosage recommendations are for adults (unless otherwise indicated) and assume normal renal function. See page 103 for abbreviations.*

TABLE 13A (7)

INFECTING ORGANISM	SUGGESTED REGIMENS		COMMENTS
	PRIMARY	ALTERNATIVE	
NEMATODES—Extraintestinal (Roundworms)/Filariasis/Body cavity *(continued)*			
Dirofilariasis: **Heartworms**			
D. immitis, dog heartworm	No effective drugs; surgical removal only option.		Can lodge in pulmonary artery → coin lesion. Eosinophilia rare.
D. tenius (raccoon), D. ursi (bear), D. repens (dogs, cats)	No effective drugs		Worms migrate to conjunctivae, subcutaneous tissue, scrotum, breasts, extremities
Gnathostoma spingicerum; eosinophilic myeloencephalitis	Surgical removal + **albendazole** 400 mg po bid or bid x21 d	**Ivermectin** 200 μg/kg/d x2 d	
Toxocariasis: *Clin Micro Rev 16:265, 2003*	**Rx directed at relief or when infection self-limited, e.g., uses of antihelmintics controversial.**		
Visceral larval migrans	**Albendazole** 400 mg po bid x5 d.	**Mebendazole** 100–200 mg po bid x5 days	Severe lung, heart or CNS disease may warrant steroids. Differential dx of larval migrans syndromes: Toxocara canis and catis, Ancylostoma spp., Gnathostoma spp., Spirometra spp.
Ocular larval migrans	First 4 wks of illness: (Oral) **prednisone** 30–60 mg po qd + subtenon **triamcinolone** 40 mg weekly) x2 weeks		Rx of little effect after 4 wks.
Trichinella spiralis (trichinosis)—muscle infection	**Albendazole** 400 mg po bid x8–14 d. Concomitant **prednisone** 40–60 mg qd	**Mebendazole** 200–400 mg po tid x3 d, then 400–500 mg po tid x10 d.	Use albendazole/mebendazole with caution during pregnancy.
TREMATODES (Flukes)			
Clonorchis sinensis (liver fluke)	**Praziquantel** 25 mg/kg po tid x1 day or **albendazole** 10 mg/kg/d, po x7 d.		Same dose in children
Fasciola buski (intestinal fluke)	**Praziquantel** 25 mg/kg po tid x1 day		Same dose in children
Fasciola hepatica (sheep liver fluke)	**Triclabendazole**[NUS] (Fasinex; Novartis Agribusiness) 10 mg/kg po x1 dose. Ref. *CID 32:1, 2007*	**Bithionol**[CDCX] Adults and children: 30–50 mg/kg (max. dose 2 gm/d) qod x10–15 doses	
Heterophyes heterophyes (intestinal fluke); Metagonimus yokogawai (intestinal fluke); Opisthorchis viverrini (liver fluke)	**Praziquantel** 25 mg/kg po tid x1 day		Same dose in children. Same regimen for Metorchis conjunctus (North American liver fluke).
Paragonimus westermani (lung fluke)	**Praziquantel** 25 mg/kg po tid x2 days or **bithionol**[CDCX] 30–40 mg/kg qod x1 day x10 d.		Same dose in children
Schistosoma haematobium; GU bilharziasis; *N/EJM 346:1212, 2002.*	**Praziquantel** 20 mg/kg po bid x1 day (2 doses)	**Oxamniquine**[NUS] single dose of 15 mg/kg po once; in North and East Africa 20 mg/kg po daily x3 d.	Same dose in children. Alternative: metrifonate 10 mg/kg/dose po q2 wks for 3 doses.
Schistosoma intercalatum	**Praziquantel** 20 mg/kg po bid x1 day (2 doses)		Same dose in children.
Schistosoma japonicum: Oriental schisto. *N/EJM 346:1212, 2002.*	**Praziquantel** 20 mg/kg po bid x1 day (2 doses)		Same dose for children.
Schistosoma mansoni (intestinal bilharziasis) *JID 176:304, 1997)* **Possible praziquantel resistance** *N/EJM 346:1212, 2002)*	**Praziquantel** 20 mg/kg po tid x1 day		Same dose for children. Cures 60–90% pts.
Toxemic schisto, Katayama fever	**Praziquantel** 25 mg/kg po tid x1 day x3 doses		Massive infection with either S. japonicum or S. mansoni
CESTODES (Tapeworms)			
Echinococcus granulosus (hydatid disease) *CID 37:1073, 2003; Ln 362:1295, 2003)*	Meta-analysis supports percutaneous aspiration-injection-reaspiration (PAIR) + albendazole. Before **and** after drainage: albendazole >60 kg, 400 mg po bid or <60 kg, 15 mg/kg/d div. bid, with meals. Then PAIR: needle aspirate (A) cyst content. If cyst content (P), absolute alcohol & wait 20–30 min., then re-aspirate (R) with final irrigation. Continue albendazole x28 d. Cure in 96% as compared to 90% pts with surgical resection.		
Echinococcus multicolularis (alveolar cyst	**Albendazole** efficacy not clearly demonstrated, can try in dosages used for hydatid disease. Wide surgical resection only reliable rx, technique evolving		

[1] **CDC** = Available from CDC Drug Service

NOTE: All dosage recommendations are for adults (unless otherwise indicated) and assume normal renal function. See page 103 for abbreviations.

TABLE 13A (8)

INFECTING ORGANISM	SUGGESTED REGIMENS		COMMENTS
disease)	PRIMARY	ALTERNATIVE	

CESTODES (Tapeworms) (continued)

Intestinal tapeworms

INFECTING ORGANISM	SUGGESTED REGIMENS		COMMENTS
	PRIMARY	ALTERNATIVE	
Diphyllobothrium latum (fish), Dipylidium caninum (dog), Taenia saginata (beef), and Hymenolepis diminuta (rats) and H. nana (humans)	Praziquantel 5–10 mg/kg po x1 dose for children and adults.		**Alternative: Niclosamide** 2 gm po x1.
Radiology 198:259, 1996)			
Cerebral (neuro) cysticercosis Larval stage of T. solium—see Comment Management refs.: *Ln 361:547, 2003 &* *Ln 12:751, 2002*	Cysticercosis outside CNS—benign—no treatment. Inside CNS—no unanimity. Expert panel: (1) If growing &/or many &/or giant cysts &/or subarachnoid disease. **Treat** (2) Calcified cysticercosis: **no treatment** (3) Disagreement: Few viable cysts, degenerating cysts	Praziquantel 25 mg/kg po x1 dose for children and adults Albendazole cheaper & more effective than praziquantel. Albendazole 15 mg/kg/d. x8 d. OR Praziquantel 50 mg/kg/d. x15 d.	**seizure meds may be needed to control rx-induced inflammation from cyst death.** **Dexamethasone ±**
Sparganosis (Spirometra mansonoides) Larval cysts; source—frogs/snakes	Surgical resection or ethanol injection of subcutaneous masses *(NEJM 330:1887, 1994).*		

ECTOPARASITES Ref.: *CID 36:1355, 2003; NEJM 346:1645, 2002*

INFECTING ORGANISM	SUGGESTED REGIMENS		COMMENTS
	PRIMARY	ALTERNATIVE	
Pediculus humanus corporis (body louse)	Treat the clothing. Organism lives in, deposits eggs in seams of clothing. Discard clothing. If not possible, treat clothing with 1% malathion powder or 10% DDT powder.	Body louse leaves clothing only for blood meal. Nits in clothing viable for 1 month. Ref.: *Med Lett 38:6, 1997.*	
P. humanus var. capitis (**head louse**, nits)	**Permethrin**, 5% prescription strength (ELIMITE). Apply entire skin from chin to toes. Leave on 8–10 hrs. Repeat in 1 week. Safe for children 2 mos. old. **Alternative: Lindane** 1% lotion. Apply as for permethrin OR ivermectin 200 µg/kg po x1 *(NEJM 333:26, 1995).* Do not use in pregnancy (see Comment)	Benefit of residual permethrin on hair reduced by shampoos or vinegar. No residual effect with lindane or pyrethrin products. Nit removal important adjunct. Use nit comb ± enzymatic egg remover (CLEAR is one example). Treat sex partners if body or pubic lice. Cost: Permethrin 60 gm $9.20; lindane 60 ml $6.35–16.40; malathion $31.25; ivermectin $9.97. For failures with 1% permethrin, repeat permethrin + po TMP/SMX 10 mg/kg/d. in 2 div. doses x10 days *(Ped 107:E30, 2001).*	
Phthirus pubis (crabs)	**Permethrin** (Nix), Wash hair, apply lotion for 10 min., rinse off; comb. 2nd treatment 7–10 days after (1st kill will kill newly hatched lice (all products). **Lindane** (Kwell) 1%, less effective (use only if failed other therapy). For head lice treatment failures, anecdotal reports of success with **ivermectin** 200 µg/kg single dose po in 2 doses 10 days apart; **does not affect nits**.	Seizures can occur from coverage of broad areas or ingestion. Another option (not in neonates/infants): **Malathion 0.5% lotion** (Ovide). Apply for 8–12 hrs. Study shows no need to comb for lice after malathion.	
Sarcoptes scabiei (**scabies**) (mites) *(CID 27:646, 1998)*			
Immunocompetent patients	**Primary: Permethrin 5% cream** (ELIMITE). Apply entire skin from chin to toes. Leave on 8–10 hrs. Repeat in 1 week. **Alternative: Lindane** (Kwell) 1%. Wash hair, apply lotion for 10 min. then rinse off; comb. (use only if failed other therapy).	Trim fingernails. Reapply to hands after handwashing. Pruritus may persist x2 wks after mites gone. Do not use lindane in pregnancy or in young children—absorbed through skin; can use 6–10% precipitated sulfur in petrolatum daily x3 days. Repeated lindane application associated with seizures in children.	
AIDS patients, CD4 <150/mm³ (Norwegian scabies—see Comments)	For Norwegian scabies: Permethrin as above on day 1, then 6% sulfur in petrolatum daily on days 2–7, then repeat x several weeks. ivermectin 200 µg/kg po x1 reported effective.	Norwegian scabies in AIDS patients: Extensive, crusted. Can mimic psoriasis. Not pruritic. ELIMITE: 60 gm $18.10; lindane 60 ml $2.60–10.50. Highly contagious—isolate!	

NOTE: All dosage recommendations are for adults (unless otherwise indicated) and assume normal renal/renal function. See page 103 for abbreviations.

TABLE 13B: DOSAGE, PRICE, AND SELECTED ADVERSE EFFECTS OF ANTIPARASITIC DRUGS

NOTE: Drugs available from CDC Drug Service indicated by "CDC." Call (404) 639-3670 (or -2888).
Doses vary with indication. For convenience, drugs divided by type of parasite; some drugs used for multiple types of parasites, e.g., albendazole.
COMMENT: Cost data represent average wholesale prices as listed in 2003 Drug Topics Red Book, Medical Economics.

CLASS, AGENT, GENERIC NAME (TRADE NAME)	USUAL ADULT DOSAGE (Cost)	ADVERSE REACTIONS/COMMENTS
Antiprotozoan Drugs		
Intestinal Parasites		
Albendazole (Albenza)	Doses vary with indication. 200–400 mg po 200 mg tab $1.37	Teratogenic. Pregnancy Cat. C; give after negative pregnancy test. Abdominal pain, nausea/vomiting, alopecia, ↑ serum transaminase. Rare leukopenia.
Dehydroemetine (CDC)*	1.5 mg/kg/d to max. of 90 mg IM	Local pain, ECG changes; cardiac arrhythmias, precordial pain, paresthesias, weakness, peripheral neuropathy. GI: nausea/vomiting, diarrhea. Avoid strenuous exercise for 4 wks after rx.
Diloxanide furoate (CDC)*	500 mg po tid	GI: flatulence, abdominal distention, nausea/vomiting. Pruritus, urticaria.
Furazolidone (Furoxone)	Peds. 6 mg/kg/d div. qid. Not for infants <1 mo. old. Liquid: 50 mg/15 ml. 473 ml $100	Only liquid antiglandiasis reaction in U.S. Disulfiram-like reaction with alcohol. Occasional side-effects: Fever, urticaria, ↓ BP, arthralgia, nausea/vomiting, headache. Hemolysis if G6PD deficient. May turn urine brown.
Iodoquinol (Yodoxin) (650 mg $0.86)	Adults: 650 mg po tid; children: 40 mg/kg/d div. tid.	Rarely causes nausea, abdominal cramps, rash, acne. Contraindicated if iodine intolerance.
Metronidazole/Ornidazole[AUS] (Tiberal)/Tinidazole[AUS] (Fasigyn)	Side-effects similar for all. See metronidazole in Table 10A, page 65, & 10B, page 72	Drug is aminoglycoside similar to neomycin; if absorbed due to concomitant inflammatory bowel disease can result in oto/nephrotoxicity. Doses >3 gm assoc. with nausea, abdominal cramps, diarrhea.
Paromomycin (Humatin) Aminosidine in U.K.	Up to 750 mg qid. 250 mg caps $1.90	
Quinacrine[AUS] (Atabrine, Mepacrine)	100 mg tid. No longer available in U.S.; 2 pharmacies will compound it: Panorama Pharm., Calif. 800-247-9767; Medical Center Pharm., Connecticut 203-785-6816. (2)	Contraindicated for pts with history of psoriasis or psoriasis. Yellow staining of skin. Dizziness, headache, vomiting, toxic psychosis (1.5%), hemolytic anemia, thrombocytopenia, urticaria, rash, fever, minor disulfiram-like reactions.
Tinidazole[AUS] (Fasigyn)	For giardiasis: 2 gm po x1 dose	Chemical structure similar to metronidazole but better tolerated. Can obtain from Panorama Pharm. 1-800-247-9767. Avoid concomitant alcohol intake.
Extraintestinal Parasites		
Antimony compounds[AUS] Stibogluconate sodium (Pentostam, Triostam) Meglumine antimoniate (Glucantime, Glucantim)—French tradenames Ref. AAC 46:1163, 2002	Solution containing 30–34% pentavalent antimony	Cough/vomiting if IV infusion too fast. Arthralgia 50%. Others: myalgia, bradycardia, cramps/diarrhea, pruritus/rash, renal toxicity, ↑ amylase. **NOTE: EKG abnormalities occur. Combination rx with, or sequential rx with, ampho B may trigger fatal arrhythmias** (Ln 351:1928, 1998).
Artesunate[AUS]	Adults: 4 mg/kg po x3 d; can give IM	Drug fever, abdominal pain, diarrhea, primary heart block. Refs. CID 33:2009, 2001; Ln 359:1365, 2002; AAC 46:778, 2002.
Atovaquone (Mepron)	Suspension: 1 tsp (750 mg) po bid 750 mg/5 ml. Cost 210 ml $709.00	No. pts stopping rx due to side-effects was 9%; heart 22%, GI 20%, headache 16%, insomnia 10%, fever 14%
Atovaquone and proguanil (Malarone) For prophylaxis of P. falciparum; little data on P. vivax	Prophylaxis: 1 tab po (250 mg + 100 mg) qd with food Treatment: 4 tabs po (1000 mg + 400 mg) once daily with food x3 days Tabs: Either 250/100 mg or 62.5/25 mg. Peds dosage: footnote 2 page 95 Cost: 250/100 mg tab $5.00	Adverse effects in rx trials: abd. pain 17%, N/V 12%, headache 10%, dizziness 5%. Rx 1.9% asymptomatic mild ↑ in ALT/AST. Children—cough, headache, anorexia, vomiting, abd. pain. See drug interactions, Table 22. Safe in G6PD-deficient pts. Can crush tabs for children and give with milk or other liquid nutrients.
Benznidazole[AUS] (Rochagan, Roche, Brazil)	Dose varies—see Malaria prophylaxis and rx. 7.5 mg/kg/d po	Photosensitivity in 50% of pts. GI: abdominal pain, nausea/vomiting/ anorexia. CNS: disorientation, insomnia, twitching/seizures, paresthesias, polyneuritis
Chloroquine phosphate (Aralen)	500 mg tabs $4.00; IM 250 mg ampule $22.00	Minor: anorexia/nausea/vomiting, headache, dizziness, blurred vision, pruritus in dark-skinned pts. Major: protracted rx in rheumatoid arthritis can lead to retinopathy. Can exacerbate psoriasis. Can block response to rabies vaccine.

All dosage recommendations are for adults

TABLE 13B (2)

CLASS, AGENT, GENERIC NAME (TRADE NAME)	USUAL ADULT DOSAGE (Cost)	ADVERSE REACTIONS/COMMENTS
Antiprotozoan Drugs/Extraintestinal Parasites (continued)		
Dapsone[AUS] Refr. CID 27:191, 1998	100 mg qd. 100 mg tabs $0.20	Usually tolerated by pts with rash after TMP/SMX. Adverse effects: nausea/vomiting, rash, oral lesions (CID 18:630, 1994). Methemoglobinemia (usually asymptomatic); if > 10–15%, stop drug. Hemolytic anemia if G6PD deficient. Sulfone syndrome: fever, rash, hemolytic anemia, atypical lymphocytes, and liver injury (West J Med 156:303, 1992).
Eflornithine[AUS] (Ornidyl)	Approved in U.S. for trypanosome infections but not marketed. Contact Hoechst Marion Roussel. (800) 552-3656.	Diarrhea in ½ pts, vomiting, abdominal pain, anemia/leucopenia in ⅓ pts, seizures, alopecia, jaundice, ↓ hearing
Fumagillin	Eyedrops + po. 20 mg po tid. Call 800-547-1392.	Adverse events: Neutropenia & thrombocytopenia
Halofantrine (Halfan)	Adults: 500 mg po q6h x3 doses Children: 8 mg/kg po q6h x3 doses 250 mg tab $9.88	Poor oral bioavailability ↑ with fatty meal. Causes delay in A-V conduction: **do not use if long QT interval or pt taking drugs known to ↑ QT interval (e.g., quinine/quinidine, astemizole, chloroquine, antidepressants, neuroleptic drugs).** Other side-effects: nausea, abdominal pain, diarrhea. Do not use in pregnancy.
Mefloquine (Lariam)	One 250 mg tab/week for malaria prophylaxis; for rx, 1250 mg x1 or 750 mg x1 & then 500 mg in 6–8 hrs. 250 mg tab $11.83. In U.S. 250 mg tab = 228 mg base; outside U.S. 275 mg tab = 250 mg base	Side-effects in roughly 3%. Minor: headache, dizziness, irritability, insomnia, weakness, diarrhea. Toxic psychoses, seizures possible, but rare. Do not use in 1st trimester of pregnancy, or in pts taking quinine, or halofantrine. Rare: Prolonged QT interval and toxic epidermal necrolysis (Ln 349:101, 1997). Not used for self-rx due to neuropsychiatric side-effects.
Melarsoprol (CDC) (Mel B, Arsobal) (Manufactured in France)	See Trypanosomiasis for adult dose. Peds dose: 0.36 mg/kg IV, then gradual ↑ to 3.6 mg/kg q1–5 days for total of 9–10 doses.	Post-rx encephalopathy (10%) with 50% mortality overall, risk of death 2° to rx 4–8%. Prednisolone 1 mg/kg/d po may ↓ encephalopathy. Other: Heart damage, albuminuria, abdominal pain, vomiting, peripheral neuropathy, Herxheimer-like reaction, pruritus.
Miltefosine[AUS] (Zentaris, Impavido)	100–150 mg (approx. 2.25 mg/kg/d.) po x28 d. Cutaneous leishmaniasis 2.25 mg/kg/d po qd x6 wks	Contact Astra Medica, Ger. **Pregnancy—No.** teratogenic. Side-effects vary kala-azar pts, vomiting in up to 40%, diarrhea in 17%; child to moderate in severity—may resolve in < 1 day.
Nifurtimox (Lampit) (CDC) (Manufactured in Germany by Bayer)	8–10 mg/kg po div. 4x/day	Side-effects in 40–70% of pts. GI: abdominal pain, nausea/vomiting. CNS: polyneuritis (1/3), disorientation, insomnia, twitching, seizures. Skin rash. Hemolysis with G6PD deficiency.
Nitazoxanide (Alinia)	Adults: 0.5–1.0 gm po bid (x14 d. if HIV+). Peds: 100–200 mg q12h x3 d.	
Pentamidine (NebuPent)	300 mg via aerosol q month. Also used IM. 300 mg $98.75 + admin. costs	Hypotension, hypocalcemia, hypoglycemia followed by hyperglycemia, pancreatitis. Neutropenia (15%), thrombocytopenia. Nephrotoxicity. Others: nausea/vomiting. ↑ liver tests, rash.
Primaquine phosphate	26.3 mg (= 15 mg base) $0.77	May G6PD def. pts, can cause hemolytic anemia with hemoglobinuria, esp. African, Asian peoples. Methemoglobinemia. With high dose, abdominal pain if not fasting.
Pyrimethamine (Daraprim, Malocide) Also combined with sulfadoxone as Fansidar	100 mg, then 25 mg qd. 25 mg $0.43. Cost of folinic acid (leucovorin) 5 mg $2.00	Major problem is hematologic: megaloblastic anemia, ↓ WBC, ↓ platelets. Can give 5 mg folinic acid/day to ↓ bone marrow depression and not interfere with antitoxoplasmosis effect. If high-dose pyrimethamine, ↑ folinic acid to 10–50 mg/d. Pyrimethamine + sulfadoxone can cause mental changes due to carnitine deficiency (AJM 95:112, 1993). Other: Rash, vomiting, diarrhea, xerostomia
Quinacrine[AUS]	For giardiasis: 100 mg po x5 d. Peds dose: 2 mg/kg po tid $0.70/100 mg.	Compounded by Med. Center Pharm., Panorama Compound. Contact Med. Center Pharm. New Haven, CT: (203) 688-6816 or Panorama Compound. (800) 247-9767.
Quinidine gluconate	Loading dose: 100 mg (equivalent to 6.2 mg of quinidine base)/kg IV over 1–2 hrs, and then constant infusion of 0.02 mg of quinidine gluconate/kg/minute. 80 mg IV $21.56	Adverse reactions of quinidine/quinine similar: (1) IV bolus injection can cause fatal hypotension (2) hyperinsulinemic hypoglycemia, esp. in pregnancy, (3) ↑ rate of infusion of IV quinidine if QT interval ↑ >25% of baseline, (4) reduce dose 30–50% after day 3 due to ↓ renal clearance and ↓ vol. of distribution.

NOTE: All dosage recommendations are for adults (unless otherwise indicated) and assume normal renal/renal function. See page 103 for abbreviations.

TABLE 13B (3)

CLASS, AGENT, GENERIC NAME (TRADE NAME)	USUAL ADULT DOSAGE (Cost)	ADVERSE REACTIONS/COMMENTS
Antiprotozoan Drugs/Extraintestinal Parasites *(continued)*		
Quinine sulfate (300 mg salt = 250 mg base)	No tabs. No IV prep. in U.S. Oral rx of chloroquine-resistant falciparum malaria: 650 mg po tid x3d, then tetracycline 250 mg po qid x7 d, 325 mg $0.16	Cinchonism: tinnitus, headache, nausea, abdominal pain, blurred vision. Rarely: blood dyscrasias, drug fever, asthma, hypoglycemia. Transient blindness in <1% of 500 pts (AnIM 136:339, 2002).
Spiramycin[1] (Rovamycine) (JAC 42:572, 1998)	Up to 3-4 gm/d	GI and allergic reactions have occurred. Not available in U.S.
Sulfadiazine	1.0-1.5 gm po q6h 500 mg $0.34	See Table 10B, page 72, for sulfonamide side-effects
Sulfadoxine and pyrimethamine combination (Fansidar)	Contains 500 mg of sulfadoxine and 25 mg of pyrimethamine One tab $3.77	Very long mean half-life of both drugs. Sulfadoxine 169 hrs, pyrimethamine 111 hrs allows weekly dosage. Fatalities reported due to Stevens-Johnson syndrome and toxic epidermal necrolysis. Renal excretion—use with caution in pts with renal impairment.
DRUGS USED TO TREAT NEMATODES, TREMATODES, AND CESTODES		
Bithionol[1] (CDC)	Adults & children: 30-40 mg/kg (to max. of 2 gm/d) po qod x10-15 doses	Photosensitivity, skin reactions, urticaria, GI upset
Diethylcarbamazine[1] (Hetrazan) (CDC)	Used to treat filariasis. Licensed (Lederle) but not available in U.S.	Headache, dizziness, nausea, fever. Host may experience inflammatory reaction to death of adult worms. Fever, urticaria, asthma, GI upset (Mazzotti reaction).
Ivermectin (Stromectol, Mectizan)	Strongyloidiasis dose: 200 μg/kg x1 dose po Onchocerciasis: 150 μg/kg x1 po Scabies: 200 μg/kg po x1 3 mg tabs $5.45	Mild side-effects: fever, pruritus, rash. In rx of onchocerciasis, can see tender lymphadenopathy, headache, bone/joint pain. Can cause Mazzotti reaction (see above).
Mebendazole (Vermox)	Doses vary with indication. 100 mg tab $5.91	Rarely causes abdominal pain, nausea, diarrhea. Contraindicated in pregnancy and children <2 yrs old.
Oxamniquine (Vansil)[NUS]	For S. mansoni. Some experts suggest 40-60 mg/kg over 2-3 days in all of Africa.	Rarely: dizziness, drowsiness, neuropsychiatric symptoms, GI upset. EKG/EEG changes. Orange/red urine.
Praziquantel (Biltricide)	Doses vary with parasite; see Table 13A, 600 mg $11.90	Mild: dizziness/drowsiness, N/V, rash, fever. Only contraindication is ocular cysticercosis. Metabolism induced by anticonvulsants and steroids, can negate effect with cimetidine 400 mg po tid.
Pyrantel pamoate (over-the-counter as Reese's Pinworm Medicine)	Oral suspension. Dose for all ages: 11 mg/kg (to max. of 1 gm) x1 dose	Rare GI upset, headache, dizziness, rash
Suramin (Germanin) (CDC)	For early trypanosomiasis. Drug powder mixed to 10% solution with 5 ml water and used within 30 minutes.	Does not cross blood-brain barrier; no effect on CNS infection. Side-effects: vomiting, pruritus, urticaria, fever, paresthesias, albuminuria (discontinue drug if casts appear). Do not use if renal/liver disease present. Deaths from vascular collapse reported.
Thiabendazole (Mintezol)	Take after meals. Dose varies with parasite; see Table 12A, 500 mg $1.25	Nausea/vomiting, headache, dizziness. Rarely: liver damage, ↓ BP, angioneurotic edema, Stevens-Johnson syndrome. May ↓ mental alertness.

Abbreviations: **Clinda** = clindamycin; **CQ** = chloroquine phosphate; **MQ** = mefloquine; **NUS** = not available in the U.S.; **PQ** = primaquine; **Pyri** = pyrimethamine; **QS** = quinine sulfate; **TMP/SMX** = trimethoprim/sulfamethoxazole

[1] Available from FDA: (301) 443-5680
[2] Available from Wyeth-Ayerst, (610) 971-5509
NOTE: All dosage recommendations are for adults (unless otherwise indicated) and assume normal renal function. See page 103 for abbreviations.

TABLE 14A: ANTIVIRAL THERAPY (Non-HIV)
(See NEJM 340:1255, 1999)

VIRUS/DISEASE	DRUG/DOSAGE	SIDE EFFECTS/COMMENTS
Adenovirus Common cause of respiratory tract infections including fatal pneumonia in young adults [outbreaks of type 4 have re-emerged in U.S. military camps (CID 35:808, 2002)]—esp. severe in immunocompromised hosts (fatality rates 50-80% survival)	**No proven rx**: case reports of possible success with ribavirin (Ped 110:e9, 2002), & cidofovir (Clin Micro Rev 16:569, 2003; PIDJ 22:928, 2003)	PCR available for adenovirus DNA (+ in 72% of children with 1st infection (JID 187:1571, 2003) & assoc. with fatal outcome in children with stem cell transplant (CID 35:526, 2002)
Coronavirus—SARS-CoV (Severe Acute Respiratory Distress Syn.) A new coronavirus, isolated in spring 2003 (NEJM 348:1953 & 1967, 2003) emerged from China (animal reservoir may be the civet cat), & spread rapidly from Hong Kong to 32 countries; by July >8000 cases, >800 deaths reported. Transmission usually by droplet aerosol spread may explain multiple cases in ICUs following intubation or bronchoscopy. Healthcare workers account for >50% of cases (>90% in Taiwan) (Ln 361:1319, 2003). Isolation of patients & use of strict infection control guidelines was likely responsible for finally controlling the epidemic (Ln 361:1519, 2003; JAMA ePub May 6, 2003).	**Therapy remains predominantly supportive care.** Therapy with drugs currently remains unproven. The following have been tried: Ribavirin—appears ineffective. Corticosteroids—methyl prednisolone 0.5 gm IV/d in a pulse dose x2 & repeated on days 3 & 4 in no response. Appears more effective in reducing hypoxemia than non-pulse methyl prednisone (AJRCCM Aug. 28, 2003) & more rather than oral prednisone (J.J. Surg., ISAAR, July 2003).	Disease presents as moderate to severe pneumonia with fever, chills, myalgias, cough & dyspnea. Leukopenia, hypocalcemia, ↑ RNH & thrombocytopenia are common (NEJM 348:1986, 2003). Initial chest x-ray abnormalities found in 80% with focal air-space opacities usually in periphery, progressing to multi focal & bilateral in 75% (Radiol, May 20, 2003). 20% require ICU care & mechanical ventilation. Diagnostic tests include PCR on respiratory secretions or ELISA & IFA on serum (± after 2-3 wks). Mortality rates 10% (↑ in elderly).
Enterovirus—Meningitis: most common cause of aseptic meningitis. PCR on CSF valuable for early dx (Scand J Inf Dis 34:359, 2003)	**No rx currently recommended**; however pleconaril (VP 63843) still under investigation. [For compassionate use call Viropharma (610) 458-7300, ext. 6297 (Donna Kolbush, RN)]	No clinical benefit demonstrated in double-blind placebo-controlled study in 21 infants with enterovirus aseptic meningitis (PIDJ 22:335, 2003)
Hemorrhagic Fever Virus Infections **Congo-Crimean Hemorrhagic Fever (HF)**	Oral **ribavirin**, **30 mg/kg** as initial loading dose & 15 mg/kg q6h x4 days & then 7.5 mg/kg x6 days (WHO recommendations). For oral drug, contact Viracole, ICN Pharmaceuticals, Costa Mesa, CA, USA.	3/3 healthcare workers in Pakistan had complete recovery (Ln 346:472, 1990) & 8/9 in Iran survived (with confirmed CCHF rx with ribavirin survived in Iran (CID 36:1613, 2003))
Ebola/Marburg HF (Central Africa) Epidemic continues to simmer in Africa (JAMA 290:317, 2003)	**No data to date on antiviral therapy** (J Virol Methods 105:89, 2002)	After infection may control viral proliferation and result in asymptomatic infection (Ln 355:2210, 2000). A vaccine in mice may be near (Nature 408:527, 2004:681, 2003).
With pulmonary syndrome: Hanta-virus. With hemorrhagic fever with renal syndrome: **"sin nombre virus"** + others now found around the world (EID 18:768, 2002)	**No benefit from ribavirin has been demonstrated** (ribavirin in progress). Refs: (Ln 262:1898, 1997; Emerg Inf Dis 3:95, 1997; Curr Inf Dis Rep 3:258, 2001.	Acute onset of fever, headache, myalgias, non-productive cough, thrombocytopenia and non-cardiogenic pulmonary edema with respiratory insufficiency following exposure to rodents. Persistent presence of myal-gias, nausea, diarrhea, dizziness, ↑ PCO₂ predicted ↑ hantavirus pulmonary syndrome (HPS) (CID 34:293, 2002). May also cause syndrome similar to other hemorrhagic fevers (CID 34:1224, 2002). Serological studies available through CDC (CID 347:739, 1996).
With renal syndrome: Lassa, Venezuelan, Junin, Machupo	**Ribavirin** IV 2 gm loading dose, then 1 gm q6h x4 days, then 0.5 gm q8h x6 d. (See Comment: Congo-Crimean HF)	Toxicity low; hemolysis reported but recovery when treatment stopped. No significant changes in WBC-, platelets, hepatic or renal function. Effective in Lassa and in 2 cases of Bolivian (CID 24:718, 1997). No data on others. Venezuelan HF may look like dengue (CID 26:308, 1998). See CID 36:1254, 2003 for management of contacts
Hemorrhagic fever viruses: Lassa HF, Bolivian HF, Junin, Machupo		
Dengue and dengue hemorrhagic fever (DHF) Aedes aegypti major vector (JID 176:313, 1997). Death rate highest in young children & elderly (Int J Inf Dis 6:118, 2002; CID 35:277, 2003)	**No proven rx to date.**	Resurgence in Southeast Asia, Central and South America and Caribbean. No vaccine; best pre-vention is to limit mosquito exposure (AnM 128:931, 1998 gives specifics). For DHF & DSS, therapy critical (Ln 352:971, 1998). Rx of DHF with colloids may be more effective than crystalloids in pts with low pulse pressures (CID 32:204, 2001; J Ped 140:629, 2002). A Brazilian pts with DHF & severe thrombocytopenia in with gamma globulin (dengue Ab-neg) 1,500 mg/kg IV had ↑ in platelet counts (CID 36:1623, 2003)
West Nile virus A flavivirus introduced into the U.S. (NYC) in 1999, transmitted by mosquitoes, blood transfusions, transplanted organs (NEJM 348: 2196, 2003). & breast-feeding (MMWR 51:877, 2002).	**No data on antiviral rx.** Ribavirin and Interferon under study: to enroll pt, see www.nyha.org/posting/mlar.html (EID 8:107, 2002) Rx of WNF (WCV from Israel (rion@pomrx.co.il) under study (www.nih.gov or CDC 800:342-6237 (Ribavirin ↓ sur-vival in hamsters & in cell culture) (EID 8:1355, 2002). Also of note: a lung transplant pt (Transpl Inf Dis 4:160, 2002). U.S. IVIG has no WNV antibody.	Dx by † PCR in serum & CSF (contact State Health Dept. (CDC). Blood supply now being tested for WNV. & in summer 2003. 150 viremic donors identified (MMWR 52:821, 2003).

NOTE: All dosage recommendations are for adults (unless otherwise indicated) and assume normal renal function.

TABLE 14A (2)

VIRUS/DISEASE	DRUG/DOSAGE	SIDE EFFECTS/COMMENTS
Hemorrhagic Fever Virus Infections (continued)	No data on antiviral rx	
Yellow fever	No therapy recommended. If within 2 wks of exposure, gamma globulin 0.02 ml/kg IM injection x1 is protective.	Reemergence across Africa (Uganda 2003) & South America (200,000 cases/yr). Vaccination effective and should be used (JAMA 276:1157, 1996).
Hepatitis Viral Infections		
Hepatitis A		For vaccine recommendations, see Table 20. 40% of pts with chronic Hep C who developed fulminant hepatic failure in 1 study (NEJM 338:286, 1998).
Acute (Ln 351:1643, 1998)	No therapy recommended	Most common cause of death from acute hepatitis in Italy (Dig Liver Dis 35:404, 2003).
Hepatitis B		**FDA-approved**
Chronic (AIM 132:296, 2000) In general, consider ↑ in pts with persistent ↑ of aminotransferase; detectable levels of HBeAg & HBV DNA in serum for at least 6 mos; hepatitis on liver bx; & compensated liver disease	For HBeAg+, 3 drugs currently Lamivudine (LAV)150 mg po qd x 12 mos. until HBeAg sero-conversion or Adefovir (ADF) 10 mg po qd x12 mos. or interferon alfa 2b 10 MU 3x/wk or 5 MU daily x16-24 wks. Repeat dosing schedule if HBeAg fails to respond but only for this indication not as with HCV once-weekly dosing makes it very attractive or PEG INF alfa 2a 180 µg sq q week (not FDA-approved) Combination therapies (not FDA-approved but probably the treatment of the future) Interferon + lamivudine or PEG INF + lamivudine or Adefovir + lamivudine For anti-HBeAb+, ↑ ALT, HBV DNA+: Rx with lamivudine as above	1st line rx: Well-tolerated & remarkably non-toxic but drug-resistant YMDD mutations emerge over time in some pts — 14-32% at 1 year, 38% at 2 years, ~67% at 4 year rx 67%. Mutants appear less virulent than wild type virus, breakthrough associated with flare of hepatitis & occ. hepatic decompensation. Thus less attractive for advanced disease. Long-term rx (yrs) improves effectiveness. Sustained Viral Response (SVR). ($156.70 for 30-day rx) Recommended for LAV failures or uncompensated disease & effective against YMDD mutants (for LAV failures but must adjust dose for renal impairment) (CrCl <50%). More expensive than LAV ($528 for 30 d.) & less than 25% show exacerbation of hepatitis after discontinuation. No resistance reported to date. (NEJM 348:800, 808, 2003). Recommended only for compensated liver disease. Do not use if ↑ bilirubin or pro time. ↓ albumin, history of ascites, encephalopathy, or variceal bleeding. As with other drugs, best response with ↓ HBV DNA (<200 pg/ml) & ↑ ALT (>3x normal). Best HBeAg seroconversion rates of the 3 drugs & shorter duration of rx but may cause bone marrow suppression, depression (severe), etc.]; subcutaneous administration & cost ($1739 for 30-day course). PEG INF alfa 2a at 90, 180 & 270 µg sq q wk was 2x more effective than standard INF 4.5 million units 3x/wk (24% sustained response vs 12%, p = .036) & will likely replace INF alfa 2b (J Viral Hepat 10:298, 2003). Multiple studies (Curr Hep Rep 2:49, 2003) suggest ↑ rate of response but conflicting study designs & failure to demonstrate superiority of a single drug combination. Difficult & recommendation of combination problematic at this time. Combination may also be less effective than LAV alone in INF-unresponsive pts (CID 36:1516, 2003; J Hepato 38:818, 2003). PEG INF & lamivudine currently being studied in Europe: reports look encouraging.

Goal of rx: ↓ liver inflammation, stop progression to cirrhosis, & prevent hepatocellular carcinoma. HBV: lamivudine (LAV), & adefovir (ADF) work; response measured by loss of HBe Ag & undetectable HBV DNA (23-32%) & return of ALT to normal (41-72%). This usually followed by appearance of HBs antibody, once appearance of HBe antibody & HBV DNA & occ. disappearance of HBe Ag with persistence of HBV DNA (SVR): lack of relapse after rx d/c) in pts with loss of both the Ag & HBV DNA with persistence of HBe antigen, seroconversion predicts viral relapse. Histological improvement seen in 50-60%. Sustained viral response (SVR) when seen with baseline HBV DNA < ULN & ALT high. The drugs work best (Hepatol 36:507, 2002), entecavir (AAC 46:2525, 2002).

Other nucleoside analogs look impressive [tenofovir (Hepatol 36:507, 2002), entecavir (AAC 46:2525, 2002)] respectively.

VIRUS/DISEASE	DRUG/DOSAGE	SIDE EFFECTS/COMMENTS
		Studies in progress
Prevention Re-infection after transplantation for hepatitis B-induced cirrhosis (See Table 15A, page 122 for post-exposure prophylaxis recommendations)	Lamivudine 100 mg/d. Start at least 4 wks pre-transplant and continue for at least 12 months post-transplant (Hpt 30: 222A, 1999; Tpt 62:1456, 1996; Ln 348: 1212, 1996)	[Based on 3 uncontrolled studies, data suggest that lamivudine reduction post-transplant. Most pts were clinically stable at 1 yr. Post-transplant recurrence of HBV was observed in some pts & YMDD variant HBV was detected in 2 pts (Hpt 30:222A, 1999; J Hpt 34:895, 2001). Lamivudine is most effective in preventing recurrence when combined with HBIG (Hpt 28:585,1994) but has been used alone in low-risk pts (J Hpt 34:888, 2001). Optimal dose and duration of HBIG unknown.

NOTE: All dosage recommendations are for adults (unless otherwise indicated) and assume normal renal function.

TABLE 14A (3)

VIRUS/DISEASE	DRUG/DOSAGE	SIDE EFFECTS/COMMENTS

Hepatitis Viral Infections *(continued)*

Hepatitis C (Up to 4 million pts in U.S.) See *NEJM 345:41, 2001; CID 33:1728, 2001; AnM 136:747, 2002.* www.hepnet.com/hep.html

Acute: Often asymptomatic (>75%). Rx of acute hepatitis C with INF alfa 2b may reduce progression to chronic Hep C infection: 43/44 pts with Hep C virus (most sympto-matic or asymptomatic (>75%), occasionally non-specific complaints such as fatigue.

Ref: www.wiki.gov.nih/hepatitis:
Rx consists of persistent elevations ALT, HCV RNA +, & findings of fibrosis & at least moderate inflammation by liver bx.

Chronic: See 2002 NIH consensus statement; http://consensus.nih.gov/cons/116/116cons_intr & Semin Liver Dis 20 Suppl 1:135, 2003 & Postgrad Med 114:48, 57, 62, 2003.

Genotype 1 is most common in U.S.
(>90%), & least responsive to rx. Once infected only 15% spontaneously clear virus, 85% have chronic infection, 10-15% progress to cirrhosis (med time 28-32 yrs), 4% hepatocellular (hrCA) carcinoma. 8-10,000 deaths in U.S./yr. Co-infection with HIV extremely common.

Consider dx in high-risk pts (see Prevention, below) with ↑ ALT. Dx made by EIA for HCV antibody, sensitivity & specificity >99% in at-risk populations & those with liver disease. Qualitative HCV PCR used for confirmation but may be neg in early HCV infection without obvious risk factors or no evidence of immunity. Immunoblot assay used as confirmatory test for pos. EIA in immunocompromised setting or neg. HCV RNA. HCV RNA (by PCR) in those with neg. EIA. Later (>90% by 3 mos). Persistent infection dx by +HCV PCR for >6 mos. Progressive liver disease associated with older pts, immunosuppressed state (HIV), alcohol use (>30 gm/d), 50% pos for serum cryo-globulins, but clinical manifestations uncommon.

When genotype 1, for 48 wks:

Pegylated INF:		Ribavirin	Wt
Alfa 2a (Pegasys)		[400 mg a.m.,	<75 Kg
180 μg sc q wk		600 mg po p.m.]	
Alfa 2b (PEG-Intron)		600 mg po bid	>75Kg
1.5 μg/kg sc q wk			

Duration of rx:
Genotype 1: check quantitative HCV RNA after 12 wks. If neg. or ≥2 log ↓, continue for 48 wks (up to 51% SVR reported). If pos. or <2 log ↓: dc rx (unlikely to respond & consider if otherwise) *(Hepato 38:645, 2003; J Hepato 39:106, 2003)*

When genotype 2 or 3 (non-1), alternatives are for 24wks:

Standard INF alfa	+	Ribavirin 400 mg
3 mIU sc 3x/wk		po bid
or		**or**
PEG INF alfa (either	+	Ribavirin 400 mg
2a or 2b as above)		po bid
(since INF alfa SVR similar to		
genotypes 2&3)		

Prevention of acute and chronic infection *(For comment on Hepatitis C prophylaxis, see Table 15, page 123)*

See *NEJM 345:1452, 2001]. 5/6 received rx 89 days to signs/symptoms of hepatitis and mean 89 days to start of rx after jaundiced [pts in Portugal w INF alfa 2b for 6 mos. had SVR (neg. HCV RNA for 1 year) (Hepatogastroenterol 50:1057, 2003). A review of published trials (206 pts) concluded that SVR following rx of acute Hep C w INF alfa 2b was 32% vs 4% with placebo (p=0.0007) (Cochrane Database Sys & Rev:CD000369, 2002)*

Obtain baseline CBC and platelet count. Follow with ribavirin.
hemolytic anemia very common with ribavirin.
Sustained viral response (neg. HCV-RNA (<50 IU/ml) at least 24 wks after end of rx) assoc. with resolution of hepatic fibrosis (Dig Dis Sci 48:1425, 2003) & lower likelihood of HCV relapse. Rx assoc. with ↓ hepatocellular carcinoma (AnIM 131:174, 1999) & at 8 yrs past INF rx: ↓ in liver-related deaths (RR 0.21 (.09–.5)) esp. in those with SVR (RR .03 (.003–.21)(Hepato 38:493, 2003).

3 large pivotal trials have demonstrated superiority of pegylated interferon + ribavirin over standard interferon-ribavirin combination or PEG-INF alone. [Sustained viral response (SVR) = 42–51% for genotype 1 after 48 wks rx or 76–82% for genotypes 2 & 3 after 24 weeks]. Rates similar with both forms of PEG-INF (alfa 2a & alfa 2b). Exceptions are genotypes 2 & 3 where PEG-INF + ribavirin similar to INF-INF-Rib-76-82% SVR after 24 wks). Factors that ↑ success: genotype other than 1, lower baseline viral levels, less fibrosis, lower body wt & surface area (J Vir Hep 10:271-75, 2002; Hepato 36:636, 2002). Serum & genetic markers (HLA class, B44) may predict ↑ response (Am J Gastro 98:1621, 2003).

Excessive alcohol consumption (>5 oz/d.) accelerates hepatic fibrosis from HCV (Ln 349:825, 1997).Occult HBV or HIV infection account for lack of response to rx in some pts (CID 32:562, 2001; J Viral 75:7864, 2001). HIV accelerates HCV disease progression (JAIDS 33:365, 2003) & HCV infection ↓ beneficial effects of HAART on HIV infection (J AIDS 33:365, 2003).

Decisions regarding re-treatment of non-responders or relapses complex. Only about 15–20% of non-responders rx with INF-Rib combination will respond to retreatment with PEG INF-Rib, whereas >60% of those with virologic relapse (w/ initial rx) had SVR w 2nd rx (Am J Gastr 98:2584, 2003). Response is independent of ribavirin dose (Clin Infec Diseases Viral 10:215, 2003). Pts with advanced liver disease/cirrhosis have ↑ risk of hepatic decompensation & should probably be retreated (2002 NIH Consensus Conference).

Side effects significant: 10–14% receiving PEG INF-Rib dc rx 2° to side effects (flu-like symptoms, hematologic & psychiatric). Psychiatric/neuropsychiatric relapse (w/ INF alfa) 10/215, 2003]. Also [Viral Hep 23:25, 2003]. Also interferon can cause or aggravate life-threatening neuropsychiatric, autoimmune, ischemic & infectious disorders—monitor closely. See drug section. Table 14B. **Ribavirin is teratogenic & must not be used if pregnancy possible in pt or partner.** Because of toxicity, rx of pts with minimal inflammation (by liver bx or low to normal ALT), is usually not recommended.

NOTE: All dosage recommendations are for adults (unless otherwise indicated) and assume normal renal function.

TABLE 14A (4)

VIRUS/DISEASE	DRUG/DOSAGE	SIDE EFFECTS/COMMENTS
Herpesvirus infections (see review: *CID 26:541, 1998*)		
Cytomegalovirus (CMV)		
Normal host	No rx indicated for acute mononucleosis syndrome and not established for congenital CMV (see Comment)	A study of newborns with symptomatic congenital CMV infection suggests 8 and 12 mg/kg/d of IV ganciclovir has limited efficacy but ↓ platelets and ↓ PMNs common (*JID 175:1080, 1997*)
Immunocompromised host	**Treatment of AIDS patients with highly active antiretroviral therapy (HAART)** is effective in suppressing CMV viremia: 16/16 pts became CMV-negative by PCR without specific CMV therapy and none developed endpoints (*AIDS 13:1203, 1999*). Monitoring of CMV DNA appears to be of value in predicting & diagnosing ganciclovir-resistant infections (*J Clin Virol 14:73, 1999; JID 177:770, 1998*). In AIDS pts with CMV retinitis, discontinuation of maintenance rx (to limit drug toxicity) seems reasonable if CD4 cell count >100–150 × several months. pp65 antigenemia predictable than for retinitis (*AJM 98:109, 1995*). Responses less predictable than for retinitis (*A/M 98:109, 1995*). **Valganciclovir** 900 mg q12h effective in 9/10 pts (*AAC 47:1587, 1988*). Responses less predictable than for retinitis (*A/M 98:109, 1995*). **Valganciclovir** also likely effective. Switch to oral valganciclovir when po tolerated.
Colitis/esophagitis	**Ganciclovir** 2.5 mg/kg q8h IV x20 days + IVIG 500 mg/kg q8h (intraventricular)/18h x20 days → IVIG 500 mg q8h IV q12h intravenous/18h x20 doses, then ganciclovir 5 mg/kg q12h x10 doses (*AnnM 109:777, 1988*)	[11/16 (the AIDS pts responded to antiviral rx (*KHNeuro1 29:139, 1991*). [11/16 made more of improvement progressed despite early antiretroviral (*CID 23:76, 1996*). In BMT recipients, serial measure of GCV antigen was useful in establishing early (*CID 23:76, 1996*). In BMT recipients, serial measure of GCV antigen was useful in establishing early CMV interstitial pneumonia with good results if GCV initiated within 6 days of antigen positivity (*Bone Marrow Transplant 26:413, 2000*). For preventive therapy, see Table 15D, page 128
CMV of the nervous system: Encephalitis & ventriculitis	**Ganciclovir:** as with retinitis. Consider combination of ganciclovir and foscarnet if prior CMV rx used. Switch to valganciclovir when possible.	Differential: HIV retinopathy, herpes simplex retinitis (*Arch Ophthal 114:834, 1996*), varicella-zoster retinitis (rare, hard to diagnose).
Lumbosacral polyradiculopathy	Treatment not defined; but disease develops while taking ganciclovir as suppressive therapy. About 50% will respond (*CID 20:747, 1995*); survival↑ (5.4 wks to 14.6 wks) (*CID 27:345, 1998*).	
Mononeuritis multiplex	Not defined	
CMV pneumonia—seen predominantly in transplants (esp bone marrow), rare in HIV	Due to vasculitis and may not be responsive to antiviral rx	Cannot use GCV ocular implant alone as approx. 50% of CMV retinitis other eye at 6 mos, and 31% risk visceral disease (*Arch Ophthal 12:155, 1994*). Risk↓ with systemic rx (*CID 24: 620, 1997; NEJM 337:83, 1997*). Similarly, intraocular injections of fomivirsen do not prevent contralateral eye or systemic visceral disease (*Am J Ophth 133:467, 475, 484, 552, 2002*). **Concurrent systemic rx recommended.** Because of unique mode of action, fomivirsen may have a role if isolates become resistant to other therapies. Watch for retinal detachments, 50–90% within 1 yr of dx of retinitis.
Retinitis (most common in AIDS)		
19/30 pts (63%) with inactive CMV retinitis who responded to HAART (↑ of >80 CD4 cells and sustained immune recovery vitreitis (vision ↓ & floaters) — with posterior segment inflammation—vitreitis, papillitis & macular changes) after ↑ of CD4 cells after rx started (*JID 179: 697, 1999*). Another reported 8/21 pts receiving HAART had inflammatory eye complications (*AIDS 14:1163, 2000*). Corticosteroid rx ↓ inflammatory reaction of immune reconstitution (*ID Abst. 751*). Antibodies to CMV glycoprotein develop rapidly following HAART, which ↓ lowering HAART (*AIM 158: 957, 1998; AIDS 16:2129, 2002*). See Guidelines of International Panel (*AIM 158: 957, 1998*).	**Induction therapy, primary:** **Valganciclovir** 900 mg po bid with food x 21 days **OR** **Ganciclovir** (GCV) 5 mg/kg IV q12h (adjust for renal function) x14–21 days **OR** **Foscarnet** (FOS) 90 mg/kg q12h (adjust for renal function) IV at constant rate (requires infusion pump) over 2 hrs x14–21 days **OR** Combination of **Intraocular ganciclovir (GCV) implant** (delivers 1–2 µg/hr x6–7 mos.) + (either concurrent **IV GCV** as above or **oral valganciclovir** 900 mg qd with food) **Induction therapy, alternative:** **Cidofovir** 5 mg/kg IV q wk x2 wks (induction dose), then 5 mg/kg q2wk (maintenance dose), 1 gm 2x2 hrs immediately before each dose, and 1 gm po 3 hrs before cidofovir dose. Give probenecid 2 gm po 3 hrs before cidofovir dose, 1 gm 2 hrs immediately after dose) and 1 liter of normal saline IV 1 hr before cidofovir infusion as above. **Fomivirsen** 330 mg by direct intravitreal injection q2wk x2, then q month q mos. (see www.aidsinfo.nih.gov for 2001 guidelines) and as above. For pts who fail monotherapy with GCV or FOS, consider combination rx with both: (1) GCV 5 mg/kg q12h or q24h and FOS 90 mg/kg q12h (up to total of 125 mg/kg/d) (*CID 34:1337, 2002*). **Suppression** (maintenance therapy): See (*CID 28:534, 1999*). With immune reconstitution from HAART, USPHS/IDSA guidelines recommend suppressive rx may be d/c if CD4 >100/mm³ after 6 mos of HAART (see www.aidsinfo.nih.gov for 2001 guidelines) and no reactivation in 35 consecutive pts (*CID 34:394, 2002*). **Primary: Valganciclovir** 900 mg po qd **OR** **GCV** 5 mg/kg IV qd x5 days/week **OR** **FOS** 90–120 mg/kg/day IV with hydration and IV hydration (dose adjusted for renal function (NOTE: oral and IV hydration found equally effective. 1700 mg/day, *Abst 298 from 4th ICAC, 1997*). **Alternative:** Combination of **GCV intraocular implant** q6 mos. + **valganciclovir** 900 mg po qd with food (as above under induction rx) **OR** **Cidofovir** 5 mg/kg IV q2 weeks.	Equal efficacy of IV GCV and FOS. GCV avoids nephrotoxicity of FOS. FOS avoids bone marrow suppression of GCV. **Oral valganciclovir should replace oral ganciclovir.** Reports indicate success of combination rx with GCV at ½ dose 5 mg/kg q24h plus FOS at 90 mg/kg/d for GCV-resistant isolates in solid organ transplant/AIDS pts with retinitis/that avoids nephrotoxicity/bone marrow suppression complication. Valganciclovir 900 mg po qd has same efficacy (17% progressed over 1 year) & toxicity profile as IV ganciclovir but with fewer IV-related events (*J AIDS 30:392, 2002*).

NOTE: All dosage recommendations are for adults (unless otherwise indicated) and assume normal renal function.

TABLE 14A (5)

VIRUS/DISEASE	DRUG/DOSAGE	SIDE EFFECTS/COMMENTS
Herpesvirus Infections (continued)		
EBV—Mononucleosis (NEJM 343:481, 2000; Ln JID 13:7,2000)	**No treatment.** Corticosteroids for tonsillar obstruction of airway or CNS complications.	Acyclovir and prednisolone inhibited oropharyngeal EBV replication but did not affect duration of symptoms (JID 174:324, 1996).
HHV-6 (see excellent review: PIDJ 21:563, 2002) [implicated as cause of roseola (exanthem subitum) & other febrile diseases of childhood. 80–90% infants infected during 1st year of life & 100% by 2 yrs.] Fever & rash documented in transplant pts (JID 179:311, 1999). 38% of 82 HHV-6 seropositive BMT pts in Japan had HHV-6 viremia 2–4 wks after transplant. ½ had rash (JID 185:847, 2002).		
HHV-7—a ubiquitous virus (>90% of the population is infected, most by age 3 yrs). No clear relationship yet to human disease. Appears to infect CD4 receptor, is probably transmitted via saliva.		
HHV-8 (probable agent of Kaposi's sarcoma and body cavity lymphoma)— may cause interstitial pneumonia (NEJM 335:351, 1996)	**No antiviral rx** currently recommended. Effective anti-HIV rx may help.	Localized lesions: radiotherapy, laser surgery or intralesional chemotherapy. Systemic: chemotherapy. Anecdotal report of remission in 5 pts given foscarnet 80 mg/kg/d (Scand J Inf Dis 26:749, 1994).
Bell's palsy (May also be caused by H. zoster, Lyme disease, HHV-6.) (CID 30:529, 2000)	**Either no rx or rx for herpesvirus** or **Acyclovir** (400 mg 5x/d for 10 days) with or without **prednisone** po (30 mg 6x/d or 1 mg/kg daily dose given bid x5 d., then taper to 5 mg 5x bid and dc after total of 10 days)	HSV-1 genomes were detected in 11/14 pts in facial nerves by PCR (AViM 124:27, 1996). In one study, 99 pts with symptoms <3 days had faster recovery and less neural degeneration when rx with acyclovir + prednisone compared to prednisone alone (Ann Oto/Rhino/Laryngol 105:371, 1996), but another study was inconclusive. More data need to support this rx recommendation (Cochrane Database Syst Rev 2:CD001869, 2001). If caused by VZV (Ramsay Hunt syndrome), acyclovir may be of value (PIDJ 21:615, 2002).
Encephalitis (Excellent reviews: CID 23:219, 1996; 25:88, 1997; CID 35:254, 2002). UK experience (CID 35:e234, 2003)	**Acyclovir** IV 10 mg/kg IV (infuse over 1 hr) q8h x14–21 days	HSV-1 is most common cause of sporadic encephalitis. **Early dx and rx imperative.** Mortality rate reduced from >70% to 19% with acyclovir rx. PCR analysis of CSF for HSV-1 DNA is 100% specific & 75–98% sensitive (CID 36:1335, 2003). All were + after 3 days; CSF IgG Ab usually appears late (>1st week). Dose: Up to 20 mg/kg q8h in children with HSV CNS disease. In adults, IV acyclovir resulted in lower fatal dose if treated early. PCR after 14 days of rx predicts outcome: only 46.2 ± 149 mg/kg, p <0.03 (CID 30:185, 2000). Use of CSF PCR should allow clinicians to more effectively utilize acyclovir rx (JDCP 11:58, 2002).
Genital, Immunocompetent		
Primary (initial episode) See excellent reviews: JID 186(Suppl):S3, 2002; Ln 357:1513, 2001 CID 35(Suppl):S173, 2002; Med Lett 46:9, 2004. Anti-HSV-2 rx, JID 186:S40, 2002 & MMWR 51 (RR-6), 2002; CDC 2002 Guidelines	**Acyclovir** (Zovirax or generic) 400 mg bid-tid x7–10 days (FDA-approved dosage is 200 mg 5x/d for 10 days). **OR** **Valacyclovir** (Valtrex) 1000 mg po bid x10 days **OR** **Famciclovir** (Famvir) 250 mg po tid x7–10 days (not FDA-approved for this indication)	An ester of acyclovir, which is well absorbed, bioavailability 3–5x greater than acyclovir. Found to be equal to acyclovir (Sex Trans Dis 24:481, 1997). Metabolized to penciclovir, which is active component. Side effects and activity similar to acyclovir.
Episodic recurrences	**Acyclovir** 400 mg po tid **x5 days** or 800 mg po bid **x2 days** **famciclovir** 125 mg po bid **x5 days** or **valacyclovir** 500 mg po bid **x3 days**	Famciclovir 250 mg po tid was found to be equal to acyclovir 200 mg 5x/d. (IDCP 6:512, 1997). All effective with few differences. Choice can be made on basis of cost & convenience (AViM 156:1729, 1996; JAMA 276:44, 1996; Genitourin Med 73:110, 1997). Trend is to a shorter course of therapy. The 2-day course of acyclovir = duration of episode & lesions from 6 to 4 days vs placebo. As well as duration of episode & lesions 4.4 days (CID 34:944, 2002). The 3-day course of valacyclovir was equivalent to 5 days; duration of episode & lesions 4.4 days (CID 34:958, 2002).
Chronic suppression (JAMA 280:928, 1998; JID 186(Suppl):S3, 2002; Med Lett 46:9, 2004) Decision to rx arbitrary, but rx sig. improves quality of life over 1 yr (Sex Trans Infect 75:398, 1999).	**Suppressive rx reduces the frequency of genital herpes recurrences** by 70–80% among pts who have frequent recurrences (i.e., >6 recurrences/yr) & many report no diminution in suppressive outcome. **Acyclovir** 400 mg po bid **OR** **Famciclovir** 250 mg po bid (cost/yr $2666), or **Valacyclovir** 1 gm po qd ($2449/yr); for pts with <9 recurrences/yr, use 500 mg po qd if breakthrough at lower dose.	Increases rate of healing but does not prevent recurrences. For severe cases only. 5 mg/kg IV q8h x5–7 days. All suppress subclinical HSV-2 shedding between episodes of active disease and ↓ symptomatic recurrences (JCI 99:1092, 1997; JAMA 280:887, 1998). Valacyclovir ↓ transmission by 75% vs placebo. Drug resistance unlikely to develop with ↑ use. 0.2% after 20 yrs of use in immunocompetent pts. However, in immunocompromised pts (HIV & BMT) 6–7% HSV are resistant (J Clin Microbiol Rev 9:427, 2000; AnIM 126:257, 1997; JIDC 18:6, 2003). Since in a large natural hx study 2/3 of pts demonstrated ↑ in recurrences between yrs 1 & 5 (glapvar, median 6 to 3 episodes/yr), daily suppressive rx should be reassessed periodically and after 3–5 yrs episodic rx may become more practical (AnIM 131:14, 1999).

NOTE: All dosage recommendations are for adults (unless otherwise indicated) and assume normal renal/renal function.

TABLE 14A (6)

VIRUS/DISEASE	DRUG/DOSAGE	SIDE EFFECTS/COMMENTS
Herpesvirus infections/Herpes simplex virus (HSV Types 1 & 2) *(continued)*		
Gingivostomatitis, primary (children)	**Acyclovir** 15 mg/kg po 5x/d 7 d.	Efficacy demonstrated in randomized double-blind placebo-controlled trial *(BMJ 315:1800, 1997)*.
Kerato-conjunctivitis and recurrent epithelial keratitis	**Trifluridine** (Viroptic), 1 drop 1% solution q2h (max. 9 drops/d.) for max. of 21 days (see *Table 1, page 9*)	In controlled trials, response % > dboxuridine. Suppressive rx with acyclovir (400 mg bid) reduced recurrences of ocular HSV from 32% to 19% over 12-month period *(NEJM 339:300, 1998)*.
Mucocutaneous		
Oral labial, "fever blisters"		
Normal host	Start rx with prodrome symptoms (tingling or burning) before lesions appear	Penciclovir *(J Derm Treat 13:67, 2002; JAMA 277:1374, 1997; AAC 46:2848, 2002). Docosanol (J Am Acad Derm 45:222, 2001). AAC (AAC 46:2238, 2002). Acyclovir (AAC 46:2238, 2002). UID 179:303, 1999)*. Topical fluocinonides (0.05% Lidex gel) q8h x5 d. in combination with famciclovir ↓ lesion size and pain when compared to famciclovir alone *(JID 181:1906, 2000)*.
	Drug	
	Oral: Valacyclovir, Famciclovir, Acyclovir[a]	**Dose** / **Cost** / **Duration Sx**
	Valacyclovir — 2 gm po q12h x1 d. — $25 — ↓ 1 day	
	Famciclovir — 500 mg po bid x7 d. — $103 — ↓ 2 days	
	Acyclovir[a] — 400 mg po 5x/d, q4h x5 d. — $50–70 — ↓ ½ day	
	Topical: Penciclovir 1% cream — q2h during day x4 d. — $23 — ↓ 1 day	
	Docosanol 10% cream — 5x/d. until healed — $13 — ↓ ½ day	
	Acyclovir 5% cream[a] — 6 x/d. (q3h) x7 d. — $78/5 gm — ↓ ½ day	
	a FDA approved only HIV	
	b Approved for immunocompromised	
	See Table 1, page 18	
Herpes Whitlow		
		Acyclovir-resistant HSV occurs, esp. in large ulcers. Most will respond to **IV foscarnet**, but recur after drug discontinued (median 6 weeks later) *(JID 189:161, 1991)*. Suppressive rx with famciclovir (500 mg bid) reduced viral shedding and clinical recurrences (total days with lesions 18% vs 5%) in HIV-infected pts *(AnIM 128:21, 1999)*, similar to findings with acyclovir & valacyclovir 500 mg q8h x5 d. in HIV-infected pts [at 6 mos. 65% of vala-rx were recurrence-free vs 26% of placebo-rx *(IDSA 2002, Abst. 653)*]. Cidofovir (topical) has been used with moderate success *(JID 176:892, 1997)*.
Oral labial or genital Immunocompromised (includes pts with AIDS and critically ill pts in ICU) Oral/Genital (See Comment)	**Acyclovir** 5 mg/kg IV (infused over 1 hr) q8h x7 d. (250 mg/M²) or 400 mg po 5x/d x14–21 d. (see *Comment if suspect acyclovir-resistant*). **Famciclovir:** In HIV-infected, 500 mg po bid for 7 d. for recurrent episodes of genital herpes. **Valacyclovir:** In HIV-infected, 500 mg po bid for 5–10 d. for recurrent genital herpes.	
	or suppressive rx.	
Perinatal (genital) in pregnancy at delivery	In 25% HSV reactivated in last month of pregnancy. Infant exposure to primary lesion 50% risk, recurrent lesion 4%, 50% mortality in infected neonates. If visible genital lesion, deliver by **C-section**, regardless of duration of membrane rupture. If visible genital HSV cultures no longer recommended. **Acyclovir** useful in dose of 10 mg/kg (20 mg/kg if premature) q8h x10–21 days *(NEJM 337:509, 1997)*.	
Herpes simiae—Monkey bite (Herpes B virus)	See *CID 35:1191, 2002; for recum. for PEP + rx*. **Postexposure prophylaxis:** Valacyclovir 1 gm po q8h x14 d. or acyclovir 800 mg po 5x/d x14 d. **Treatment of disease:** (1) CNS symptoms present. Ganciclovir 5 mg/kg IV q8h or ganciclovir 5 mg/kg IV q12h. (2) CNS symptoms absent: Acyclovir 12.5–15 mg/kg IV q8h or ganciclovir 5 mg/kg IV q12h	Fatal human cases of myelitis and hemorrhagic encephalitis have been reported following bites, scratches, or eye inoculation of saliva from monkeys. Initial sx include fever, headache, myalgias and diffuse adenopathy. Incubation period of 2–14 days *(EID 9:246, 2003)*.
Herpes Varicella-Zoster Virus (VZV)		
Varicella		
Normal host (chickenpox)		
Child (2–12 years)	**Rx not recommended** by American Academy of Pediatrics. Oral acyclovir recommended for healthy persons at ↑ risk for moderate to severe varicella, i.e., >12 yrs of age, chronic cutaneous or pulmonary diseases, chronic salicylate rx (↑ risk of Reye syndrome), use acyclovir **20 mg/kg** po qid x5 days (start rx within 24 hrs of rash).	Modest response to acyclovir. Slowed development and ↓ number of new lesions; duration of disease ↓ in children receiving acyclovir in Europe. ↑ 6 vs 9.0 days *(PIDJ 17:39, 2002)*. Analgesic requirements decreased *(J Pediatr 116:633, 1990)*. IV dose of acyclovir in children should not exceed 80 mg/kg/d or 3200 mg/d.

NOTE: All dosage recommendations are for adults (unless otherwise indicated) and assume normal renal function.

TABLE 14A (7)

VIRUS/DISEASE	DRUG/DOSAGE	SIDE EFFECTS/COMMENTS
Herpesvirus Infections/Herpes Varicella-Zoster Virus (VZV)/Varicella (continued)		
Normal host (chickenpox) (continued) Adolescents; young adults	**Acyclovir** 800 mg po 5x/d x5–7 days (start within 24 hrs of rash) or **valacyclovir**[APDA*] 1000 mg po 3x/d; x5 d. **Famciclovir**[APDA] 500 mg po 3x/d: also probably effective but data lacking (AVIM 130:922, 1999).	↓ duration of fever, time to healing, and symptoms (AVIM 117:358, 1992).
Pneumonia or chicken-pox in 3rd trimester of pregnancy	**Acyclovir** 800 mg po 5x/d or 10 mg/kg IV q8h x5 days. Risks and benefits to fetus and mother still unknown. Many experts recommend Rx, especially in 3rd trimester. Some would add VZIG (varicella-zoster immune globulin).	Varicella pneumonia severe in pregnancy (41% mortality, Ob Gyn 25:734, 1965) and **acyclovir** incidence and severity (JID 185:422, 2002). If varicella-susceptible mother exposed and respiratory symptoms develop within 10 days after exposure, start acyclovir (CCTID 13:123, 1993). Acyclovir in pregnancy category B, no evidence of ↑ birth defects (MMWR 42:806, 1993).
Immunocompromised host	**Acyclovir** 10–12 mg/kg IV (infused over 1 hr) q8h x7 days (500 mg/M²)	Continuous infusion of high-dose acyclovir (2 mg/kg/hr) was used successfully in 1 pt with severe hemorrhagic varicella (NEJM 336:732, 1997). Mortality high (43%) in AIDS pts (Int J Infect Dis 6:6, 2002).
Prevention	**CDC Recommendations for Prevention:** Since <6% of cases of varicella-related deaths occur in adults >20 yrs of age, the CDC recommends a more aggressive approach in this age group. **1st, varicella-zoster immune globulin (VZIG)** (125 U/10 kg (22 lbs) body weight IM up to a max. of 625 U; minimum dose is 125 U) is recommended for post-exposure prophylaxis in susceptible persons at greater risk for complications (immunocompromised such as HIV, malignancies, pregnancy, and steroids) as soon as possible after exposure (<96 hrs). If varicella develops, initiate rx quickly (<24 hrs of rash) with **acyclovir**. **2nd,** susceptible adults should be vaccinated. Check antibody in adults with negative or uncertain hx of varicella (10–30% will be Ab-neg.) and vaccinate those who are Ab-neg, and susceptible children should receive vaccine/post-exposure. Recommended routinely before age 12–18 mos. OK at any age (MMWR 4:410, 19 May 1997). Varicella is the leading cause of vaccine-preventable deaths in the U.S. (MMWR 47:365, 1998).	
Herpes zoster (shingles) (See NEJM 342:635, 2000 & 347:340, 2002) **Normal host** Effective rx most evident in pts >50 yrs. (For rx of post-herpetic neuralgia, see p. 113 [JAMA 280:1837, 1998; JID 188:1396, 2003]) 25-fold ↑ in zoster after immunization (MMWR 48:R-6, 1999)	**[NOTE: Trials showing benefit of rx only in pts treated within 3 days of onset of rash]** **Valacyclovir** (Valtrex) 1000 mg po bid x7 days (adjust dose for renal failure) or **Famciclovir** [Famvir] 500 mg po q8h x7 days. Adjust for renal failure (see Table 17) or **Acyclovir** 800 mg po 5x/d x7–10 days [**Prednisone** po 30 mg bid days 1–7, 15 mg bid days 8–14 and 7.5 mg bid days 15–21 also recommended by some authorities in pts >50 yrs of age (NEJM 335:32, 1996) and especially when pt has large number of lesions (>21) and/or severe pain at presentation (JID 179:9, 1999).]	Valacyclovir ↓ post-herpetic neuralgia more rapidly than acyclovir in pts >50 yrs of age: median duration of zoster-associated pain was 38 days on acyclovir vs 51 days on acyclovir (AAC 39:1546, 1995). Toxicity of both drugs similar (Arch Fam Med 9:863, 2000). Time to healing more rapid. Reduced post-herpetic neuralgia (PHN) vs placebo in pts >50 yrs of age: duration of PHN reduced by 2-fold (NEJM 330:896, 1994; placebo 163 days). Famciclovir similar to acyclovir in reduction of acute pain and PHN (Ant J Antimicrob Agents 4:21, 1994; AnM 123:89, 1995). A meta-analysis of 4 placebo-controlled trials (691 pts) demonstrated that acyclovir accelerated by approx. 2-fold pain resolution by all measures employed and reduced post-herpetic neuralgia at 3 & 6 mos (CID 22:341, 1996). med. time to resolution of pain 41 days vs 101 days in placebo >50 yrs. Prednisone added to acyclovir improved quality of life measurements and accelerated return to normal activity (AnM 125:376, 1996). Placebo-controlled trials demonstrated effectiveness of gabapentin in controlling pain, the lidocaine patch (5%), & opioid analgesic in controlling pain. Nortriptyline & amitriptyline are equally effective but nortriptyline is better tolerated (CID 36:877, 2003).
Immunocompromised host Not severe Severe: >1 dermatome, trigeminal nerve or disseminated	**Acyclovir** 800 mg po 5x/d x7 days (famciclovir and valacyclovir not FDA-approved for this indication). [If progression, switch to IV] **Acyclovir** 10–12 mg/kg IV (infusion over 1 hr) q8h x7–14 days. ↓ to 5 mg/kg, ↓ to 7.5 mg/kg. If nephrotoxicity and pt improving, ↓ to 5 mg/kg q8h.	[If progression, switch to IV] Rx must be begun within 72 hrs. Acyclovir-resistant VZV occurs in HIV+ pts previously treated with acyclovir. Foscarnet (40 mg/kg IV q8h for 14–26 days) successful in 4/5 pts but 2 relapsed in 7 and 14 days (AnM 115:19, 1991).

NOTE: All dosage recommendations are for adults (unless otherwise indicated) and assume normal renal function.

TABLE 14A (8)

VIRUS/DISEASE	DRUG/DOSAGE	SIDE EFFECTS/COMMENTS
Influenza (A & B) JAMA 287:1016 & 1051, 2000; NEJM 343:1778, 2000; CID 31:1166, 2000; CID 35:729, 2002; Surveillance in acute respiratory illness. Rapid diagnostic tests available (J Clin Virol 25:15, 2002). antiviral rx cost-effective without viral testing in febrile pts with typical symptoms during influenza A season (Am J Med 113:200, 2002). **Prevention.** See MMWR 52:RR-8, 2003. Annual vaccination is recommended (preferably Oct–Nov.) for the following who are at ↑ risk for complications from influenza: >65 yrs, residents of nursing homes or chronic care facilities that house persons with chronic medical conditions, those with chronic pulmonary or cardiac disorders (asthma), chronic metabolic diseases (diabetes, renal failure, etc.), immunosuppression, children on chronic ASA, women in 2nd or 3rd trimester or persons who can transmit virus to above (HCWs, etc.)	**If influenza A & B cough; known community influenza activity; and 1st 48 hrs of illness, consider:** **For influenza A & B only:** **Oseltamivir** 75 mg po bid x5 d. (also approved for rx of children age 1–12 yrs. dose 2 mg/kg up to a total of 75 mg bid x5 d.) OR **Zanamivir** 2 inhalations (2x5 mg) bid x5 d. **For influenza A only: Rimantadine or amantadine:** 1–9 yrs, 5 mg/kg/d to max. of 75 mg po bid; 10–65 yrs, 100 mg po bid; >65 yrs, 100 mg po (adjust for ↓ renal function) for 3–5 d. and 1–2 after the disappearance of symptoms. **Prevention of influenza A & B:** give vaccine and if ≥13 yrs age, consider **oseltamivir** 75 mg po for duration of peak influenza in community. (Consider for similar populations as immunization recommendations.) **Prevention of influenza A:** give influenza vaccine followed by **rimantadine** or **amantadine** (dosages as above) for duration of influenza A activity in community. (Consider for similar populations as immunization recommendations.)	Pts with ↑ risk of asthma and/or ↑ inherent risk of bronchospasm with **zanamivir** should have rapid-acting bronchodilator. Use before dose of zanamivir. Amantadine & rimantadine equally effective, but rimantadine ↓ side effects (Cochrane Database Sys Rev CD 001169, 2002). All 3 drugs reduce duration of symptoms by approx. 50% (1–2 d.) if given within 30–36 hrs after onset of symptoms (JID 137:125, 2002; AIM 30:585, 2002). If reviewed benefit dramatically influenced by duration of osetamivir within 1st 12 hrs after fever onset + total median illness duration by 74.6 hrs (3.1 days) if given >48 hrs after onset of symptoms. fever onset + 1 total median illness duration by 74.6 hrs (3.1 days) if given >48 hrs after onset of symptoms. Influenza immunization contraindicated in those with hypersensitivity to hen's eggs. Both amantadine and rimantadine are about 70–90% effective against influenza A. Both osetamivir and zanamivir reported efficacious (82 and 84% respectively) in clinical trials (JAMA 285:748, 2001; JID 186:1582, 2002).
Measles		After incubation period of 12 days, symptoms are fever, headache, cough, adeno-
Children	No therapy. ↓ **vitamin A** 200,000 i.u. po x2 days	↓ severity of measles (NEJM 323:160, 1990), not in others.
Adults	No rx. If **ribavirin** IV (J) 20–35 mg/kg/d x7 d.	↓ severity of illness in adults (CID 20:454, 1994).
Metapneumovirus (HMPV) [See JID 186(Suppl 1):S37, 1999] isolated from pts with ↑ illnesses ranging from mild bronchiolitis/bronchospasm to pneumonia. All persons in the Netherlands had antibody to HMPV by age 5 yrs.	No therapy recommended	HMPV accounted for 2.3% of all respiratory viral isolates in Canada over the winter of 2000–2001. Similar to parainfluenza 2.3%, adenovirus 3.4%, RSV 4.8%, while influenza A & B was 20% (JID 186:1330, 2002).
Monkey pox (orthopox virus) In 2003, 72 pts contracted monkey pox from contact with ill prairie dogs. The index source is likely Gambian giant rats imported to Texas in April 2003 (MMWR 42:642, 2003).	No therapy recommended. Cidofovir is active in vitro & in mouse model (AAC 46:1329, 2002; Antivira Res 57:13, 2003)	
Norovirus (Norwalk-like virus, or NLV) Leading cause of outbreaks of acute gastroenteritis (AGE) (93% of 233 outbreaks of non-bacterial gastroenteritis reported to CDC between 1997 & 2000). 23 million cases of norovirus AGE occur each year in the U.S. (JID 186:1, 2002) & account for 2/3 of all food-borne illnesses (MMWR 52:41, 2003). Transmission is fecal-oral contact (often raw or undercooked), food (often contaminated), contaminated surfaces, or fomites. Commonly causes outbreaks on cruise ships.	No antiviral therapy shown to be effective. Elderly, children, pts with co-morbid conditions may need volume repletion.	Incubation period 12–48 hrs, followed by sudden onset of nausea, vomiting, & watery diarrhea lasting 12–60 hours.
Papillomaviruses		
Anogenital Warts: Condyloma acuminatum [See CID 28(Suppl 1):S37, 1999] Recurrences common after all treatments	See JAMA 27:796, 1998, for consensus statement: **Podofilox** (Condylox) 2x daily application with cotton swab for 3 days followed by 4 days no therapy; repeat cycle 4x as necessary **OR podophyllin** in tincture of benzoin (Podocon-25) apply once weekly for up to 6 wks, wash after 1–4 hrs.| If no response after 4 weekly applications, use alternate rx. **Interferon alfa-n3** (Intron A); **alfa-n3** (Alferon N): 1 million units (0.1 ml) into lesion 3x/week x3 weeks Cryotherapy or electrosurgery	Podofilox: Local reactions—pain, burning, inflammation in 50%. Efficacy in warts 74% vs placebo 0%. Recurrences 55% vs 100% with placebo. (Podocon-25 15 ml $32.40, Condylox 3.5 ml $56.64.) Warts recur in 1/3 with either agent within 1st month after rx. Podophyllin: dilute to 10 million units/1 ml. Painful; wash 1 hr. Use when other rx fails, resp. in AIDS. Podophyllin: Other concentrations are hypertonic (CID 28:S37, 1999).

NOTE: All dosage recommendations are for adults (unless otherwise indicated) and assume normal renal function.

TABLE 14A (9)

VIRUS/DISEASE	DRUG/DOSAGE	SIDE EFFECTS/COMMENTS
Papillomavirus/Anogenital Warts (continued)	Imiquimod (5% cream). Apply 3x/week prior to sleep; remove 6–10 hrs later when awake. Continue until cleared or max. 16 wks.	When applied 3x/wk overnight for up to 16 wks or until warts completely cured, produced clearance rates of 52% vs 14% for controls (AAC 43:1,998). Cost of 1–4 wks rx: $108–432. Imiquimod: Local reactions—mild erythema 60%, erosion 30% (AJM 102(5A):34, 1997)
Parvo B19 Virus (Erythrovirus B19)		
Uncomplicated or self-limited acute arthritis. May be chronic in children.	No treatment recommended	Bone marrow shows selective erythrocyte maturation arrest with giant pronormoblasts. IgM antibody available for diagnosis. Specialty Labs, Santa Monica, CA. Parvo B19 also associated with respiratory distress syndrome (CID 27:900, 1998) and myocarditis/myocarditis (CID 28:1,343, 1999).
Acute profound anemia, e.g., sickle in hemolytic anemia, in HIV	IVIG 0.4 gm/kg IV qd x5 d in immune deficient states with severe anemia	IVIG contains anti-parvo B19 antibody. In pts with pre-existing hemolytic anemia, parvo B19-induced bone marrow arrest can result in sudden severe anemia. See Am J Hematol 61:16, 1999 for new suggestions on management.
Papovavirus/Polyomavirus		
Progressive multifocal leucoencephalopathy (PML)/(JC virus) Usually in pts with advanced HIV disease & organ transplant (CID 55:1081, 2002)	See Sanford Guide to HIV/AIDS Therapy. **HAART** ↑ survival (545 d. vs 60 d., p < 0.0001) and either improved (50%) or stabilized (50%) neurological deficits in 12 pts (AIDS 12:2467, 1999). Others less optimistic (CID 28:1152, 1999).	Cytarabine of no value in controlled trial (NEJM 338:1,345, 1998). Camptothecin, a human topoisomerase I inhibitor, was administered to a single pt with slowing of progression (Ln 349:1366, 1997). Use of cidofovir controversial (Clin Micro Rev 16:569, 2003).
Polyomavirus-associated nephropathy	Due to BK virus post renal transplant.	Possible rx roles for cidofovir (UID 3:611, 2003).
Rabies (see Table 20C, pages 139–140)		
Rabid dogs account for 50,000 cases/yr worldwide. Most cases in the U.S. are due to unimmunized animals; no documented evidence of bite or contact with a rabid animal (CID 35:738, 2003). Recently, in most U.S. cases, the eastern pipistrella in the southeast & the silver-hair bat in the northwest (EID 9:151, 2003). These viruses appear to exhibit ↑ infectivity.	**Mortality 100% with only wildlife virus those who receive rabies vaccine before the onset of illness/symptoms** (CID 36:61, 2003). Therapies that have failed in human cases after symptoms develop include rabies vaccine, rabies immunoglobulin, rabies virus neutralizing antibody, ribavirin, alfa interferon, & ketamine.	Corticosteroids ↑ mortality rate and ↓ incubation in mice.
Respiratory Syncytial Virus Major cause of morbidity in neonates/infants (JID 179:25, 1999), now documented recognition in adults: 2–9% of pts >65 yrs of age with pneumonia requiring hospitalization are due to RSV (JID 179:25, 1999).	Rapid dx by antigen detection on nasopharyngeal wash. **No rx.**	Ribavirin reported to ↓ fever and other symptoms and signs. However, in controlled studies, **ribavirin had no beneficial effect** (J Ped 126: 422, 1994; AJRCCM 160:829, 1999). Still recommended by some authorities in immunocompromised children (PID 19:253, 2000) & still controversial (PIDJ 22:599, 2003). RSV-IVIG very expensive—estimated cost per infusion $1,175. See conventional opinion for details. Ped Inf Dis J 15:1059, 1996. See Ln 354:847, 1999 for updated review.
Prevention (1) Children <24 mos. old with bronchopulmonary dysplasia (BPD) requiring supplemental O₂. (2) Perhaps premature infants (<26 wks gestation) and <6 mos. old at start of RSV season.	RSV immune globulin intravenous (RSV-IG) 100 mg/kg IV once monthly Nov. through April (for northern hemisphere) 1st year of life for prematures. Perhaps up to 60 months of age for pts with BPD. **OR** Palivizumab 15 mg/kg IM q month Nov–April as above (Scand J Inf Dis 33:323, 2001).	Palivizumab reduced hospitalization rates for RSV in 1500 premature infants & children with chronic lung disease from 10.6% to 4.8% (Pediatrics 102:531, 1998). Cost: $3000–5000/yr
Rhinovirus (Colds) See Ln 361:51, 2003	No antiviral rx indicated. Symptomatic: • ipratropium bromide nasal (2 sprays/nostril tid) • clemastine 1.34 mg 1–2 tab po bid–tid (OTC)	Sx relief: ipratropium nasal spray + rhinorrhea and sneezing vs placebo (AnIM 125:89, 1996). Clemastine (an antihistamine) improved sx of rhinorrhea but associated with dry nose, mouth & throat in 6–19% (CID 22:656, 1996). Zinc lozenges were ineffective in reducing the severity of symptoms in 2 studies of natural colds (CID 31:1202, 2000). Intranasal zinc of no benefit (CID 33:1865, 2007). Oral **pleconaril** (an experimental oral antiviral) reduced duration (1 day) & severity of "cold symptoms" in double-blind placebo-controlled trial (p < 001) (CID 36:1523, 2003). 4% intranasal sodium cromoglycate of no value (CID 35:9-25, 2002). A combination of intranasal interferon alfa-2b, oral chlorpheniramine & ibuprofen + symptoms by 33–73% vs placebo when started 24 hrs after intranasal rhinovirus (JID 186:147, 2002).
Smallpox (NEJM 346:1300, 2002) **Contact vaccinia** (JAMA 288:1901, 2002)	Smallpox vaccine (if within 4 days of exposure) + cidofovir (dosage uncertain) contact CDC: 770-488-7100. From vaccination. Progressive vaccinia—vaccinia immune globulin may be of benefit. To obtain immune globulin, contact CDC: 770-488-7100.	

NOTE: All dosage recommendations are for adults (unless otherwise indicated) and assume normal renal function.

TABLE 14B: ANTIVIRAL DRUGS (Other Than Retroviral)

DRUG NAME(S) GENERIC (TRADE)	DOSAGE/ROUTE/COST*	COMMENTS/ADVERSE EFFECTS
CMV (See *SANFORD GUIDE* TO HIV/AIDS THERAPY)		
Cidofovir (Vistide)	5 mg/kg IV q week x2, then q2 weeks. (375 mg \$888) Properly timed IV prehydration with normal saline and oral probenecid **must be used with each cidofovir infusion** (see *pkg insert* for details). Renal function (serum creatinine and urine protein) must be monitored prior to each dose (see *pkg insert*).	**Adverse effects: Nephrotoxicity;** dose-dependent proximal tubular injury (Fanconi-like syndrome): proteinuria, glycosuria, bicarbonaturia, phosphaturia, polyuria (nephrogenic diabetic insipidus now reported, *Ln 350:413, 1997*), ↑ creatinine. Concomitant saline prehydration, probenecid, extended dosing intervals allowed use: 25% of pts IV cidofovir due to nephrotoxicity. Other toxicities: nausea 48%, fever 31%, alopecia 16%, myalgia 18%, probenecid hypersensitivity 16%, neutropenia 25%. No effect on hearing seen. **Comment:** Recommended dosage, frequency or infusion rate of cidofovir must be exceeded. Dose must be reduced or discontinued if changes in renal function occur during rx. For ↑ of 0.3-0.4 mg/dl in serum creatinine, cidofovir dose must be ↓ from 5 to 3 mg/kg; discontinue cidofovir if ↑ of 0.5 mg/dl above baseline or 3+ proteinuria develops (for 2+ proteinuria, observe pts carefully and consider discontinuation).
Fomivirsen (Vitravene)	330 µg by direct intravitreal injection q2 wks x2, then q 4 wks (6.6 mg \$4000)	This is an antisense drug approved for local treatment of CMV retinitis in AIDS who are intolerant of, have a contraindica- tion to or were unresponsive to other treatments for CMV. It inhibits production of proteins responsible for regulation of viral gene expression essential for virulence. **Adverse effects:** ocular inflammation (uveitis), iritis and vitreitis, ↑ intraocular pressure, abnormal vision, anterior chamber inflammation and cataracts. Do not give if pt had received IV or intravitreal cidofovir (Vistide) within last 2-4 wks, may exaggerate ocular inflammation (*Priority Pharmacy 3, #8, Oct. 30, 1998*).
Foscarnet (Foscavir)	90 mg/kg q12h IV (induction) 90 mg/kg qd (maintenance) Dosage adjust. with renal dysfunction (see *Table 17*) (6 gm \$76)	**Adverse effects: Major clinical toxicity is renal impairment (1/3 of patients):** ↑ creatinine, proteinuria, nephrogenic diabetes insipidus. ↓ K⁺, Ca²⁺ → Mg²⁺. Toxicity ↑ with other nephrotoxic drugs [amphotericin B, aminoglycosides (+), pentamidine (especially severe ↓ Ca²⁺), etc.]. Adequate hydration may ↓ toxicity. Other: headache, mild (100%), fatigue (100%). Penile ulcers, nausea (80%), fever (25%). CNS: seizures. Hemato.: ↓ WBC, ↓ Hgb. Hepatic: liver function tests ↑. Neuropathy. ↓ WBC, ↓ platelets.
Ganciclovir (Cytovene)	IV: 5 mg/kg q12h x14 days (induction) 5 mg/kg IV qd or q od 5x/wk (maintenance) Dosage adjust. with renal dysfunction (see *Table 17*) (500 mg IV \$37) Oral: 1.0 gm tid with food (fatty meal) (250 mg cap \$4.62)	**Adverse effects:** Absolute neutrophil count dropped below 500/mm³ in 15%, thrombocytopenia 21%, anemia 6%. Fever 48%. GI 50%: nausea, vomiting, diarrhea, abdominal pain 19%, rash 10%. Retinal detachment 11% (relationship to ganciclovir ?). Confusion, headache, psychiatric disturbances and seizures. Neutropenia may respond to granulocyte colony-stimulating factor (G-CSF) and GM-CSF. Hematologic myelosuppression may be ↑ with coadministration of zidovudine or azathioprine. 32% dc/interrupted IV, principally Gl. Hematologic: less frequent than with IV. Granulocytopenia 18%, anemia 12%, thrombocytopenia 6%. GI: skin same as with IV. Retinal detachment 7%.
Ganciclovir (Vitraset)	Intraocular implant (~\$5000/device + cost of surgery)	**Adverse effects:** Late retinal detachment (7/30 eyes). Does not prevent CMV retinitis in good eye or visceral dissemination. **Comment:** Replacement every 6 months recommended.
Valganciclovir (Valcyte)	900 mg (two 450 mg tabs) po bid x21 d for induction, followed by 900 mg po qd. Take with food. (450 mg tab) Doses: see *Table 14A*	A prodrug of ganciclovir with better bioavailability.: 60% with food. **Adverse effects:** Similar to ganciclovir.
Herpesvirus (non-CMV)		
Acyclovir (Zovirax) or generic	**po:** See *Table 14A* 400 mg tab NB \$2.07 G \$0.70 IV \$500 mg NB \$46 G \$4.75 Suspension 200 mg/5 ml: 1 gm \$3.00 amount 5%, 15 gm \$62.41	po: Generally well-tolerated with occ. diarrhea, vertigo, arthralgia. Less frequent rash, fatigue, insomnia, fever, menstrual abnormalities, acne, sore throat, muscle cramps, lymphadenopathy. IV: Phlebitis, caustic with vesicular lesions with IV infiltration. CNS (1%): lethargy, tremors, confusion, hallucinations, delirium, seizures, coma (*CID 21:435, 1995*). Improve 1-2 weeks after rx stopped. Renal (5%): ↑ creatinine, hematuria. With high doses may crystallize in renal tubules → obstructive uropathy (rapid infusion, dehydration, renal insufficiency) (*CID 20:1557, 1995*), rash. Adequate pre-hydration such as nausea, vomiting. Hepatic.
Famciclovir (Famvir)	250 mg cap \$3.66 500 mg cap \$7.36	Metabolized to penciclovir. **Adverse effects:** similar to acyclovir; included headache, nausea, diarrhea, and dizziness but incidence did not differ from placebo (*JAMA 276:47, 1996*). May be taken without regard to meals. Dose should be reduced if CrCl <60 ml/min (see *package insert & Table 14, page 108 & Table 17, page 133*)
Penciclovir (Denavir) (Viroptic)	Topical 1% cream 1.5 gm \$24	Apply to area of recurrence of herpes labialis with start of sx, then q2h while awake x4 d. Well tolerated
Trifluridine (Viroptic)	1 drop 1% solution q2h (max. 9 drops/d.) for max of 21 d. (7.5 ml) 1% solution \$99)	Mild burning (5%), palpebral edema (3%), punctate keratopathy, stromal edema

NOTE: All dosage recommendations are for adults (unless otherwise indicated) and assume normal renal function.

TABLE 14B (2)

DRUG NAME(S) GENERIC (TRADE)	DOSAGE/ROUTE/COST*	COMMENTS/ADVERSE EFFECTS
Herpesvirus (non-CMV) *(continued)*		
Valacyclovir (Valtrex)	500 mg cap $4.52	An ester pro-drug of acyclovir that is well-absorbed, bioavailability 3–5x greater than acyclovir. **Adverse effects** similar to acyclovir (see *AID 1:240, 2000*). Thrombotic thrombocytopenic purpura/hemolytic uremic syndrome reported in pts with advanced HIV disease and transplant recipients participating in clinical trials at doses of 8 gm/day.
Hepatitis		
Adefovir dipivoxil (Hepsera) Each tab/cap 10 mg ($17.60)	10 mg po qd (with normal CrCl) 20–50 CrCl: 10 mg q48h 10–19 CrCl: 10 mg q72h Hemodialysis: 10 mg q7 days following dialysis	Adefovir dipivoxil is a diester prodrug of the active moiety adefovir. It is an acyclic nucleotide analog with activity against hepatitis B (HBV) at 0.2–2.5 mM (IC$_{50}$). Peak plasma concentration after 10 mg po was 18.4 ± 6.26 ng/ml. 1–4 hrs after dose. Terminal elimination t½ was 7.48 ±1.65 hrs. Primarily renal excretion—adjust dose. No food interactions. Generally remarkably few side effects. Nephrotoxicity was found with higher doses in HIV with 60 & 120 mg/d & early studies in Hep B with 30 mg/d. Not yet reported at 10 mg/d, but important to monitor renal function, esp. with pre-existing or other risks for renal impairment. Lactic acidosis reported with nucleoside analogs. Pregnancy Category C. Hepatitis may exacerbate when no dc. 6–25% of pts developed ALT ↑ 10x normal within 12 wks; usually respond to retreatment or are self-limited, but hepatic decompensation has occurred.
Interferon alfa is available as alfa-2a (Roferon-A), alfa-2b (Intron-A)	3 million units (Roferon $37, Intron $43; Infergen 9 μg $39)	**Adverse effects:** Flu-like syndrome is common, esp. during 1st week of rx: fever 98%, fatigue 89%, myalgia 73%, headache 71%, GI: anorexia 46%, diarrhea 29%, CNS: dizziness 21%, Hash rash later profound fatigue & psychiatric symptoms in up to ⅓ of pts (*J Clin Psych 64:708, 2003*) (depression, anxiety, emotional lability and agitation), alopecia, ↓ TSH, autoimmune thyroid disorders in pts with history. ↓ WBC 49%, ↓ Hgb 27%, ↓ platelets 35%. Consider prophylactic antidepressant in pts with history. Acute reversible hearing loss and/or tinnitus in up to 46% developing chronic rx for HBV.
PEG interferon alfa-2b (PEG-Intron)	0.5–1.5 μg/kg sc q wk (100 μg) $351)	Attachment of INF to polyethylene glycol (PEG) prolongs half-life and allows weekly dosing. Better efficacy data with similar adverse effects profile compared to regular formulation.
Pegylated-40k interferon alfa-2a (Pegasys)	180 μg sc q wk x48 wks (180 μg $363)	
Lamivudine (3TC) (Epivir-HBV)	100 mg po qd x1 yr for hepatitis B. NOTE: 100 mg po qd x1 yr for hepatitis B. (100 mg cap $6.05)	
Ribavirin + Interferon alfa-2b combination pack (Rebetron)	**Adverse effects:** See Table 14D, page 120. Combination kit contains 2 wk supply of INF and 42, 70, or 84 caps of 200 mg ribavirin. **Dose:** INF 3 million U sc tiw AND ribavirin 400 mg po q a.m. + 600 mg po q p.m. (<75 kg) or 600 mg po bid (>75 kg) Rebetron (1000 mg/d ribavirin dose pack): ($8207/24 wk course)	See *interferon alfa* above. Hemolytic anemia common (mean reduction in Hgb >50%) but usually responds to ↓ ribavirin dose (see package insert). Severe psychiatric effects, esp. depression, most common (23–36%) reason for discontinuation reported (*Mayo Clin Proc 74:367, 1999*). **Since ribavirin is teratogenic, drug must not be used during pregnancy or within 6 months of pregnancy.** Also should not be used in pts with endstage renal failure, severe heart disease, or hemoglobinopathies. ARDS reported (*Chest 124:406, 2003*). Dose changes: <table><tr><td></td><td>Ribavirin</td><td>Interferon</td></tr><tr><td>Hgb <10</td><td>↓ to 200 mg q a.m. 400 mg q p.m.</td><td>No change</td></tr><tr><td> <8.5</td><td>DC</td><td>DC</td></tr><tr><td>WBC <1500</td><td>No change</td><td>↓ to 1.5 mIU sc 3x/wk</td></tr><tr><td> <1000</td><td></td><td>DC</td></tr><tr><td>Abs. PMNs <750</td><td>No change</td><td>↓ to 1.5 mIU sc 3x/wk</td></tr><tr><td> <500</td><td></td><td>DC</td></tr><tr><td>Platelets <50,000</td><td>No change</td><td>↓ to 1.5 mIU sc 3x/wk</td></tr><tr><td> <25,000</td><td>DC</td><td>DC</td></tr></table>Response of immune complex renal disease: *AJM 106:347, 1999.*

NOTE: *All dosage recommendations are for adults (unless otherwise indicated) and assume normal renal function.*

* From 2003 Drug Topics Red Book, Medical Economics. Price is average wholesale price (AWP). **NB** = name brand, **G** = generic.

TABLE 14B (3)

DRUG NAME(S) GENERIC (TRADE)	DOSAGE/ROUTE/COST*	COMMENTS/ADVERSE EFFECTS
Hepatitis (continued)		
Ribavirin (Rebetol)	For use with an interferon for hepatitis C & was unbundled from the combination Rebetron (see above) mostly for use with the pegylated interferons (alfa-2a & 2b). Available as 200 mg capsules. Dose: <75 kg BW = 2 caps a.m. & 3 caps p.m.; >75 kg BW 3 caps in a.m. & 3 caps p.m. Cost: 200 mg \$11.04	Side-effects as above, esp. hemolytic anemia (during 1st 1-2 wks of rx) with hemoglobin ↓ 3-4 gm. Should not be used with CrCl <50 ml/min & cautiously with cardiac disease.
Influenza A		
Amantadine (Symmetrel) or Rimantadine (Flumadine)	Amantadine and rimantadine doses are the same (rimantadine approved only for prophylaxis in children, not treatment). Amantadine 100 mg po bid; >65 y.o. 100 mg qd. G: 100 mg cap \$0.20; 100 mg/10 ml soln. \$1.50. Rimantadine 100 mg tab/syrup \$2	**Side-effects/toxicity:** CNS (nervousness, anxiety, difficulty concentrating, and lightheadedness). Symptoms occurred in 6% on rimantadine vs 14% on amantadine. They usually ↓ after 1st week and disappear when drug dc. Some serious side-effects—delirium, hallucinations, and seizures—are associated with high plasma drug levels resulting from potential renal insufficiency, esp. in older pts, those with prior seizure disorders, or psychiatric disorders. In pts with impaired renal function, dosage of both drugs should be reduced (amantadine: creatinine clearance <50 ml/min, imantadine: CrCl <10 ml/min); see package inserts and *Table 17, pages 133 & 134.* Both drugs teratogenic in animals and contraindicated during pregnancy (*Med Lett 39:72, 1997*).
Influenza A and B—For both drugs, initiate within 48 hrs of symptom onset		
Zanamivir (Relenza) For pts ≥12 yrs of age	2 inhalations (2 x 5 mg) bid x5 d. Powders inhaled using a specially designed breath-activated device. Each medication-containing blister contains 5 mg of zanamivir. \$48/course	Active by inhalation against neuraminidase of both influenza A and B and inhibits release of virus from epithelial cells of respiratory tract. Approx. 4-17% of inhaled dose absorbed into plasma. Excreted by kidney but with low absorption, dose reduction not necessary in renal impairment. Minimal side-effects: <3% cough, sinusitis, diarrhea, nausea and vomiting. **Reports of respiratory adverse events in pts with or without h/o airways disease, should be avoided in pts with respiratory disease.**
Oseltamivir (Tamiflu)	75 mg po bid for treatment (pediatric suspension [12 mg/ml] approved for treatment, not prevention, in children age 1-12 at dose of 2 mg/kg up to 75 mg total bid x5 d). For prevention: 75 mg po qd for duration of peak of flu epidemic. \$70/5 day course	Well absorbed (80% bioavailable) from GI tract as ethyl ester of active compound GS 4071. T½ 6-10 hrs; excreted unchanged by kidney. Adverse effects in 15% include diarrhea 1.6%, nausea 0.5%, vomiting, headache (*J Am Ger Soc 50:608, 2002*). Nausea ↓ with food. Also available as 12 mg/ml oral suspension.
Respiratory Syncytial Virus (RSV) and other		
Palivizumab (Synagis) (*See Med Lett 41:1, 1999*) Used only for prevention of RSV infection in high-risk children (*Ped 102:1211, 1998*)	15 mg/kg IM q month 100 mg/ml vial (for 1 injection) \$1369	A monoclonal antibody directed against the F glycoprotein on surface of virus; side-effects are normal; occ. ↑ ALT (*JID 176:1215, 1997*).
Ribavirin (Virazole)	1.1 gm/day (6 gm vial for inhalation [\$1374])	**Ribavirin side-effects:** Anemia, rash, conjunctivitis. Read package insert. Avoid procedures that lead to drug precipitation in ventilator tubing with subsequent dysfunction. Significant teratogenicity in animals. **Contraindicated in pregnant women and partners.** Pregnant health care workers should avoid direct care of pts receiving aerosolized ribavirin. RespiGam side-effects rare but include fatal anaphylaxis, pruritus, rash, wheezing, fever, joint pain.
RSV-iV immunoglobulin (RG) (RespiGam)	100 mg/kg IV q month (50 ml) \$816)	
Warts (*See CID 28:S37, 1999*)		
Interferon alfa-2b or alfa-n3	Apply 1 million units into lesion	Interferon alfa-2b 3 million units/0.5 ml; interferon alfa-n3 5 mU/1 ml. Cost: \$10
Podofilox (Condylox)	3.5% for topical application; \$110	Side-effects: Local reactions—pain, burning, inflammation in 50%. No systemic effects.
Imiquimod (Aldara)	Cream applied 3x/week to maximum of 16 wks. 250 mg packets \$12	Mild erythema, rash, itching and burning

NOTE: *All dosage recommendations are for adults (unless otherwise indicated) and assume normal renal function.*
* From 2003 DRUG TOPICS RED BOOK, Medical Economics. Price is average wholesale price (AWP). **NB** = name brand, **G** = generic

TABLE 14C: ANTIRETROVIRAL THERAPY IN ADULTS

(See the SANFORD GUIDE TO HIV/AIDS THERAPY, Table 5, for background, concepts, and metabolic complications)

2003 continued to bring enormous changes to the care of the HIV-infected individual. With increased experience in clinical practice, a reduction in cost and a better understanding of the meaning of quantitative measures of viral RNA and increased experience of utilizing **Highly Active Antiretroviral Therapy (HAART)**, clinicians have gained valuable lessons in managing this increasingly complex disease. The current practice is moving towards later (but before CD4 counts get below 200mm³) initiation of HAART, more liberal use of resistance testing, more attention to adherence (with construction of less frequent dosing schedules) and more time spent on managing toxicities. See www.aidsinfo.nih.gov

A. When to start therapy? (www.aidsinfo.nih.gov)

• HIV Symptoms	CD4 cells/μl	Start Treatment	Comment
Yes	<350, usually <200	Yes	
No	<200	Yes	
No	>350	No (see Comment)	Maybe if CD4 decreasing rapidly and/or viral load > 100,000 copies/ml

• Acute retroviral syndrome

B. Suggested Initial Therapy Regimens for Untreated Chronic HIV Infection

1. Preferred Regimens

	Regimen	Capsule (pill size, mg)	Daily Regimen	No. pills/day	Cost/month (AWP)[1]	Comment
a.	**(Zidovudine + Lamivudine)**	(300 + 150)	(Combination—Combivir® 1 tab po bid)[2]	3	$1193	Good efficacy; low pill burden; low AE profile
	Efavirenz	600	1 tab po qd hs, empty stomach[2]			
b.	**Tenofovir + Lamivudine +**	300 + 300 +	1 tab po qd with high-fat meal 1 tab po qd	3	$1235	Tenofovir: expensive & emerging renal toxicity
	Efavirenz	600	1 tab po qd			
c.	**(Zidovudine + Lamivudine)**	(300 + 150)	(Combination—Combivir® 1 tab po bid)	8	$1434	Good efficacy and durable effect. Tolerable AEs. Possible elevated triglycerides. Some data suggest slower rate of accumulation of resistance mutations than nelfinavir regimens (Abst. 600, 10ᵗʰ CROI, 2003).[3]
	Ritonavir/Lopinavir*	133.3/33.3	3 tabs po bid with food			

2. Alternative Regimens[4]

	Regimen	Capsule (pill size, mg)	Daily Regimen	No. pills/day	Cost/month (AWP)[1]	Comment
a.	**Didanosine EC + Lamivudine +**	400 + 300 +	1 cap po daily hs, fasting + 1 tab po daily[2] +	3	$1100	Efficacy and durability under study. Potential didanosine AEs. Low pill burden.
	Efavirenz	600	1 tab po daily hs, empty stomach[2]			
	(Zidovudine + Lamivudine)	(300 + 150)	(Combination—Combivir® 1 tab po bid)[2]			
	+ Nelfinavir	625	2 tabs po bid, with food	6	$1579	Good efficacy. Nelfinavir-associated diarrhea in 20%. Large pill burden.
b.	**Didanosine EC + Stavudine +**	400 + *Stavudine extended release dose: >60 kg, 100 mg qd; <60 kg, 75 mg qd*	1 cap po hs, fasting + 1 cap po qd +	3	$1107	Efficacy and durability under study. Potential didanosine & stavudine AEs. Low pill burden. ↑ risk of lactic acidosis/hepatic steatosis when used in pregnant 9. Stavudine toxicity emerging as a problem.
	Efavirenz	600	1 tab po qd hs, empty stomach[2]			
d.	**(Zidovudine + Lamivudine) + Indinavir +**	(300 + 150) 400 +	(Combination—Combivir® 1 tab po bid) 2 caps po q12h +	8	$1213	Indinavir can be administered with or without food when combined with ritonavir
	Ritonavir	100	1 cap po q12h			

[1] **AWP** = average wholesale price.
[2] Food may inactivate medication, which can lead to ↑ in the risk of adverse events.
[3] **CROI** = Conference on Retroviruses and Opportunistic Infections.
[4] Subject to new data, the authors do not, at this time, recommend the fixed combination of abacavir-zidovudine-lamivudine (Trizivir®) alone as a treatment regimen.

TABLE 14C (2)

B. Suggested Initial Therapy Regimens for Untreated Chronic HIV Infection *(continued)*

	Regimen	Capsule (pill size, mg)	Daily Regimen	No. pills/day	Cost/month (AWP)[1]	Comment
2.	**Alternative Regimens** *(continued)*					
e.	**(Zidovudine + Lamivudine) + Saquinavir + Ritonavir**	(300 + 150) 200 100	(Combination—Combivir® 1 tab po bid) 5 caps po q12h with food 1 cap po q12h with food.	14	$1264	
f.	**Stavudine + Lamivudine + Atazanavir**	100 mg extended release 300 mg 200 mg	1 tab po qd 1 tab po qd 2 tabs po qd	4	$1558	

C. Suggested Regimen for Acute Primary HIV Infection (mono-like syndrome)

	Regimen	Capsule (pill size, mg)	Daily Regimen	No. pills/day	Cost/month (AWP)[1]	Comment
	(Zidovudine + Lamivudine) (Combivir®)	Zidovudine 300 mg + Lamivudine 150 mg	1 tab po bid	3	$1193	Appropriate duration of therapy is unknown. Many experts suggest 6 months–2 years
	Efavirenz (Sustiva)	600 mg tab	1 tab po hs, empty stomach[2]			

D. Characteristics of Antiretroviral Drugs
1. Selected Characteristics of Nucleoside or Nucleotide Reverse Transcriptase Inhibitors (NRTIs)

Generic/Trade Name	Pharmaceutical Prep.	Usual Dosage	% Absorbed, po	Serum T½, hrs	Intracellular T½, hrs	Elimination	Major Adverse Events/Comments
Abacavir (Ziagen)	300 mg tabs or 20 mg/ml oral solution ($425/month)	300 mg po bid. Food OK	83	1.5	3.3	Liver metab, renal excretion of metabolites, 82%	Hypersensitivity reaction: fever, rash, N/V, diarrhea, abdominal pain, respiratory symptoms. **Do not rechallenge!** Report to 800-270-0425
Didanosine (ddI; Videx) or Videx EC——**Dose reduction with tenofovir**	25, 50, 100, 150, 200 mg chewable tabs; 100, 167, 250 mg packets for oral solution; 125, 200, 250, 400 enteric-coated tabs ($321/month)	≥60 kg: Usually 400 mg po qd ½ hr before or 2 hrs after meal See Comment	30–40	1.6	25–40	Renal excretion, 50%	Pancreatitis, peripheral neuropathy, lactic acidosis & hepatic steatosis (rare but life-threatening). **Reduce dose to 250 mg EC if used with tenofovir**
Emtricitabine (FTC; Emtriva)	200 mg caps ($303/month)	200 mg po qd. No significant effect of food	50–95% in animal studies	Approx. 10		Extent of liver metabolism unknown; 14% excreted in feces, 86% in urine	Well tolerated, headache 20%, nausea, vomiting & diarrhea occasionally, skin rash rarely. Differs only slightly in structure from lamivudine (5-fluoro substitution). Also active vs hepatitis B. Exacerbation of Hep B reported in pts after DC of FTC.
Lamivudine (3TC; Epivir)	150, 300 mg tabs; 10 mg/ml oral solution ($316/month)	150 mg po bid or 300 mg po qd. Food OK	86	3–6	16	Renal excretion, unchanged	Safest of NRTIs. Rare life-threatening lactic acidosis.
Stavudine (d4T; Zerit, Zerit XR)	15, 20, 30, 40, 60 mg capsules or 75, 100 mg extended-release (XR) caps; 1 mg/ml oral solution ($323/month)	≥60 kg: 40 mg cap bid or 100 mg XR cap qd. <60 kg: 30 mg cap bid or 75 mg XR cap qd. Food OK	86	1	3.5	Renal excretion, 50%	Pancreatitis, peripheral neuropathy, lactic acidosis with hepatic steatosis and/or neuromuscular weakness.
Tenofovir disoproxil fumarate (Viread)—a nucleotide	300 mg tabs ($456/month)	300 mg po qd with high-fat meal. **Do not use if CrCl <60** See Comment	39	17	10–50	Renal excretion	Asthenia, headache, N/V, rarely hepatic steatosis & lactic acidosis if combined with didanosine, lower didanosine dose.

[1] **AWP** = average wholesale price
[2] Food may ↑ serum concentration, which can lead to ↑ in the risk of adverse events.

TABLE 14C (3)

1. Selected Characteristics of Nucleoside or Nucleotide Reverse Transcriptase Inhibitors (NRTIs) (continued)

Generic/Trade Name	Pharmaceutical Prep. (AWP)	Usual Dosage	% Absorbed, po	Serum T½, hrs		Elimination	Major Adverse Events/Comments
Zalcitabine (ddC; Hivid)	0.375, 0.75 tabs ($235/month)	0.75 mg po tid. Food OK.	85	1.2	3	Renal excretion, 70%	Peripheral neuropathy, stomatitis, rarely life-threatening lactic acidosis, pancreatitis.
Zidovudine (ZDV, AZT; Retrovir)	100 mg caps, 300 mg tabs; 10 mg/ml IV solution; 10 mg/ml oral solution ($319/month)	300 mg po bid. Food OK.	60	1.1	3	Metabolized to glucuronide & excreted in urine	Anemia, marrow suppression, GI intolerance, headache, insomnia, weakness, rarely lactic acidosis

2. Selected Characteristics of Non-Nucleoside Reverse Transcriptase Inhibitors (NNRTIs)

Generic/Trade Name	Pharmaceutical Prep. (AWP)	Usual Dosage	% Absorbed, po	Serum T½, hrs	Elimination	Major Adverse Events/Comments
Delavirdine (Rescriptor)	100, 200 mg tabs ($292/month)	400 mg po tid. Food OK.	85	5.8	Cytochrome P450 (3A inhibitor), 51% excreted in urine (<5% unchanged), 44% in feces	Rash severe enough to dc use of drug in 4.3%.
Efavirenz (Sustiva)	50, 100, 200 mg capsules; 600 mg tablet ($463/month)	600 mg po hs, without food[1]	42	40-55	Cytochrome P450 (3A mixed inducer/inhibitor). 14-34% of dose excreted in urine as glucuronidated metabolites, 16-61% in feces	Rash severe enough to dc use of drug in 1.7%. High frequency of diverse CNS AEs: somnolence, dreams, confusion, agitation; false-positive cannabinoid test
Nevirapine (Viramune)	200 mg tabs; 50 mg/5 ml oral suspension ($307/month)	200 mg po x14 d. & then 200 mg po bid. Food OK.	>90	25-30	Cytochrome P450 (3A) inducer: 80% of dose excreted in urine as glucuronidated metabolites, 10% in feces	Rash severe enough to dc use of drug in 7%. Hepatitis reported

3. Selected Characteristics of Protease Inhibitors (PIs)

Generic/Trade Name	Pharmaceutical Prep. (AWP)[2]	Usual Dosage	% Absorbed, po	Serum T½, hrs	Elimination	Major Adverse Events/Comments
Amprenavir (Agenerase)	50, 150 mg capsules; 15 mg/ml oral solution. (For oral solution dosage, see package insert or PDR) ($634/month)	1200 mg (Eight 150 mg caps) po bid. OR With ritonavir [600 mg amprenavir (4 caps) + ritonavir 100 mg po bid] (1200 mg amprenavir caps + 200 mg ritonavir) po qd	No data Food OK; avoid high-fat meal	7.1–10.6	Cytochrome P450 (3A4 inhibitor)	Nausea/vomiting, diarrhea, rash, oral paresthesias; ↑ SGOT/SGPT; glucose/lipid abnormalities.* Oral solution contains propylene glycol; do not use in pregnancy, children <4 y/o, renal/hepatic failure, with disulfiram or metronidazole. Possible hemophilia bleeding
Fosamprenavir (Lexiva)	700 mg tablets (contains 600 mg amprenavir)	Rx naive: 1400 mg (2 tabs) bid or 1400 mg (2 tabs) + ritonavir 200 mg qd or 700 mg (1 tab) + ritonavir 100 mg bid. PI-experienced: 700 mg (1 tab) + ritonavir 100 mg bid. Child Pugh Class B—700 mg bid. Child Pugh Class C—avoid.	Good oral bioavailability; food enhances bioavailability & ↓ pharmacokinetic variability	Approx. 7	Cytochrome P450 (3A4 inhibitor). UGT1A1 inhibitor. 13% excreted in urine (7% unchanged) & in feces (20% unchanged)	A prodrug of amprenavir, rapidly converted to parent drug in gut. Good absorption without propylene glycol. Same properties as amprenavir.
Atazanavir (Reyataz)	100, 150, 200 mg capsules ($828/month)	400 mg qd with food (exception is atazanavir 300 mg qd + ritonavir 100 mg qd when combined with efavirenz 600 mg qd). Take 2 hr pre or 1 hr post buffered ddI. Dosage adjustment in hepatic insufficiency: Child Pugh Class B—300 mg qd. Child Pugh Class C—avoid.				No ↑ lipids in available studies. Asymptomatic unconjugated hyperbilirubinemia in up to 60% of pts, grade 3 & 4 in 5–9% of pts, jaundice in 17%. Diarrhea 2%, nausea & abdominal pain 20%, headache 25%, rash 20%. Prolongation of PR interval (1st degree AV block) reported. Caution in pre-existing conduction system disease.

[1] Food may ↑ serum concentration, which can lead to ↑ in the risk of adverse events.
[2] AWP = average wholesale price

TABLE 14C (4)

3. Selected Characteristics of Protease Inhibitors (PIs) (continued)

Generic/Trade Name	Pharmaceutical Prep. (AWP)	Usual Dosage	% Absorbed, po	Serum T½, hrs	Elimination	Major Adverse Events/Comments
Indinavir (Crixivan)	200, 333, 400 mg capsules ($549/month)	Two 400 mg caps (800 mg) po q8h. Without food or with light meal. Can take with enteric-coated Videx. (If taken with ritonavir, no food restrictions)	65	1.2-2	Cytochrome P450 (3A4 inhibitor)	Nephrolithiasis, inconsequential ↑ of indirect bilirubin, ↑ SGOT/SGPT, glucose/fat abnormalities.* headache, asthenia, blurred vision, metallic taste. Possible hemophilia bleeding
Lopinavir + ritonavir (Kaletra) Can be kept at room temperature x2 mos.	133.3 mg lopinavir + 33.3 mg ritonavir capsules. Oral solution: (80 mg lopinavir + 20 mg ritonavir)/ml. Refrigerate. ($703/month)	(400 mg lopinavir + 100 mg ritonavir)—3 caps po bid, with food	No data in humans	5-6	Cytochrome P450 (3A4 inhibitor)	Nausea/vomiting/diarrhea, asthenia, ↑ SGOT/SGPT, glucose/fat abnormalities.* Oral solution 42% alcohol. Possible hemophilia bleeding
Nelfinavir (Viracept)	250, 625 mg tabs; 50 mg/gm oral powder ($849/month)	2 tabs (1250 mg) po bid, with food	20-80	3.5-5	Cytochrome P450 (3A4 inhibitor)	Diarrhea, glucose/fat abnormalities.* ↑ SGOT/SGPT. Possible hemophilia bleeding
Ritonavir (Norvir) Can be kept at room temperature x1 mo.	100 mg capsules, 600 mg/7.5 ml solution. Refrigerate ($702/month)	Full dose: 6 caps (600 mg) po q12h, with food. Escalate to full dose: 300 mg bid x2 d; 400 mg bid x3 d; 500 mg bid x7 d.; then full dose	Approx. 65	3-5	Cytochrome P450. Potent 3A4 inhibitor	Nausea/vomiting/diarrhea, extremity & circumoral paresthesias, hepatitis, pancreatitis, taste perversion, ↑ CPK & uric acid, glucose/fat abnormalities.* Possible hemophilia bleeding
Saquinavir mesylate (Invirase) hard gel caps + ritonavir	Saquinavir 200 mg caps: ritonavir 100 mg caps ($711/month)	2 caps saquinavir (400 mg) + 4 caps ritonavir (400 mg) po bid, with food	Erratic, 4	1-2	Cytochrome P450 (3A4 inhibitor)	Nausea, diarrhea, headache, ↑ SGOT/SGPT glucose/fat abnormalities.* Possible hemophilia bleeding
Saquinavir (Fortovase) softgel caps	Refrigerate (can be kept at room temperature x3 mos.) ($751/month)	6 caps (1200 mg) po tid, with food	Not known	1-2	Cytochrome P450 (3A4 inhibitor)	Nausea, diarrhea, abdominal pain, headache, Possible hemophilia bleeding
Tipranavir (Texega) FDA action Pending 01/04		500 mg with ritonavir 200 mg bid in Phase III studies.	30% in animal studies. ↑ AUC & peak plasma conc. in presence of food & if combined with ritonavir		Cytochrome P450 (3A4 mixed inducer/inhibitor)	Nausea & vomiting, diarrhea, abdominal pain

* All PIs: Glucose metabolism: new diabetes mellitus or deterioration of glucose control
Hypertriglyceridemia or hypercholesterolemia

4. Selected Characteristics of Fusion Inhibitors

Generic/Trade Name	Pharmaceutical Prep.	Usual Dosage	% Absorbed, po	Serum T½, hrs	Elimination	Major Adverse Events/Comments
Enfuvirtide (T20, Fuzeon)	Single-use vials of 90 mg/ml when reconstituted. Vials should be stored at room temperature. Reconstituted vials can be refrigerated for 24 hrs. (~$20,000/year)	90 mg (1 ml) sc bid	84.3 ± 15.5	3.8 ± 0.6	Catabolism to its constituent amino acids with subsequent recycling of the amino acids in the body pool. Elimination pathway(s) have not been performed in humans. Does not alter the metabolism of CYP3A4, CYP2D6, CYP1A2, CYP2C19 or CYP2E1 substrates.	Local injection site reactions 98% (premedication with antihistamine reduces symptoms), <3% DC (erythema 87%, induration 84%, nodules/cysts 82%). Peripheral neuropathy 8.9%, insomnia 11.3%, ↓ appetite 6.3%, myalgia 5%, lymphadenopathy 2.3%, eosinophilia 11.2%. Incidence of bacterial pneumonia & other infections. Don't add to failing regimen. Need 2 other active drugs!

¹ AWP = average wholesale price

TABLE 14D: ANTIRETROVIRAL DRUGS AND ADVERSE EFFECTS (Ln 358:1322, 2001)

DRUG NAME(S): GENERIC (TRADE)	ADVERSE EFFECTS
Nucleoside Reverse Transcriptase Inhibitors (NRTI)	
Abacavir (Ziagen) (Clin Ther 23:1603, 2001)	**Most common:** Headache 16%, nausea/vomiting 16%, diarrhea 12%, loss of appetite/anorexia 11%, malaise **Most significant: Hypersensitivity reaction** in 5% with malaise, fever, GI upset, rash, lethargy, & respiratory symptoms most commonly reported; myalgia, arthralgia, edema, paresthesia less commonly reported. **Rechallenge contraindicated; may be life-threatening.**
Didanosine (ddI) (Videx)	**Most common:** Diarrhea 28%, nausea 6%, rash 9%, headache 7%, fever 12%, hyperuricemia 2% **Most significant: Pancreatitis 1–9%.** Cases of fatal & nonfatal pancreatitis have occurred in pts receiving ddI, especially when used in combination with d4T or d4T + hydroxyurea. Peripheral neuropathy in 20%, 12% required dose reduction.
Emtricitabine (FTC, Emtriva)	**Most common:** Diarrhea 20%, nausea 20%, diarrhea, nausea, rash **Most significant:** Lactic acidosis
Lamivudine (3TC), (Epivir)	Well tolerated. Headache 35%, nausea 33%, diarrhea 18%, abdominal pain 9%, insomnia 11% (in combination with ZDV). Pancreatitis more common in pediatrics (15%).
Stavudine (d4T) (Zerit)	**Most common:** Diarrhea, nausea, vomiting, headache **Most significant: Peripheral neuropathy** 15–20%. Pancreatitis 1%. Appears to produce lactic acidosis more commonly than other NRTIs. Fatal lactic acidosis/steatosis in pregnant women receiving d4T + ddI. Motor weakness in the setting of lactic acidosis mimicking the clinical presentation of Guillain-Barre syndrome (including respiratory failure) (rare).
Zalcitabine (ddC) (Hivid)	**Most common:** Oral ulcers 1%, rash 8% **Most significant: Peripheral neuropathy** 22–35%. Severe continuous pain, slowly reversible when ddC is discontinued, ↑ risk with diabetes mellitus.
Zidovudine (ZDV, AZT) (Retrovir)	**Most common:** Nausea 50%, anorexia 20%, vomiting 17%, headache 53%, fatigue 53%, pigmentation of nails, asthenia, insomnia, myalgias. Macrocytosis expected with all dosage regimens. **Most significant: Anemia** (<8 gm 1%), granulocytopenia (<750 1.8%). Anemia may respond to epoetin alfa if endogenous serum erythropoietin levels are <500 mU/ml.
Nucleotide Reverse Transcriptase Inhibitor (NRTI)	
Tenofovir (Viread)	**Most common:** Nausea 11%, diarrhea 9%, vomiting 5%, flatulence 4% (generally well tolerated) **Most significant:** Lactic acidosis with hepatic steatosis. Affinity of tenofovir for polymerase gamma is lower than for other NRTI. Several reports of Fanconi syndrome & renal failure induced by tenofovir (Ann J Kidney Dis 35:1331, 2002; CID 35:1070 & 1082, 2003).
Non-Nucleoside Reverse Transcriptase Inhibitors (NNRTI)	
Delavirdine (Rescriptor)	**Most common:** Nausea, diarrhea, vomiting, headache **Most significant: Skin rash** has occurred in 18%, can continue or restart drug in most cases. Stevens-Johnson syndrome and erythema multiforme have been reported rarely. ↑ in liver enzymes in <5% of cases.
Efavirenz (Sustiva)	**Most common: CNS side-effects 52%;** symptoms include dizziness, insomnia, somnolence, impaired concentration, and abnormal dreams; symptoms are worse after 1st or 2nd dose and improve over 2–4 weeks; discontinuation rate 2.6%. Rash 26%; improves with oral antihistamines; discontinuation rate 1.7%. Can cause false-positive urine test results for cannabinoid with EMIT-DAU multi-level THC assay. **Most significant:** Elevation in liver function tests. **Teratogenicity in primates; not recommended in pregnant women** (see Table 7).
Nevirapine (Viramune)	**Most common: Rash 37%;** occurs during 1st 6 weeks of therapy. Women experience 7-fold ↑ in risk of severe rash (CID 32:124, 2001). 50% resolve within 2 wks of dc drug and 80% by 1 month. 6.7% discontinuation rate. Severe life-threatening skin reactions reported. Stevens-Johnson syndrome, toxic epidermal necrolysis, and hypersensitivity reaction or drug rash with eosinophilia and systemic symptoms (DRESS) (AVM 161:2501, 2001). For severe rashes, dc drug immediately and do not restart. In a clinical trial, the use of prednisone ↑ the risk of rash. **Most significant: Life-threatening hepatotoxicity reported,** 2/3 during the first 12 wks of rx. Overall 1% develop hepatitis. Pts with pre-existing ↑ in ALT or AST &/or history of clinical Hep B or C are at increased risk of developing Hep (Hepatol 35:182, 2002). Monitor pts monthly (clinical and LFTs), esp. during the first 12 wks of rx. If clinical hepatotoxicity occurs, dc drug and never rechallenge. A cohort study of nevirapine tolerance in French Aquitaine has been reported (CID 35:1231, 2002).
Protease inhibitors (PI)	
Amprenavir (Agenerase) and fosamprenavir (Lexiva)	Spontaneous bleeding episodes have been reported in HIV+ pts with hemophilia being treated with PI. All PIs may be associated with hyperglycemia and/or hyperlipidemia. Rheumatoid complications have been reported with the use of PIs (An Rheum Dis 61:82, 2002). Pts taking PI may be at increased risk for developing osteopenias and osteoporosis. **Most common:** Nausea 43–74%, vomiting 24–34%, diarrhea 39–60%, paresthesias 26–31% **Most significant: Skin rash** 28%. Most maculopapular of mild–moderate intensity, some with pruritus. Severe or life-threatening rash, including Stevens-Johnson syndrome, in 1% of pts. Rash onset 7–73 days, median 11 days.

TABLE 14D (2)

DRUG NAME(S): GENERIC (TRADE)	ADVERSE EFFECTS
Protease Inhibitors (PI) *(continued)*	
Atazanavir ((Reyataz)	**Most common:** Asymptomatic unconjugated hyperbilirubinemia in up to 60% of pts, grade 3 & 4 in 5–9% of pts, jaundice in 17% (should probably discontinue drug if persistent elevation of >5x normal bilirubin). Diarrhea 20–25%, nausea & abdominal pain 20%, headache 25%, rash 20%. **Most significant:** Prolongation of PR interval (1° degree AV block) reported.
Indinavir (Crixivan)	**Most common:** ↑ In indirect bilirubin 10–15% (≥2.5 mg/dl), due to a drug-induced Gilbert's syndrome (of no clinical significance). Severe hepatitis reported in 3 cases (*Ln* 349:924, 1997). Nausea 12%, vomiting 4%, diarrhea 5%. Paronychia of big toe reported (*AIDS 14:296, 1997*); 12/174 (6.9%) developed nephrolithiasis within 4 months of starting indinavir; 5/8 who continued rx had a 2nd episode (*ICAAC Abst. 183, 1997*). **Most significant: Kidney stones** Due to indinavir crystals in collecting system (2–3% on 2.4 gm/d but higher in "hot climates" (*CID 32:142, 2001*). Prevent (minimize) by good hydration (at least 48 oz. water/day) (*AAC 42:332, 1998*).
Nelfinavir (Viracept)	**Most common:** Mild to moderate **diarrhea** 14–52%. Oat bran tabs, calcium, or oral anti-diarrheal agents (e.g., loperamide, diphenoxylate/atropine sulfate) can be used to manage diarrhea.
Ritonavir (Norvir)	**Most common:** GI: bitter aftertaste ↓ by taking with chocolate milk, Ensure, or Advera; nausea 23%, ↓ by initial dose escalation (titration) regimen; vomiting 13%, diarrhea 13%. Circumoral paresthesias 5–6%. ↑ dose >100 mg bid assoc. with ↑ GI side-effects & ↑ in lipid abnormalities. **Most significant:** Hepatic failure (*AnIM 129:670, 1998*). Many important drug-drug interactions—inhibits P450 CYP3A system *(see Table 22)*.
Saquinavir (Invirase, hard cap) (Fortovase softgel cap)	**Most common:** GI: **diarrhea** 16–20%, abdominal discomfort 9–13%, nausea 11–18%. Headache 5–9%.
Tipranavir (Texapa)	**Most common:** Nausea & vomiting, diarrhea, abdominal pain.
Lopinavir/Ritonavir (Kaletra)	**Most common:** GI: **diarrhea** 14–24%, nausea 2–16%, lipid abnormalities in up to 30% **Most significant:** Pancreatitis, inflammatory edema of the legs (*AIDS 16:673, 2002*)
Fusion Inhibitor	
Enfuvirtide (T20, Fuzeon)	**Most common:** local injection site reactions (98% at least 1 local ISR, 3% dc because of ISR (pain & discomfort, induration, erythema, nodules & cysts, pruritus, & ecchymosis). Diarrhea 27%, nausea 20%, fatigue 16%. Local injection site reactions 98%, <3% DC (erythema 87%, induration 84%, nodules/cysts 82%). **Most significant:** ↑ rate of bacterial pneumonia (4.68 pneumonia events/100 pt yrs), hypersensitivity reactions <1% (rash, fever, nausea & vomiting, chills, rigors, hypotension, & ↑ serum liver transaminases)

TABLE 15A

ANTIMICROBIAL PROPHYLAXIS FOR SELECTED BACTERIAL AND VIRAL INFECTIONS

CLASS OF ETIOLOGIC AGENT/DOSE/CONDITION	PROPHYLAXIS: AGENT/DOSE/ROUTE/DURATION	COMMENTS
Group B streptococcal disease (GBS), neonatal: Approaches to management [CDC Guidelines, MMWR 51(RR-11):1, 2002]:		
Pregnant women—intrapartum antimicrobial prophylaxis—The use of standard orders and forms correlates with ↑ in prophylaxis administration (AJOG 184:1177, 2001)	**Intrapartum prophylaxis indicated** (culture positive or risk factors dictate prophylaxis (but not if pre-labor, planned C-section without labor or ruptured membranes))	
▶ a ↓ in neonatal disease (NEJM 347:233, 2000).	**Rx mother during labor with pen G** 5 MU IV (load) then 2.5 MU IV q4h until delivery.	
• Screen all pregnant women with vaginal & rectal swab for GBS at 35–37 wks gestation (unless other indications for prophylaxis exist: GBS bacteriuria during this pregnancy or previously delivered infant with invasive GBS disease; even then cultures may be useful for susceptibility testing). Use transport medium; GBS survive at room temp. up to 96 hrs. Rx during labor if swab culture positive.	Alternate if **Ampicillin** 2 gm IV (load) then give 1 gm IV q4h until delivery. **Pen-allergic: Pts not at high risk for anaphylaxis: Cefazolin** 2 gm IV (load) then 1 gm IV q8h until delivery. **Pts at high risk for anaphylaxis:** GBS susceptible to clinda & erythro: **Clindamycin** 900 mg IV q8h until delivery or **erythromycin** 500 mg IV q6h until delivery. Vancomycin needed for pts at high risk for anaphylaxis to clindamycin or erythromycin needed (e.g., GBS-resistant or unknown susceptibility) [MMWR 51(RR-11):1, 2002].	
• On admission in labor if previously delivered infant with invasive GBS infection, or if GBS bacteriuria during this pregnancy.		
• Rx if GBS status unknown but if any of the following are present: (a) delivery at <37 wks gestation [see MMWR 51(RR-11):1, 2002 algorithm for threatened preterm delivery]; or (b) duration of ruptured membranes ≥18 hrs; or (c) intrapartum fever ≥100.4°F (≥38.0°C) [see MMWR 51(RR-11):1, 2002 re: broadening spectrum if amnionitis suspected].		
Neonate of mother before prophylaxis	Careful observation of signs & symptoms; 95% of infants who will show clinical signs of infection during the 1st 24 hrs whether mother received intrapartum antibiotics (or not (Pediatrics 106:244, 2000).	
Preterm, premature rupture of the membranes in Group B strep-negative women (JAMA 278:989, 1997)	(IV **ampicillin** 2 gm q6h + IV **erythromycin** 250 mg q6h for 48 hrs) then followed by po **amoxicillin** 250 mg q8h + po **erythromycin** base 333 mg q8h x5 d. Effective in ↓ infant morbidity.	Antibiotic rx reduced infant respiratory distress syndrome (50.6% to 40.8%, p = 0.03), necrotizing enterocolitis (5.8% to 2.3%, p = 0.03) and prolonged pregnancy (2.9 to 6.1 days, p < 0.001) vs placebo. In 1 large study (4809 pts), po erythromycin rx improved neonatal outcomes vs placebo (11.2% vs 14.4% poor outcomes, p =0.02 for single births) but not co-AMCL (Lt 357:979, 2001).
Influenza (see Table 14, page 111, & Table 20, pages 136–137)		
Meningitis: Hemophilus and Neisseria meningitidis—See Table 1, pages 5, 6		
Neutropenic patients, afebrile, e.g., post-chemotherapy	**Routine antibacterial prophylaxis not recommended**—even though TMP/SMX 2 double strength tablets po bid	Addition of penicillin, vancomycin, macrolide or rifampin reduced Gm+ bacteremia (OR = 0.46) but had no impact on fever-related morbidity (OR = 0.3) or infection-related mortality (OR = 0.74) (CID 23:795, 1996; AnIM 125:183, 1996). Fluconazole prophylaxis recommended in HSCT (CID 33:1399, 2001).
See CID 34:730, 2002	or **Ciprofloxacin** 500 mg po bid has been shown to reduce febrile episodes. No reduction in mortality and ↑ resistance prompt this recommendation.	
Management of Exposure to Blood, Vaginal/Penile Secretions With Risk of Transmission of Hepatitis B/C and/or HIV (Needlestick Injury) (Refs. MMWR 50:RR-11, 2001; NEJM 348:826, 2003).		
General steps in management: For free consultation for clinicians treating occupational exposures, call CDC PEPLine 1-888-HIV-4911 or website. http://www.cdc.gov/ncidod/.		
1. Wash clean wound/flush mucous membranes immediately (use of caustic agents or squeezing the wound or expressing fluid is discouraged; data lacking regarding antiseptics).		
2. Assess risk by doing the following: (a) Characterize exposure. (b) Determine/evaluate **source of exposure** by medical history, risk behavior, & testing for hepatitis B/C, HIV; (c) Evaluate and test post-exposed individual for B, C & HIV		

Hepatitis B Exposure [See CDC recommendations: MMWR 50(RR-11), 2001]

Exposed Person		Exposure Source	
	HBs Ag+	**HBs Ag–**	**Status Unknown**
Unvaccinated	Give HBIG 0.06 mL/kg IM & initiate HB vaccine	Initiate HB vaccine	Initiate HB vaccine. If possible, check HBs Ag of source person
Vaccinated (antibody status unknown)	Do anti-HBs on exposed person: If titer ≥10 MIU/ml, no rx If titer <10 MIU/ml, give HBIG + 1 dose HB vaccine	No rx necessary	Do anti-HBs on exposed person: If titer ≥10 MIU/ml, no rx If titer <10 MIU/ml, give 1 dose of HB vaccine (plus 1 dose HBIG if source high risk)

For known vaccine series responder (titer ≥10 MIU/ml), monitoring of levels or booster doses not currently recommended. For non-responder (<10 MIU/ml) to 1° series HB vaccine, a 2nd course (a complete 2nd series) with high-dose—rx with HBIG & 1-dose vaccine series or give 2 doses HBIG 1 month apart. For non-responders after a 2nd vaccine series, 2 doses HBIG 1 month apart is preferred approach to new exposure [MMWR 40(13):21, 2001].

TABLE 15A (2)

Hepatitis C Exposure
Determine antibody to hepatitis C for both exposed person and, if possible, exposure source. If source +, follow-up HCV testing advised. **No recommended prophylaxis; immune serum globulin not effective.** Monitor for early infection, as therapy may ↓ risk of progression to chronic hepatitis. *See Table 14A.*

HIV: Occupational exposure management *(for sexual exposure to HIV, see page 124)*
- The decision to initiate post-exposure prophylaxis (PEP) for HIV is a clinical judgment that should be made in concert with the exposed healthcare worker (HCW). It is based on:
  1. Likelihood of the source patient having HIV infection: 1 with history of high-risk activity—injection drug use, sexual activity with multiple partners (either hetero- or homosexual), receipt of blood products 1978–1985, 1 with clinical signs suggestive of advanced HIV (unexplained wasting, night sweats, thrush, seborrheic dermatitis, etc.).
     Remember, the vast majority of persons are **not** infected with HIV (1/200 women infected in larger U.S. cities) and likelihood of infection **extremely rare** if not in above risk groups.
  2. Type of exposure (approx. 1 in 300–400 needlesticks from infected source will transmit HIV).
  3. Limited data regarding efficacy of PEP (PEP with ZDV alone reduced transmission by >80% in 1 retrospective case-controlled study—*NEJM 337:1485, 1997*).
  4. Significant adverse effects of PEP drugs.
- If source person is **known positive for HIV** or **likely to be infected** and **status of exposure warrants PEP**, antiretroviral drugs should be started **immediately** (at least within 72 hrs). If ELISA for HIV is negative, drugs can be stopped. Availability of rapid HIV testing has potential to ↓ unnecessary PEP use (*NEJM 384:826, 2003*). The HCW should be re-tested at **3-4 weeks, 3 & 6 months** whether **PEP is used or not** (the vast majority of seroconversions will occur by 3 months; delayed conversions after 6 months are exceedingly rare).
- PEP for HIV is usually given for **4 weeks** and monitoring of adverse effects recommended: baseline **complete blood count, renal and hepatic panel** to be repeated at 2 weeks. 50–75% of HCW on PEP have side-effects while mild (nausea, diarrhea, myalgia, headache, etc.) but in up to ⅓ severe enough to discontinue PEP (*Antivir Ther 3:195, 2000*). Consultation with infectious diseases/HIV specialist valuable when questions regarding PEP arise. Seek expert help in special situations, such as pregnancy, renal impairment.

3 Steps to HIV Post-Exposure Prophylaxis (PEP) After Occupational Exposure: *(MMWR 50:RR-11, 2001)*

Step 1: Determine the exposure code (EC)

Is source material blood, bloody fluid, semen/vaginal fluid or other normally sterile fluid or tissue?

Yes		No → No PEP

What type of exposure occurred?

Mucous membrane or skin integrity compromised (e.g., dermatitis, open wound) → Volume

Intact skin → No PEP

Percutaneous exposure → Severity

Volume:
- Small: Few drops → EC1
- Large: Major splash and/or long duration → EC2

Severity:
- Less severe: Solid needle, scratch → EC2
- More severe: Large-bore hollow needle, deep puncture, visible blood, needle used in vein of source (risk 1:300/400) → EC3

Step 2: Determine the HIV Status Code (HIV SC)

What is the HIV status of the exposure source?

HIV negative → No PEP

HIV positive:
- Low titer exposure: asymptomatic & high CD4 count → HIV SC 1
- High titer exposure: advanced AIDS, prim. HIV high viral load or low CD4 count → HIV SC 2

Status unknown → HIV SC unknown

Source unknown → HIV SC unknown

Step 3: Determine Post-Exposure Prophylaxis (PEP) Recommendation

EC	HIV SC	Recommendation
1	1	Consider basic regimen[1]
1	2	Recommend basic regimen[1]
2	1	Recommend basic regimen[1]
2	2	Recommend expanded regimen[1]
3	1,2	Recommend expanded regimen[1]
2,3	Unknown	If exposure setting suggests risks of HIV exposure, consider basic regimen[1]

Regimens:
Treat for 4 weeks: Monitor for drug side-effects q2 weeks
Basic regimen: ZDV + 3TC, or d4T + 3TC. Best to avoid ddI + d4T (↑ side effects)
Expanded regimen: Basic regimen + one of the following: indinavir, nelfinavir, abacavir, or efavirenz. (Do not use nevirapine: 22 HCWs receiving drug for PEP had serious adverse events, including hepatic necrosis with one requiring liver transplant (*MMWR 49:1153, 2001*))
If possible, use two antiretroviral drugs that the source pt is not currently taking or for which resistance is unlikely.
NOTE: Some authorities feel that an expanded regimen should be employed whenever PEP is used. See *NEJM 348:826, 2003*.

Post-Exposure Prophylaxis (after high-risk sex or parenteral drug exposure) (*JID 183:707, 2001*) *[Adapted from MMWR 47:RR-17, 1998; also see Int J STD AIDS 11:424, 2000; NEJM 336:1097, 1997]*
Since the probability of transmission of HIV via sexual contact may approach that of a needlestick, it is reasonable to consider PEP in persons who have had a sexual encounter with an HIV+ person. Currently there are no data on effectiveness of PEP in this setting. The same assessment as suggested above for occupational exposure might be followed in an attempt to determine relative risk. It has been **estimated that transmission of HIV following an episode of HIV following receptive penile-anal sexual exposure is 0.1–3%, for receptive vaginal exposure 0.1–0.2%**, and unknown for receptive oral intercourse (although less risky than others).
PEP should be used for low-risk exposures (potentially infected body fluids on intact skin) or for persons who have had casual low per-act probability of transmission against **given for PEP when risk is high, PEP can be initiated promptly, and adherence is likely**. It is prudent to weigh risk relative low per-act probability of transmission against uncertain effectiveness, potential toxicities, and cost (approx. $800–1000/course).
Management and drug selection as above. Patient should also be screened for other sexually transmitted diseases. Approaches to the evaluation & treatment of sexual & other non-occupational exposures to HIV are discussed in *Arch Intern Med 126:306, 1998; Peds 111:1475, 2003;* and in Brown University/Rhode Island Dept. of Health guidelines at www.brown.edu/Departments/BRUNAP/package.htm.

CLASS OF ETIOLOGIC AGENT/DISEASE/CONDITION	PROPHYLAXIS AGENT/DOSE/ROUTE/DURATION	COMMENTS
HIV transmission from mother to neonate (vertical transmission) (*JID 187, page 41*) Mother should not breast-feed if possible. See USPHS Task Force recommendations & supplement (Sept. 22, 2003) for discussion & options, use of antiretrovirals (ART) in pregnancy, & risks/benefits of scheduled C-section if RNA >1000 copies before delivery (http://aidsinfo.nih.gov).	**Standard for developed countries with prenatal care:** **Zidovudine (ZDV)** 300 mg bid on starting 1wk 14 of pregnancy, then 1 mg/kg (load during labor & then 2 mg/kg po q6h to baby beginning 8–12 hrs after birth for 6 weeks (dose adjustments needed in preterm infants (http://aidsinfo.nih.gov). [Cost: $200/mother-baby pair] 1 mother already receiving ART (↑x, consult with HIV/ID specialist). **ART rx during or before delivery:** ZDV 2 mg/kg po q6h to baby 8–12 hrs after birth for 6 wks. **Alternative regimen for less-developed countries:** **Nevirapine** 200 mg po to mother at onset of labor & a single 2 mg/kg dose to baby within 72 hrs of birth (not FDA-approved indication). [Cost: $4.00/mother-baby pair]. **See Comment**	ACTG 076 trial (402 mother-baby pairs) showed reduced infection in neonate from **7.6% vs 22.6%** with ZDV regimen. No evidence of fetal abnormalities in neonates attributed to drug. None of the mothers breast-fed (*NEJM 331:1173, 1994; NEJM 335:1621, 1996*). Standard course for mother (starting at 28th wk of gestation) superior to short course (starting at 35th wk). Shorter course to infant (3 d.) similar to standard 6 wks if mother at 28th wk (*NEJM 343:982, 2000*). Observational study of 900 births showed ZDV rx to infant reduced transmission from 30% to 10% (*NEJM 339:1409, 1998*). In specific circumstances, some may use broader ART rx (http://aidsinfo.nih.gov). Nevirapine efficacy compared favorably to ZDV (*Ln 354:795, 1999*) and ZDV + 3TC (*JID 187: 725, 2003*). Nevirapine + ZDV somewhat better (*Ln 362:1171, 2003*). **There is concern over potential life-threatening hepatotoxicity & severe skin reactions.** esp. in resource-poor environments (*AIDS Reader 13:459, 2003*).
Lyme Disease (see *Table 1, page 39*)		
Otitis media (see *Table 1, page 7*)		
Rheumatic fever, acute (see *Table 1, page 41*)		
Sickle-cell disease, prevent bacteremia, likely agents: Pneumococcus (90%), meningococci, H. influenzae type b (also at ↑ risk of fatal malaria, severe babesiosis) (immunization important, see *Comments*)	**Penicillin V** Children—Age < 5 yrs 125 mg po bid, > 5 yrs 250 mg po bid. Adults 250 mg po bid. (Alternatives: **Amoxicillin, TMP/SMX** (also ↑ pneumo. resistance) NOTE: Repeat pneumococcal vaccine every 6 years	Daily antimicrobial prophylaxis effective with sickle-cell disease, but should also be considered for asplenic children < 5 yrs. Also recommended in children and adolescents for 3 yrs post splenectomy. **Adjunct measures for all ages: meningococcal A, C, Y & W-135, pneumococcal AM/CL vaccines before elective splenectomy**. Some authorities prescribe AM/CL for self-administration with onset of any fever for all ages. Compliance with recommendations poor (*J Clin Path 54:214, 2001*). See *Curr Clin Top Inf Dis 22:78, 2002*.

TABLE 15A (4)

CLASS OF ETIOLOGIC AGENT/DISEASE/CONDITION	PROPHYLAXIS: AGENT/DOSE/ROUTE/DURATION	COMMENTS
Sexual Exposure		
Sexual assault victim [likely agents and risks, see *JAMA* 322:713, 1990 & *MMWR* 51 (RR-6):1, 2002]	(**Ceftriaxone** 125 mg IM) + (**metronidazole** 2 gm po single dose) + (**azithromycin** 1 gm po single dose) or (**doxycycline** 100 mg po bid x 7 d)] (*MMWR* 51 (RR-6):1, 2002)	Obtain expert advice re: forensic exam & specimens, pregnancy, physical trauma, psychological issues, HIV risk evaluation. Culture for gonococcus & chlamydia (if available), wet mount for T. vaginalis, serologic test for syphilis & hepatitis B surface antigen, HIV serology at 6, 12, 24 wks if appropriate. Initiate HIV post-exposure protocols & Hep B vaccine as appropriate; follow-up exam for STD at 1–2 wks. Retest syphilis & HIV serology at 6, 12, 24 wks if negative earlier.
Sexual contacts, likely agents: N. gonorrhoeae, C. trachomatis	[(**Ceftriaxone** 125 mg IM) + **doxycycline** 100 mg po bid, po x7 d)] or (**cefixime** 400 mg po) + (**azithromycin** 1 gm po), each as single dose)	Be sure to check for syphilis (all regimens may not eradicate incubating syphilis (*JID* 170:689, 1994). Identify & tx contacts as appropriate to suspected STD (*MMWR* 51(RR-6):1, 2002).
Syphilis exposure		Rx for syphilis within 3 months. Make effort to check.
Sickle-cell disease Likely agent: S. pneumoniae (see *post-splenectomy, above*)	3 mos.–5 yrs: **Amoxicillin** 125 mg po bid >5 yrs: **Penicillin V** 250 mg po bid	Start prophylaxis before age 4 mos (*Am Acad Ped Red Book 1994, p. 375*). Children with SCD should receive vaccines: DTP, OPV, MMR, Hep B, Hib, pneumococcus, influenza ± meningococcal. Treat febrile episodes with ceftriaxone (50 mg/kg IV) (*NEJM 329:472,1993*).
Varicella-Zoster (see *Table 14, page 110*)		
Wegener's granulomatosis	TMP/SMX 800/160 tab po bid	Reduced relapses of pts in remission (18% (TMP/SMX) vs 40% (placebo)) (*NEJM 335:16, 1996*).

TABLE 15B: SURGICAL ANTIBIOTIC PROPHYLAXIS (*MMWR 48(15):316, 1999; ED 7:220, 2001*)

Surgical Procedures: To be optimally effective, antibiotics must be started in the interval: 2 hrs before time of surgical incision (NEJM 326:281, 1992). For most procedures the number of doses for optimal coverage has not been defined. Current practice is to give a single dose (*Ln 344:1547, 1994; Med Lett 43:92, 2001*) when FDA-approved product labeling is often for 2 or more doses. Antibiotic selection influenced by local factors—lasts 2–3 hrs; intraoperative doses should be given at approx. 3-hr intervals. (Note: The dose/route/durations listed below for adults are for the most part those approved by the FDA for product labeling. For single dose regimens they are the same.)

TYPE OF SURGERY	PROPHYLAXIS	COMMENTS
Cardiovascular Surgery Antibiotic prophylaxis in cardiovascular surgery has been proven beneficial only in the following procedures: • Reconstruction of abdominal aorta • Procedures on the leg that involve a groin incision • Any vascular procedure that inserts prosthesis/foreign body • Lower extremity amputation for ischemia • Cardiac surgery • Perhaps permanent pacemakers (see *Comment*)	**Cefazolin** 1 gm IV, as a single dose or **cefuroxime** 1.5 gm IV as a single dose or q12h for total of 6 gm. Consider **intranasal mupirocin** evening before, day of surgery add bid x5 days post-op in pts with pos. nasal culture for S. aureus.	Single intravenous dose before surgery probably as effective as multiple doses (*Eur J Cardiothor Surg 18:440, 2000*). Not recommended for cardiac catheterization. For prosthetic heart valves, customary to stop prophylaxis either after removal of retrosternal drainage catheters or just a 2nd dose after coming off bypass. Vancomycin may be preferable in hospitals with high frequency of MRSA but no coverage vs gram-neg bacilli, therefore would add cefazolin for groin incisions. A meta-analysis of 7 placebo-controlled studies of antimicrobial prophylaxis for implantation of permanent pacemakers, sig. ↓ in incidence of infection (*Circ 97:1796, 1998*). Intranasal mupirocin ↓ sternal wound infections from S. aureus in 1850 pts; used historical controls (*Ann Thoracic Surg 71:1572, 2001*). In another trial, it reduced nosocomial S. aureus infections only in nasal carriers (*NEJM 346:1871, 2002*).
Gastric, Biliary and Colonic Surgery **Gastroduodenal** Gastroduodenal, includes percutaneous endoscopic gastrostomy (high-risk only, see *Comments*)	**Cefazolin** or **cefoxitin** or **cefotetan** or **ceftizoxime** 1 gm IV as a single dose (some give additional doses q12h x2–3 d).	Gastroduodenal: High-risk is marked obesity, obstruction, ↓ gastric acid or ↓ GI motility. Biliary: Oral/cholecystectomy not active vs enterococci yet clinically effective as prophylaxis in biliary surgery. When percutaneous endoscopic gastrostomy performed AMB 123:442, 1996, cefazolin 1 gm, treat as infection, not prophylaxis. TC-CL 3.1 gm q4–8h IV or (PIP-TZ 3.375 gm q6h or 4.5 gm q8h IV or AM/SB 3.0 gm q8h IV. Biliary high-risk: age >70, acute cholecystitis, non-functioning gallbladder, obstructive jaundice or common duct stones. Meta-analysis supports use in percutaneous endoscopic gastrostomy (*Am J Gastro 95:3133, 2000*).
Biliary, includes laparoscopic cholecystectomy (high-risk only, see *Comments*)	In biliary surgery, cefazolin 1 gm & cefoxitin 1 gm (± repeat dosing at 12 & 24 hrs) were equivalent (*AAC 40:70, 1996*).	
Endoscopic retrograde cholangiopancreatography (ERCP)	No tx without obstruction. If obstruction: **Ciprofloxacin** 500 mg–1 gm po 2 hr prior to procedure	Most studies show that achieving adequate drainage will prevent postprocedural cholangitis or sepsis and no further benefit from prophylactic antibiotics. With inadequate drainage, antibiotics may be of value. American Society for GI Endoscopy recommends use for known or suspected biliary obstruction.
[Controversial: No benefit from single dose piperacillin in randomized placebo-controlled trial. *AnIM 125:442, 1996* (see *Comment*)]	**Ceftizoxime** 1.5 gm IV 1 hr prior to procedure or **Piperacillin** 4 gm IV 1 hr prior to procedure	Oral CIP as effective as cephalosporins in 2 studies & less expensive (*CID 23:380, 1996*).

TABLE 15B (2)

TYPE OF SURGERY	PROPHYLAXIS	COMMENTS
Colorectal, includes appendectomy		Elective colorectal prep. Pre-op day: (1) 10 am 4 L polyethylene glycol electrolyte solution po over 2h OR (2) X-Prep LY 1 pm enema, (3) clear liquid diet only (3) 1 pm, 2 pm and 11 pm NPO after midnight. There are alternative
Elective surgery	**Neomycin + erythromycin** po (see Comment for dose) **Cefazolin** 1-2 gm IV + **metronidazole** 0.5 gm IV (single dose)	regimens which have been less well studied. Go LYTELY 1-6 pm, then neomycin 2 gm po + metronidazole 2 gm po at 7 pm and 11 pm. Oral regimen as effective as parenteral; parenteral in addition to oral not required. For emergency colorectal surgery, use parenteral. [CID 15
Emergency surgery	**Cefoxitin** 1-2 gm IV or **cefotetan** 1-2 gm IV	Suppl. 1:S313, 1992]
Ruptured viscus: See Peritonitis (Ann Otol Rhinol Laryngol 101 Suppl 16, 1992)	**Cefotetan** 2 gm IV, then 1.0 gm IV q8h x 5 d. (Base on clinical signs) or **clindamycin** 600 mg IV q6h + **gentamicin** 1.5 mg/kg IV q8h) x 5 d	
Head and Neck Surgery (Ann Otol Rhinol Laryngol 107 Suppl 16, 1992) Antimicrobial prophylaxis only for procedures involving oral/pharyngeal mucosa (i.e., laryngeal or pharyngeal tumor) but even with prophylaxis, wound infection rate high (41% in 1 center) (Head Neck 39:447, 2001). Uncontaminated head & neck surgery does not require prophylaxis		**Cefazolin** 2 gm IV (single dose) or **clindamycin** 1.5 mg/kg IV + IV (single dose) or **clindamycin** 600 mg IV q6h + **gentamicin** 1.5 mg/kg IV q8h) x 5 d
Neurosurgical Procedures [Prophylaxis not effective in ↓ infection rate in ↑ infection rate with intracranial pressure monitors in retrospective analysis of 215 pts (J Neurol Neurosurg Psych 69:381, 2000)]		Reference: Ln 344:1547, 1994
Clean, non-implant, e.g., craniotomy	**Cefazolin** 1 gm IV x1. Alternative **vanco** 1 gm IV x1	British recommend amoxicillin/clavulanate 1.2 gm IV[M4] or (cefuroxime 1.5 gm IV +
Clean, contaminated (cross sinuses, or naso/oropharynx)	**Clindamycin** 900 mg IV (single dose)	metronidazole 0.5 gm IV)
CSF shunt surgery: controversial (Meta-analysis CID 17:98, 1993)	**Vancomycin** 10 mg into cerebral ventricles + **gentami-cin** 3 mg into cerebral ventricles (Ln 344:1547, 1994)	Efficacy when infection rate >16%. Alternative: TMP (160 mg) + SMx (800 mg) IV q12h x 5 doses
Obstetric/Gynecologic Surgery		
Vaginal or abdominal hysterectomy	**Cefazolin** 1-2 gm IV or **cefotetan** 1-2 gm IV or **cefuroxime** 1.5 gm IV all IV 30 min. before surgery	1 study found cefotetan superior to cefazolin (CID 20:677, 1995). For prolonged procedures, doses can be repeated q3-4h for duration of procedure
Cesarean section for premature rupture of membranes or active labor	**Cefazolin** x1, administer IV as soon as umbilical cord clamped	For prolonged procedures, a large prospective double-blind randomized trial (BJOG 108:143, 2001). However, meta-analysis of
Abortion	**pen G** 2 mU IV or **doxycycline** 300 mg po. 2nd trimester: **Cefazolin** 1 gm IV	Not effective in [in Comments] aqueous (Drugs 41:19, 1991). High-risk: Pts with previous pelvic inflammatory disease, gonorrhea or multiple sexual partners
Orthopedic Surgery (Generally do not require antibiotic for dental procedures. Individual considerations prevail (J Am Dental Assn 128:1004, 1997). See Table 1, pages 21, 22		
joints do not require prophylaxis for dental procedures		Customarily stopped after 1st dose. Post-op: some would give no further Rx [Med Lett 39:98, 1997]
Hip arthroplasty, spinal fusion	Same as cardiac	
Total joint replacement (other than hip)	**Cefazolin** 1-2 gm IV pre-op 1-2nd dose) or **vancomycin** 1 gm IV on call to OR	
Open reduction of closed fracture with internal fixation	**Ceftriaxone** 2 gm IV or IM x1 dose	3.6% vs 8.3% (for placebo) infection found in Dutch trauma trial [Lancet 347:1133, 1996]
Peritoneal Dialysis Catheter Placement	**Vancomycin** single 1000 mg dose 12 hrs prior to procedure	Effectively reduced peritonitis during 14 days post-placement in 221 pts. vanco 1%, cefazolin 7%, placebo 12% (p=0.02) (Am J Kidney Dis 36:1014, 2000)
Urologic Surgery/Procedures	Recommended antibiotic for pts with pre-operative bacteriuria. **Cefazolin** 1 gm IV q8h x1-3 doses perioperatively, followed by oral antibiotics (**nitrofurantoin** or TMP/SMX) until catheter is removed or 10 d. Modify based on susceptibility test results	
Antimicrobials not recommended in pts with sterile urine. Pts with pre-operative bacteriuria should be treated.		
Transrectal prostate biopsy	**Ciprofloxacin** 500 mg po 12 hrs prior to biopsy and repeated 12 hrs after biopsy (levo, norflox should work)	CIP reduced bacteremia from 37% (in gentamicin-rx group) to 0% (Urology 38:84, 1991; and J UAC 19:15, 1997)
Others		
Breast surgery, herniorrhaphy	**IP Ceph 1,2**, dosage as C-section above	
Traumatic (non-bile) wound	Either **cefazolin** 1 gm IV q8h or **ceftriaxone** 2 gm IV q24h x 5 d. (Base on clinical signs)	

[1] Gentamicin (12.5 mg/gm of acrylic bone cement) is released for at least 3 weeks. Usefulness not proven.

TABLE 15C: ANTIMICROBIAL PROPHYLAXIS FOR THE PREVENTION OF BACTERIAL ENDOCARDITIS IN PATIENTS WITH UNDERLYING CARDIAC CONDITIONS

[These are the recommendations of the American Heart Association (JAMA 277:1794, 1997). However, a population-based prospective case-controlled study brings into serious question whether dental procedures predispose to endocarditis and whether antibiotic prophylaxis is of any value (see AnIM 129:761, 1998; Br Dent J 189:610, 2000).]

Cardiac conditions associated with endocarditis

ENDOCARDITIS PROPHYLAXIS RECOMMENDED	ENDOCARDITIS PROPHYLAXIS NOT RECOMMENDED
High-risk conditions: Prosthetic valves—bioprosthetic and homograft, as well as mechanical Previous bacterial endocarditis Complex cyanotic congenital heart disease (CHD), e.g., single ventricle, transposition, tetralogy of Fallot Surgically constructed systemic pulmonic shunts or conduits **Moderate-risk conditions:** Most other CHD; hypertrophic cardiac myopathy; mitral prolapse with regurgitation	Negligible-risk (same as general population): Atrial septal defect (secundum), or repaired ASD/VSD, or PDA (beyond 6 months) Mitral valve prolapse without MI (see discussion JAMA 277:1794, 1997) Physiologic, functional, or innocent heart murmurs Previous Kawasaki or rheumatic fever without valve dysfunction Cardiac pacemakers (all) and implanted defibrillators

Dental and other procedures where prophylaxis is considered for patients with moderate- or high-risk cardiac conditions:

ENDOCARDITIS PROPHYLAXIS RECOMMENDED	ENDOCARDITIS PROPHYLAXIS NOT RECOMMENDED
Dental: Extractions, periodontal procedures[1] Implants, root canal, subgingival antibiotic fibers/strips Initial orthodontic bands (not brackets); intrabigumentary local anesthetic Cleaning of teeth/implants if bleeding anticipated Respiratory: T&A, surgery on respiratory mucosa, rigid bronchoscopy GI: Sclerotherapy of esophageal varices; dilation of esophageal stricture; ERCP with biliary obstruction GU: D&C, surgery on prostate, cystoscopy, urethral dilatation	Dental: Filling cavities with local anesthetic Placement of rubber dams, suture removal, orthodontic removal Orthodontic adjustments, dental x-rays Shedding of primary teeth Respiratory: Intubation, flexible bronchoscopy[2] tympanostomy tube GI: Transesophageal cardiac echo[2]; ERCP without biopsy Vaginal hysterectomy,[2] vaginal delivery,[2] C-section GU: Uncomplicated urinary catheterization, therapeutic abortion, tubal ligation, insert/remove IUD Other: Cardiac cath, balloon angioplasty, implanted pacemaker, defibrillators, coronary stents Skin biopsy, circumcision

Abbreviations: CHD = cyanotic heart disease, **T&A** = tonsillectomy/adenoidectomy **ERCP** = endoscopic retrograde cholangiography, **ASD/VSD** = atrial septal defect/ventricular septal defect, **PDA** = patent ductus arteriosus. **EGD** = esophagogastroduodenoscopy, **D&C** = dilation and curettage

PROPHYLACTIC REGIMENS FOR DENTAL, ORAL, RESPIRATORY TRACT, OR ESOPHAGEAL PROCEDURES

SITUATION	AGENT	REGIMEN[3]
Standard general prophylaxis	Amoxicillin	Adults 2 gm; children 50 mg/kg orally 1 hr before procedure
Unable to take oral medications	Ampicillin	Adults 2 gm IV or IV; children 50 mg/kg IM or IV within 30 min. before procedure
Allergic to penicillin	Clindamycin OR (Cephalexin[4] or cefadroxil[4]), OR Azithromycin or clarithromycin	Adults 600 mg; children 20 mg/kg orally 1 hr before procedure Adults 2 gm; children 50 mg/kg orally 1 hr before procedure Adults 500 mg; children 15 mg/kg orally 1 hr before procedure
Allergic to penicillin and unable to take oral medications	Clindamycin OR Cefazolin[4]	Adults 600 mg; children 20 mg/kg IV within 30 min. before procedure Adults 1 gm; children 25 mg/kg IM or IV within 30 min. before procedure

[1] Some now recommend that prophylaxis prior to dental procedures should be used for **only** be used for patients with **extractions** and **gingival surgery** (including implant replacement) and **only** for patients with **prosthetic cardiac valves** or **previous endocarditis** (AnIM 129:829, 1998). If any of these 4 conditions exist = prophylactic antibiotics according to American Heart Association are recommended.
[2] Prophylaxis optional for high-risk patients
[3] Total children's dose should not exceed adult dose
[4] Cephalosporins should not be used in individuals with immediate-type hypersensitivity reaction (urticaria, angioedema, or anaphylaxis) to penicillins.

TABLE 15C (2)

SITUATION	AGENT[a]	REGIMEN
High-risk patients	Ampicillin + gentamicin	**Adults: ampicillin** 2 gm IM or IV + **gentamicin** 1.5 mg/kg (not to exceed 120 mg) within 30 min. of starting the procedure; 6 hr later, **ampicillin** 1 gm IM or IV, or **amoxicillin** 1 gm orally. **Children: ampicillin** 50 mg/kg IM or IV (not to exceed 2.0 gm) + **gentamicin** 1.5 mg/kg within 30 min. of starting the procedure; 6 hrs later, **ampicillin** 25 mg/kg IM/IV or **amoxicillin** 25 mg/kg orally
High-risk patients allergic to ampicillin/amoxicillin	Vancomycin + gentamicin	**Adults: vancomycin** 1 gm IV over 1-2 hrs + **gentamicin** 1.5 mg/kg IV/IM (not to exceed 120 mg); complete injection/infusion within 30 min. of starting the procedure. **Children: vancomycin** 20 mg/kg IV over 1-2 hrs + **gentamicin** 1.5 mg/kg IV/IM; complete injection/infusion within 30 min. of starting the procedure
Moderate-risk patients	Amoxicillin or ampicillin	**Adults: amoxicillin** 2 gm orally 1 hr before procedure, or **ampicillin** 2 gm IM/IV within 30 min. of starting the procedure **Children: amoxicillin** 50 mg/kg orally 1 hr before procedure, or **ampicillin** 50 mg/kg IM/IV within 30 min. of starting the procedure
Moderate-risk patients allergic to ampicillin/ amoxicillin	Vancomycin	**Adults: vancomycin** 1 gm IV over 1-2 hrs; complete infusion within 30 min. of starting the procedure **Children: vancomycin** 20 mg/kg IV over 1-2 hrs; complete infusion within 30 min. of starting the procedure

TABLE 15D: PREVENTION OF OPPORTUNISTIC INFECTION IN HUMAN STEM CELL TRANSPLANTATION (HSCT) OR SOLID ORGAN TRANSPLANTATION (SOT)

General comments: See Table 1C, page 47 for typical timing of infections post-transplant. References: *MMWR 49(RR-10):1, 2000; CID 33:526, 2001*

OPPORTUNISTIC INFECTION (at risk)	TYPE OF TRANSPLANT	PROPHYLACTIC REGIMENS	COMMENTS/REFERENCES
Herpes simplex (seropositive)	HSCT	Acyclovir 200 mg po 3x/d, from conditioning to engraftment or resolution of mucositis	Do not need acyclovir if receiving CMV prophylaxis
	SOT	Acyclovir 200 mg po 3x/d.—start early post-transplant	
CMV (Recipient + OR Donor +, Recipient –) Ref.: *Clin Micro Rev 16:647, 2003*	HSCT	Universal (Recipient +): Ganciclovir 5 mg/kg IV q12h x5–7d, then 5–6 mg/kg 1 x/d. x100 days. Preemptive (Donor +, recipient neg.): 1–2 x/wk screen plasma for either (1) CMV antigen or (2) CMV-DNA by PCR—when positive, start ganciclovir as for Universal, above	
	SOT	Kidney, kidney/pancreas, heart: Valganciclovir 900 mg po 1x/d. by day 10 to day 100 post-transplant Liver: Ganciclovir 1000 mg po tid by day 10 to day 100 post-transplant Lung: Ganciclovir 5 mg/kg IV q12h x5–7 d. + CMV-immune globulin 150 mg/kg IV within 72 hrs, then at 2, 4, 6 & 8 wks post-transplant, then 100 mg/kg at wks 12 & 16), then valganciclovir 900 mg po 1x/d. x6 months	Some have combined with HBIG (*Hepato 28:585, 1998*)
Hepatitis B-induced cirrhosis	Liver	Lamivudine 100 mg po 1x/d. 4 wks pre-transplant & 12 months post-transplant	
Candida sp.	Liver, HSCT	Fluconazole 200–400 mg IV/po 1x/d. starting before transplant & continuing up to 3 mos. in high-risk pts. Optimal duration unknown.	
		Fluconazole 400 mg po 1x/d. from day 0 to engraftment or ANC >1000	
Aspergillus sp.	Lung/Heart-lung	No controlled trials.	
Coccidioides immitis	All	Reasonable: Fluconazole 400 mg po 1x/d.	
Pneumocystis carinii (P. jiroveci) & Toxoplasma gondii	All	TMP/SMX-SS or –DS, 1 tab po 1x/d. Duration: 4 mos.–1 yr renal; ≥6 mos for allogenic HSCT; ≥1 yr to lifetime for heart, lung, liver	
Trypanosoma cruzi	Heart	If known Chagas' disease in donor or recipient, contact CDC for nifurtimox	

TABLE 16: PEDIATRIC DOSAGES OF SELECTED ANTIBACTERIAL AGENTS
[Adapted from: (1) Nelson's Pocket Book of Pediatric Antimicrobial Therapy, 2002-2003, 15th Ed., J. Bradley & J. Nelson, eds., Lippincott Williams and Wilkins, and (2) 2003 Red Book, 26th Ed., American Academy of Pediatrics, pages 700–718

DRUG	DOSES IN MG/KG/D OR MG/KG AT FREQUENCY INDICATED[1]				>28 DAYS OLD
	BODY WEIGHT <2000 gm		BODY WEIGHT >2000 gm		
	0–7 days old	8–28 days old	0–7 days old	8–28 days old	
Aminoglycosides, IV or IM (check levels; some dose by gestational age + wks of life; see Nelson's Pocket Book, page 19)					
Amikacin	7.5 q18–24h	7.5 q12h	10 q12h	10 q12h	10 q8h
Gent/tobra	2.5 q18–24h	2.5 q12h	2.5 q12h	2.5 q12h	2.5 q8h
Aztreonam, IV	30 q12h	30 q8h	30 q8h	30 q6h	30 q6h
Cephalosporins					
Cefaclor					20–40 div tid
Cefadroxil					30 bid (max 2 g/d)
Cefazolin	20 q12h	20 q12h	20 q12h	20 q8h	20 q8h
Cefdinir					7 q12h or 14 qd
Cefepime					150 div q8h
Cefixime					8 as qd or div bid
Cefotaxime	50 q12h	50 q8h	50 q12h	50 q8h	50 q6h (75 q6h for meningitis)
Cefoxitin		20 q12h			80–160 div q6h
Cefpodoxime					10 div bid (max 400 mg/d)
Cefprozil					15–30 div bid (max 1 g/d)
Ceftazidime	50 q12h	50 q8h	50 q12h	50 q8h	50 q8h
Ceftibuten					4.5 bid
Ceftizoxime					33–66 q8h
Ceftriaxone	50 qd	50 qd	50 qd	75 qd	50–75 qd (meningitis 100)
Cefuroxime IV	50 q12h	50 q8h	50 q8h	50 q8h	50 q8h (80 q8h for meningitis)
po					10–15 div bid (max 1 g/d)
Cephalexin					25–50 div 4x/d (max 4 g/d)
Loracarbef					15–30 div bid (max 0.8 g/d)
Chloramphen. IV	25 q24h	25 q24h	25 q24h	15 q12h	12.5–25 q6h (max 2–4 g/d)
Clindamycin IV	5 q12h	5 q8h	5 q8h	5 q6h	7.5 q6h
po					5–6 q8h
Ciprofloxacin po[2]					20–30 div bid (max 1.5 g/d)
Imipenem[3] IV			25 q12h	25 q8h	15–25 q6h (max 2 g/d)
Linezolid	No data	10 q8h	No data	10 q8h	10 q8h to age 12
Macrolides					
Erythro IV & po	10 q12h	10 q12h	10 q12h	13 q8h	10 q6h
Azithro po					10–12 day 1, then 5/d[4]
Clarithro po					7.5 q12h (max. 1 g/d)
Meropenem IV	20 q12h	20 q8h	20 q12h	20 q8h	60–120 div q8h (120 for meningitis)
Metro IV & po	7.5 q24h	7.5 q12h	7.5 q12h	15 q12h	7.5 q6h
Penicillins					
Ampicillin	50 q12h	50 q8h	50 q8h	50 q6h	50 q6h
Amp-sulbactam					100–300 div q6h
Amoxicillin po			30 div bid		25–50 div tid
Amox-Clav po	30 div bid	30 div bid	30 div bid	30 div bid	45 or 90 (AM/CL-HD) div bid if over 12 wks of age
Cloxacillin					50–100 div 4x/d
Dicloxacillin					12–25 div 4x/d
Mezlocillin	75 q12h	75 q8h	75 q12h	75 q8h	75 q6h
Nafcillin, oxacillin IV	25 q12h	25 q8h	37 q8h	37 q6h	37 q6h (to max. 8–12 gm/d)
Piperacillin, PIP/tazo IV	75 mg/kg q12h	75 mg/kg q12h	75 mg/kg q12h	75 mg/kg q12h	100–300 div q4–6h
Ticarcillin, T.clav IV	75 q12h	75 q8h	75 q12h	75 q8h	75 q6h
Penicillin G, U/kg IV	50,000 q12h	75,000 q8h	50,000 q8h	50,000 q6h	50,000 U/kg/d
Penicillin V					25–50 mg/kg/d div 3–4x/d
Rifampin			10, single dose	20, single dose	20, single dose (max. 600 mg)
Sulfisoxazole po				120–150	120–150 mg/kg/d div q4–6h
TMP/SMX po,IV; UTI: 8–12 TMP component div bid; Pneumocystis: 20 TMP component div 4x/d					
Tetracycline po (age 8 or older)					25–50 div 4x/d
Doxycycline po,IV (age 8 or older)					2–4 div bid
Vancomycin IV	12.5 q12h	15 q12h	18 q12h	22 q12h	40–60 div q6h

Abbreviations: **Chloramphen.** = chloramphenicol, **Clav** = clavulanate, **div** = divided, **Gent/tobra** = gentamicin/tobramycin, **Metro** = metronidazole, **Tazo** = tazobactam; **TMP** = trimethoprim; **TMP/SMX** = trimethoprim/sulfamethoxazole, **UTI** = urinary tract infection

[1] May need higher doses in patients with meningitis
[2] With exception of cystic fibrosis, not approved for use under age 18.
[3] Not recommended in children with CNS infections due to risk of seizures.
[4] Dose for otitis; for pharyngitis, 12 mg/kg x5 d.

TABLE 17A: DOSAGE OF ANTIMICROBIAL DRUGS IN ADULT PATIENTS WITH RENAL IMPAIRMENT

Adapted from DRUG PRESCRIBING IN RENAL FAILURE, 4th Edn. Aronoff et al (Eds.), American College of Physicians, 1999 and Bennett et al, Renal Aspects of Antimicrobial Therapy for HIV Infection. In: P. Kenimel & J. Bennett, Eds., HIV INFECTION AND THE KIDNEY. Churchill-Livingstone, 1995, pp 195-236.

UNLESS STATED, ADJUSTED DOSES ARE % OF DOSE FOR NORMAL RENAL FUNCTION.

Drug adjustments are based on the patient's estimated endogenous creatinine clearance, which can be calculated as:

(140–age)(ideal body weight in kg) for men (x 0.85 for women)

Ideal body weight for men: 50.0 kg + 2.3 kg per inch over 5 feet

Ideal body weight for women: 45.5 kg + 2.3 kg per inch over 5 feet

(72)(serum creatinine, mg/dL)

For alternative method to calculate estimated CrCl, see AnIM 130:461, 1999.

NOTE: For summary of drugs requiring **no** dosage adjustment with renal insufficiency, see Table 17B, page 135.

ANTIMICROBIAL	HALF-LIFE (NORMAL/ESRD) hr	DOSE FOR NORMAL RENAL FUNCTION[1]	METHOD* (see footnote)	ADJUSTMENT FOR RENAL FAILURE Estimated creatinine clearance (CrCl), ml/min			SUPPLEMENT FOR HEMODIALYSIS, CAPD[2] (see footnote)	COMMENTS AND DOSAGE FOR CAVH
				>50-90	10-50	<10		
ANTIBACTERIAL ANTIBIOTICS **Aminoglycoside Antibiotics:**		**Traditional multiple daily doses—adjustment for renal disease**						High-flux hemodialysis membranes lead to unpredictable aminoglycoside clearance, measure post-dialysis drug levels for efficacy and toxicity. With CAPD, pharmacokinetics highly variable—check serum levels. Usual method for CAPD: 2 liters of dialysis fluid placed qid or 6 liters/day (give 8U20 mg lost/L = 160 mg of amikacin supplement IV per liter).
Amikacin	1.4–2.3/17–150	7.5 mg/kg q12h	D&I	60–90% q12h	30–70% q12-18h **Same dose for CAVH[F]**	20–30% q24-48h	HEMO: Extra ½ of normal renal function dose AD[a] CAPD: 15–20 mg lost/L dialysate/day[b] (see Comment)	
Gentamicin, Tobramycin	2–3/20–60	1.7 mg/kg q8h	D&I	60–90% q8-12h	30–70% q12h **Same dose for CAVH[F]**	20–30% q24-48h	HEMO: Extra ⅔ of normal renal function dose AD[a] CAPD: 3–4 mg lost/L dialysate/day	
Netilmicin[ALB]	2–3/35–72	2.0 mg/kg q8h	D&I	50–90% q8-12h	20–60% q12h **Same dose for CAVH[F]**	10–20% q24-48h	HEMO: Extra ⅔ of normal renal function dose AD[a] CAPD: 3–4 mg lost/L dialysate/day	
Streptomycin	2–3/30-80	15 mg/kg (max. of 1.0 gm) q24h	I	50% q24h	q24-72h **Same dose for CAVH[F]**	q72-96h	HEMO: Extra ½ of normal renal function dose AD[a] CAPD: 20-40 mg lost/L dialysate/day	Adjust dosing weight for obesity: ideal body weight + 0.4(actual body weight – ideal body weight) C/D 25:112, 1997.

ONCE-DAILY AMINOGLYCOSIDE THERAPY: ADJUSTMENT IN RENAL INSUFFICIENCY (see Table 10C for OD dosing/normal renal function)

Creatinine Clearance (ml/min): Drug	4/>4	>80 60- Dose q24h (mg/kg)		60-90	40-60 Dose q24h (mg/kg)	30-40	20-30 Dose q48h (mg/kg)	10-20	<10
Gentamicin/Tobramycin		5.1			4	3.5	4	3	2
Amikacin/Kanamycin/streptomycin		15			12	7.5	7.5	4	3
Isepamicin[†]		8			8	8 q48h	8 q72h	8 q96h	
Netilmicin[‡]		6.5			5	4	3	2.5	2.0

Carbapenem Antibiotics									
Ertapenem	4/>4	1.0 gm q24h	D	1.0 gm q24h	0.5 gm q24h (CrCl <30)	0.5 gm q24h	HEMO: Dose as for CrCl <10; if dosed <6 hrs prior to HD, give150 mg supplement AD		
Imipenem (see Comment)	1/4	0.5 gm q6h	D&I	250–500 mg q6-8h	250 mg q6-12h (CrCl <30)	125–250 mg q12h	HEMO: Dose AD CAPD: Dose for CrCl <10		potential for seizures if recommended doses exceeded in pts with CrCl <20 ml/min. See pkg insert, esp. for pts <70 kg.
Meropenem	1/6-8	1.0 gm q8h	D&I	1.0 gm q8h **Same dose for CAVH**	1.0 gm q12h	0.5 gm q24h	HEMO: Dose AD CAPD: Dose for CrCl <10		

[1] **CAVH** = continuous arteriovenous hemofiltration (NEJM 336:1303, 1997) usually results in CrCl of approx. 30 ml/min.; AD = after dialysis. "**Dose AD**" refers only to timing of dose with **NO** extra drug.

See page 134 for other footnotes and abbreviations. **Supplement is to replace drug lost via dialysis; extra drug is to replace continuation of regimen used for CrCl <10 ml/min.**

TABLE 17A (2)

ANTIMICROBIAL	HALF-LIFE (NORMAL/ESRD) hr	DOSE FOR NORMAL RENAL FUNCTION	METHOD* (see footnote)	ADJUSTMENT FOR RENAL FAILURE — Estimated creatinine clearance (CrCl), ml/min			SUPPLEMENT FOR HEMODIALYSIS, CAPD† (see footnote)	COMMENTS AND DOSAGE FOR CAVH
				>50-90	10-50	<10		
Cephalosporin Antibiotics: DATA ON SELECTED PARENTERAL CEPHALOSPORINS								
Cefazolin	1.9/40-70	1.0-2.0 gm q8h	I	q8h	q12h	q24-48h	HEMO: Extra 0.5-1 gm AD / CAPD: 0.5 gm q12h	CAVH not recommended
Cefepime	2.2/18	2.0 gm q8h (max. dose)	I	2 gm q8h	**Same dose for CAVH** / 2 gm q12-24h	1 gm q24h	HEMO: Extra 1 gm AD / CAPD: 1-2 gm q48h	
Cefotaxime, Ceftizoxime	1.7/15-35	2.0 gm q8h	I	q8-12h	q12-24h / **Same dose for CAVH**	q24h	HEMO: Extra 1 gm AD / CAPD: 0.5-1 gm qd	Active metabolite of cefotaxime in ESRD, ↓ dose further for hepatic &
Cefotetan	3.5/13-25	1-2 gm q12h	D	100%	50%	25%	HEMO: Extra 1 gm AD / CAPD: 1 gm qd	CAVH: 750 mg q12h
Cefoxitin	0.8/13-23	2.0 gm q8h	I	q8h	q8-12h / **Same dose for CAVH**	q24-48h	HEMO: Extra 1 gm AD / CAPD: 1 gm qd	May falsely increase serum creatinine by interference with assay.
Ceftazidime	1.2/13-25	2 gm q8h	I	q8-12h	q24-48h / **Same dose for CAVH**	q48h	HEMO: Extra 1 gm AD / CAPD: 0.5 gm qd	Volume of distribution increases with infection.
Cefuroxime sodium	1.2/17	0.75-1.5 gm q8h	I	q8h	q8-12h	q24h	HEMO: Dose AD / CAPD: Dose for CrCl <10	For CAVH: 1.5 gm, then 750 mg IV q24h
Fluoroquinolone Antibiotics								
Ciprofloxacin	4/6-9	500-750 mg po (or 400 mg IV) q12h	D	100%	50-75%	50%	HEMO: 250 mg q12h or 200 mg IV q12h / CAPD: 250 mg q8h or 200 mg IV q8h	CAVH: 200 mg IV q12h
Gatifloxacin	7-14/36	400 mg po/IV q24h	D	400 mg q24h	200 mg q24h	200 mg q24h	HEMO: 200 mg q24h AD / CAPD: 200 mg q24h	CAVH: As for CrCl 10-50
Gemifloxacin	7/>7	320 mg po qd	D	320 mg po qd	160 mg qd	160 mg qd	HEMO: 160 mg qd AD / CAPD: 160 mg qd	CAVH: As for CrCl 10-50
Levofloxacin	4-8/76	500 mg qd IV, PO	D*	100%	500 mg x1, then 250 mg q24-48h	500 mg x1, then 250 mg q48h	HEMO/CAPD: Dose for CrCl <10	CAVH: As for CrCl 10-50
Ofloxacin	7.0/28-37	400 mg po/IV q12h	D&I	100%	200-400 mg q12h	200 mg q24h	HEMO: 100-200 mg AD / CAPD: Dose for CrCl <10	CAVH: 300 mg/d
Macrolide Antibiotics								
Clarithromycin	5-7/22	0.5-1.0 gm q12h	D	100%	75%	50-75%	HEMO: Dose AD* / CAPD: None	ESRD dosing recommendations based on extrapolation
Erythromycin	1.4/5-6	250-500 mg q6h	D	100%	50-75%	50-75%	HEMO: None / CAPD: None	Ototoxicity with high doses in ESRD. Vol. of distribution increases in ESRD.
Miscellaneous Antibacterial Antibiotics								
Colistin	?	2.5 mg/kg q12h	D	2.5 mg/kg q24h	2.5 mg/kg q24h	1.5 mg/kg q24h		
Daptomycin	9.4/30	4 mg/kg/d	None	4 mg/kg q24h	CrCl <30, 4 mg/kg q48h	4 mg/kg q48h	HEMO & CAPD: 4 mg/kg q48h (after dialysis)	CAVH: No data
Linezolid	6.4/7.1	600 mg po/IV q12h		600 mg q12h	600 mg q12h	600 mg q12h	HEMO: Dose for CrCl <10 / CAPD: No data	CAVH. Accumulation of 2 metabolites—risk unknown.
Metronidazole	6-14/7-21	7.5 mg/kg q8h	D	100%	100%	50%	HEMO: Dose AD / CAPD: Dose for CrCl <10	Hemo clears metronidazole and its metabolites (AAC 29:235, 1986)
Nitrofurantoin	0.5/1	50-100 mg	D	100% q12h	Avoid	Avoid	HEMO: Not applicable	
Sulfamethoxazole	10/20-50	1.0 gm q8h	D&I	q12h	q18h / **Same dose for CAVH**	q24h	HEMO: Extra 1 gm AD / CAPD: 1 gm AD	

¹ Regardless of CrCl, 1st dose is 500 mg, and then adjust dose and interval
† CAVH = continuous arteriovenous hemofiltration (NEJM 336:1303, 1997) usually results in CrCl of approx. 30 ml/min; **AD** = after dialysis
‡ **Supplement is to replace drug lost via dialysis; extra drug beyond continuation of regimen used for CrCl <10 ml/min. "Dose AD" refers only to timing of dose with NO extra drug.**
See page 134 for other footnotes and abbreviations.

TABLE 17A (3)

ANTIMICROBIAL	HALF-LIFE (NORMAL/ESRD) hr	DOSE FOR NORMAL RENAL FUNCTION (continued)	METHOD* (see footnote)	ADJUSTMENT FOR RENAL FAILURE Estimated creatinine clearance (CrCl), ml/min >50-90	10-50	<10	SUPPLEMENT FOR HEMODIALYSIS, CAPD† (see footnote)	COMMENTS AND DOSAGE FOR CAVH
Miscellaneous Antibacterial Antibiotics								
Teicoplanin[3,6]	45/62-230	6 mg/kg/day	I	q48h	**Same dose for CAVH** q48h (30 ml/min)	q72h	HEMO: Dose for CrCl <10 / CAPD: Dose for CrCl <10	IV amoxicillin not available in the U.S.
Telithromycin	10/15	800 mg qd	D	800 mg qd	400 mg qd (if <30 ml/min)	400 mg qd	HEMO 800 mg qd AD / CAPD: No data	
Trimethoprim	11/20-49	100-200 mg q12h	I	q12h	q18h	q24h	HEMO: Dose AD / CAPD: Dose AD	
Vancomycin[1]	6/200-250	1 gm q12h	D&I	1 gm q12h	1 gm q24-96h	1 gm q4-7 d.	HEMO: Dose AD/Dose for CrCl <10 / CAPD: Dose AD/Dose for CrCl <10	CAVH: 500 mg q24-48h. New hemodialysis membranes ↑ clear. of vanco; check levels.
Penicillins								
Amoxicillin	1.0/5-20	250-500 mg q8h	I	q8h	q8-12h	q24h	HEMO: Dose AD* / CAPD: Dose for CrCl <10	
Ampicillin	1.07/7-20	250 mg-2 gm q6h	I	q6h	q6-12h	q12-24h	HEMO: Dose AD / CAPD: 250 mg q12h	
Amoxicillin/ Clavulanate	1.3 AM/1.0 ... 5-20/4.0 ...	500/125 mg q8h (see Comments)	I	500/125 mg q8h	250-500 mg AM component q12h	250-500 mg AM component q24h	HEMO: As for CrCl <10; extra dose after dialysis / CAPD: Dose for CrCl <10	**If CrCl <30/ml, do not use 875/125 or 1000/62.5 AM/CL products**
Ampicillin/ Sulbactam(SB)	1.0 (AM)/1.0 (SB) ... 9.0 (AM)/10.0 (SB)	2 gm AM + 1.0 gm SB q6h	I	q6h	q8-12h	q24h	HEMO: 2 gm AM/1 gm SB q24h / CAPD: 2 gm AM/1 gm SB q12h	CAVH: 1.5 AM/0.75 SB q12h
Aztreonam	2.0/6-8	2 gm q8h	D	100%	50-75%	25%	HEMO: Extra 0.5 gm AD / CAPD: Dose for CrCl <10	Technically is a β-lactam antibiotic.
Penicillin G	0.5/6-20	0.5-4 million U q4h	D	100%	75%	20-50%	HEMO: Dose AD / CAPD: Dose for CrCl <10	1.7 mEq potassium/mU. * potential for seizures; 6 mU/d upper limit dose in ESRD.
Piperacillin	1.0/3.3-5.1	3-4 gm q4-6h	I	q4-6h	q6-8h	q8h	HEMO: Dose AD / CAPD: Dose for CrCl <10	1.9 mEq sodium/gm
Pip (P)/Tazo(T)[6]	1.0 P/1.0 T ... 3.0 P/4.0 T	3.375 gm q6h	D&I	3.375 gm q6h	2.25 gm q6h	2.25 gm q8h	HEMO: Dose for CrCl <10 + 0.75 gm AD / CAPD: Dose for CrCl <10	
Ticarcillin	1.2/13	3 gm q4h	D&I	1-2 gm q4h	1-2 gm q8h	1-2 gm q12h	HEMO: Extra 3.0 gm AD / CAPD: Dose for CrCl <10	5.2 mEq sodium/gm
Ticarcillin/ Clavulanate	1.0 (TC)/1.0 (CL) ... 13 (TC)/4.0 (CL)	3.1 gm q4h	D&I	3.1 gm q4h	2.0 gm q8h	2.0 gm q12h	HEMO: Extra 3.1 gm AD / CAPD: 3.1 gm q12h	
Tetracycline Antibiotics								
Tetracycline	6-10/57-108	250-500 mg qid	I	q8-12h	q12-24h	q24h	HEMO: None / CAPD: None	Avoid in ESRD
ANTIFUNGAL ANTIBIOTICS								
Amphotericin B & ampho B lipid complex	24/unchanged	Non-lipid: 0.4-1.0 mg/kg/d, ABLC† 3-4.6 mg/kg/d, ABCD‡ 3-6 mg/kg/d, LAB 3-5 mg/kg/d	I	q24h	q24h	q24-48h	HEMO: None / CAPD: Dose for CrCl <10	For ampho B, toxicity lessened by saline loading; risk amplified by concomitant cyclosporine A, aminoglycosides, or pentamidine
Fluconazole	37/100	200-400 mg q24h	D	200-400 mg	100-200 mg q24h	100-200 mg q24h	HEMO: 100% of recommended dose AD / CAPD: Dose for CrCl <10	
Flucytosine	3-6/75-200	37.5 mg/kg q6h	I	q12h	q12-24h	q24h	HEMO: Dose AD* / CAPD: 0.5-1.0 gm q24h	Goal is peak serum level >25 μg/ml and <100 μg/ml

[1] Vancomycin serum levels may be overestimated in renal failure if measured by either fluorescence polarization immunoassay or radioimmunoassay; vanco breakdown products interfere. EMIT method OK.

[2] ABCC = ampho B cholesteryl complex; ABLC = ampho B lipid complex; LAB = liposomal ampho B

[3] CAVH = continuous arteriovenous hemofiltration (NEJM 336:1303, 1997) usually results in CrCl of approx. 30 ml/min.; AD = after dialysis. Supplement is to replace drug lost via dialysis; extra drug lost beyond continuation of regimen used for CrCl <10 ml/min. drugs.

See page 134 for other footnotes and abbreviations.

TABLE 17A (4)

ANTIMICROBIAL	HALF-LIFE (NORMAL/ESRD) hr	DOSE FOR NORMAL RENAL FUNCTION†	METHOD* (see footnote)	ADJUSTMENT FOR RENAL FAILURE Estimated creatinine clearance (CrCl), ml/min			SUPPLEMENT FOR HEMODIALYSIS, CAPD† (see footnote)	COMMENTS AND DOSAGE FOR CAVH
				>50-90	10-50	<10		
ANTIFUNGAL ANTIBIOTICS (continued)								
Itraconazole, po soln	35/–	100-200 mg q12h	–	100%	100%	100%	HEMO/CAPD/CAVH: No adjustment with oral solution	
Itraconazole, IV	35/–	200 mg IV q12h	–	200 mg IV bid		Do not use IV if CrCl <30 due to accumulation of carrier cyclodextrin		
Terbinafine	36-200?	250 mg po/day	–	q24h		Use has not been studied. Recommend avoidance of drug.		
Voriconazole, **IV**	Non-linear kinetics	6 mg/kg IV q12h x2, then 4 mg/kg q12h	–	No change		If CrCl <50 ml/min, accum. of IV vehicle (cyclodextrin). Switch to po or DC		
ANTIPARASITIC ANTIBIOTICS								
Pentamidine	29/118	4 mg/kg/d	I	q24h	q24-36h	q48h	HEMO/CAPD/CAVH: None	Marked tissue accumulation
Quinine	5-16/5-16	650 mg q8h	I	q8h **Same dose for CAVH**	650 mg q8-12h **Same dose for CAVH**	650 mg q24h	HEMO: Dose AD‡ CAPD: Dose for CrCl <10	
ANTITUBERCULOUS ANTIBIOTICS (Excellent review: Nephron 64:169, 1993)								
Ethambutol	4/7-15	15-25 mg/kg q24h	I	q24h **Same dose for CAVH**	q24-36h	q48h	HEMO: Dose AD‡ CAPD: Dose for CrCl <10	25 mg/kg 4-6 hr prior to dialysis for usual 3x/wk dialysis. Streptomycin recommended in lieu of ethambutol in renal failure.
Ethionamide	2.1/?	250-500 mg q12h	D	100%	100%	50%	HEMO/CAPD/CAVH: None	
Isoniazid	0.7-4/8-17	5 mg/kg/d (max. 300 mg)	D	100%	100%	100%	HEMO: Dose AD CAPD/CAVH: Dose for CrCl <10	
Pyrazinamide	9/26	25 mg/kg q24h (max. dose 2.5 gm qd)	D*	25 mg/kg q24h	25 mg/kg q24h	12-25 mg/kg q24h	HEMO: 25-35 mg/kg after each dialysis CAPD: No reduction, CAVH: No data	
Rifampin	1.5-5/1.8-11	600 mg qd	D	600 mg q24h	300-600 mg q24h	300-600 mg q24h	HEMO/CAPD/CAVH: Dose for CrCl <10	Biologically active metabolite
ANTIVIRAL AGENTS								
Acyclovir, IV	2.5/20	5-12.4 mg/kg q8h	D&I	5-12.4 mg/kg q8h	5-12.4 mg/kg q12-24h	2.5-12.4 mg/kg q24h	HEMO: Dose AD‡ CAPD: Dose for CrCl <10	Rapid IV infusion can cause renal failure. CAVH: 3.5 mg/kg/d
Adefovir	2.5/unknown	10 mg po qd	I	10 mg q24h	10 mg q48-72h	10 mg q7 days	HEMO: q7d AD	
Amantadine	12/500	100 mg po bid	I	100 mg po bid	q48-72h	q7/d	HEMO/CAPD/CAVH: None	
Cidofovir: Complicated dosing—see package insert								
Induction	2.5/unknown	5 mg/kg 1x/wk for 2 wks	–	5 mg/kg 1x/wk	0.5-2 mg/kg 1x/wk	0.5 mg/kg 1x/wk	No data	Major toxicity is renal. No efficacy, safety, or pharmacokinetic data in pts with moderate/severe renal disease.
Maintenance	2.5/unknown	5 mg/kg q2wks	–	5 mg/kg q2wks	0.5-2 mg/kg q2wks	0.5 mg/kg q2wks	No data	
Didanosine tablets³	0.6-1.6/4.5	125-200 mg q12h buffered fabs	D	200 mg q12h	200 mg q24h	<60 kg: 150 mg q24h >60 kg: 100 mg q24h	HEMO: Dose AD‡ CAPD/CAVH: Dose for CrCl <10	Based on incomplete data. Data are estimates.
		400 mg qd enteric-coated fabs		400 mg qd	125-200 mg qd	**Do not use EC tabs**	HEMO: Dose AD CAPD: No data	**If <60 kg & CrCl <10 ml/min, do not use EC tabs**
Famciclovir	2.3-3.0/10-22	500 mg q8h	D&I	500 mg q8h	500 mg q12-24h	250 mg q24h	HEMO: Dose AD CAPD: No data	CAVH: Dose for CrCl 10-50

† Ref. for NRTIs and NNRTIs: *Kidney International* 60:821, 2001
‡ **CAVH** = continuous arteriovenous hemofiltration (*NEJM* 336:1303, 1997) usually results in CrCl of approx. 30 ml/min. **AD** = after dialysis. **"Dose AD"** refers only to timing of dose with NO extra drug.
Supplement is to replace drug lost via dialysis; extra drug lost beyond continuation of regimen used for CrCl <10 ml/min.
* See page 134 for other footnotes and abbreviations.

TABLE 17A (5)

ANTIMICROBIAL	HALF-LIFE (NORMAL/ESRD) hr	DOSE FOR NORMAL RENAL FUNCTION[†]	METHOD* (see footnote†)	ADJUSTMENT FOR RENAL FAILURE — Estimated creatinine clearance (CrCl), ml/min >50-90	10-50	<10	SUPPLEMENT FOR HEMODIALYSIS, CAPD[§] (see footnote)	COMMENTS AND DOSAGE FOR CAVH
ANTIVIRAL AGENTS (continued)								
Foscarnet (CMV) — Dosage adjustment based on est. CrCl (ml/min) div. by pt's kg	Normal half-life (T½) 3 hrs with terminal T½ of 18-88 hrs. T½ very long with ESRD	Induction: 60 mg/kg q8h, x2-3 wks IV; Maintenance: 90-120 mg/kg IV	*see foscarnet sub-table below (CrCl as ml/min/kg body weight—ONLY FOR FOSCARNET)*					See package insert for further details
Ganciclovir	2.9/30	Induction 5 mg/kg q12h IV	D&I	5 mg/kg q12h	1.25-2.5 mg/kg q24h	1.25 mg/kg 3x/wk	HEMO: Dose AD; CAPD: Dose for CrCl <10	CAVH: Dose for CrCl 10-50
	IV:	Maintenance 5 mg/kg q24h IV	D&I	2.5-5.0 mg/kg q24h	0.6-1.25 mg/kg q24h	0.625 mg/kg 3x/week	HEMO: 0.6 mg/kg AD; CAPD: Dose for CrCl <10	CAPD/CAVH: No data
	po:	1.0 gm tid po	D&I	0.5-1.0 gm tid	0.5-1.0 gm qd	0.5 gm 3x/wk	HEMO: 0.5 gm AD; CAPD: 0.5 gm qd	No data
Indinavir/nelfinavir		No data on influence of renal insufficiency. Less than 20% excreted unchanged in urine. Probably no dose reduction.						
Lamivudine[†]	5-7/15-35	150 mg bid po	D&I	150 mg bid	150 mg qd	50-150 mg qd	HEMO: Dose AD; CAPD/CAVH: No data	CAVH: No data. Dose for CrCl 10-50
Oseltamivir	1-3/no data	75 mg po bid	I	75 mg bid	75 mg qd	No data	No data	CAVH: No data
Ribavirin		Use with caution in patients with creatinine clearance <10 ml/min.						
Rimantadine	13-65/Prolonged	100 mg bid po		100 mg bid	100 mg qd-bid	100 mg qd	HEMO/CAPD: No data	Use with caution, little data
Ritonavir & Saquinavir, SGC				Negligible renal clearance, no patient data				
Stavudine, po[†]	1-1.4/5.5-8	30-40 mg q12h	D&I	100%	50% q12-24h		HEMO: Dose as for CrCl <10 AD; CAPD: No data	CAVH: Dose for CrCl 10-50
Tenofovir	2.5-3.3/14	300 mg q24h		300 mg q24h	**DO NOT USE IF CrCl <60 ml/min.**			
Valacyclovir		1.0 gm q8h	D&I	1.0 gm q8h	1.0 gm q12-24h	0.5 gm q24h	HEMO: Dose AD; CAPD: Dose for CrCl <10	CAVH: No data. Dose for CrCl 10-50
Valganciclovir	4/67	900 mg po bid	D&I	900 mg po bid	450 mg qd to 450 mg qod	DO NOT USE	HEMO: Dose AD; CAPD: Dose for CrCl <10	CAVH: Dose for CrCl 10-50
Zalcitabine[†]	2.0/>8	0.75 mg q8h	D&I	0.75 mg q8h	0.75 mg q12h	0.75 mg q24h	HEMO: Dose AD; CAPD: Dose for CrCl <10	CAVH: Dose for CrCl 10-50
Zidovudine[†]	1.1-1.4/1.4-3	200 mg q8h or 300 mg q12h	D&I	200 mg q8h or 300 mg q12h	200 mg q8h or 300 mg q12h	100 mg q8h, if hemo, AD	HEMO: Dose for CrCl <10; CAPD: Dose for CrCl <10	CAVH: 100 mg q8h

Foscarnet — CrCl as ml/min/kg body weight (ONLY FOR FOSCARNET):

CrCl (ml/min/kg)	>1.4	>1-1.4	>0.8-1.0	>0.6-0.8	>0.5-0.6	>0.4-0.5	<0.4
Induction (60 mg/kg q8h)	60 q8h	45 q8h	50 q12h	40 q12h	60 q24h	50 q24h	Do not use
Maintenance (120 mg/kg q24h)	120 q24h	90 q24h	65 q24h	106 q48h	80 q48h	65 q48h	Do not use

¹ CAVH = continuous arteriovenous hemofiltration (NEJM 336:1303, 1997). AD = after dialysis.
§ **Supplement is to replace drug lost via dialysis; extra drug beyond continuation of dose with NO other drug.**
§ Dosages are for life-threatening infections. *Method: D = dosage reduction, I = interval extension; **Per cent refers to % change from dose for normal function. **"Dose AD" refers only to timing of dose with NO other drug.**
Abbreviations: HEMO = hemodialysis, CAPD = chronic ambulatory peritoneal dialysis; ESRD = endstage renal disease; NUS = not available in the U.S.

† Ref. for NRTIs and NNRTIs: Kidney International 60:821, 2001

TABLE 17B: NO DOSAGE ADJUSTMENT WITH RENAL INSUFFICIENCY, BY CATEGORY:

Antibacterials		Antifungals	Anti-TBc	Antivirals	
				Non-HIV	Anti-HIV Drugs
Azithromycin	Doxycycline	Amphotericin B	Rifabutin	None	Abacavir
Ceftriaxone	Linezolid	Caspofungin	Rifapentine		Amprenavir;
Chloramphenicol	Minocycline	Itraconazole oral solution			fosamprenavir
Ciprofloxacin XL	Moxifloxacin	Voriconazole, **po only**			Delavirdine
Clindamycin	Nafcillin				Efavirenz
Dirithromycin	Pyrimethamine				Lopinavir
					Nevirapine

TABLE 18: ANTIMICROBIALS AND HEPATIC DISEASE DOSAGE ADJUSTMENT

The following alphabetical list indicates antibacterials excreted/metabolized by the liver **wherein a dosage adjustment may be indicated** in the presence of hepatic disease. Space precludes details; consult the PDR or package inserts for details. List is **not** all-inclusive:

Amprenavir; fosamprenavir	Delavirdine	Nafcillin
Atazanavir	Efavirenz	Nevirapine
Caspofungin (Table 11B)	Indinavir	Rifabutin
Ceftriaxone	Isoniazid	Rifampin
Chloramphenicol	Itraconazole solution	Rimantadine
Clindamycin	Metronidazole	Voriconazole

TABLE 19: TREATMENT OF CAPD PERITONITIS IN ADULTS[1]
(Periton Dial Intl 20:396, 2000)

EMPIRIC Intraperitoneal Therapy:[2] Culture Results Pending

Drug		Residual Urine Output	
		<100 ml/day	>100 ml/day
Cefazolin +	Can mix in same bag	1 gm/bag, qd	20 mg/kg BW/bag, qd
Ceftazidime		1 gm/bag, qd	20 mg/kg BW/bag, qd

Drug Doses for SPECIFIC Intraperitoneal Therapy—Culture Results Known. NOTE: Few po drugs indicated

Drug	Intermittent Dosing (once/day)		Continuous Dosing (per liter exchange)	
	Anuric	Non-Anuric	Anuric	Non-Anuric
Gentamicin	0.6 mg/kg	↑ dose 25%	MD 8 mg	↑ MD by 25%
Cefazolin	15 mg/kg	20 mg/kg	LD 500 mg, MD 125 mg	LD 500 mg, ↑ MD 25%
Ceftazidime	1000–1500 mg	ND	LD 250 mg, MD 125 mg	ND
Ampicillin	250–500 mg po bid	ND	250–500 mg po bid	ND
Ciprofloxacin	500 mg po bid	ND	LD 50 mg, MD 25 mg	ND
Vancomycin	15–30 mg/kg q5–7 d	↑ dose 25%	MD 30–50 mg/L	↑ MD 25%
Metronidazole	250 mg po bid	ND	250 mg po bid	ND
Amphotericin B	NA	NA	MD 1.5 mg	NA
Fluconazole	200 mg qd	ND	200 mg qd	ND
Itraconazole	100 mg q12h	100 mg q12h	100 mg q12h	100 mg q12h
Amp/sulbactam	2 gm q12h	ND	LD 1.0 gm, MD 100 mg	ND
TMP/SMX	320/1600 mg po q1–2 d	ND	LD 320/1600 mg po, MD 80/400 mg po qd	ND

[1] All doses IP unless indicated otherwise.
  LD = loading dose, **MD** = maintenance dose, **ND** = no data; **NA** = not applicable—dose as normal renal function. **Anuric** = <100 ml/d, **non-anuric** = >100 ml/d.

[2] Does not provide treatment for MRSA. If Gram-positive cocci on Gram stain, include vancomycin.

TABLE 20A: RECOMMENDED CHILDHOOD AND ADOLESCENT IMMUNIZATION SCHEDULE[1]: UNITED STATES, 2003 (MMWR 52:Q1, 2003) (For overall recommendations, see MMWR 51:RR-2, 2002)

VACCINE	Birth	1 mo	2 mos	4 mos	6 mos	12 mos	15 mos	18 mos	24 mos	4-6 yrs	11-12 yrs	13-18 yrs
		Range of recommended ages							**Catch-up vaccination**		**Preadolescent assessment**	
Hepatitis B[2,9]	HepB #1 only if mother HBsAg(−)										HepB series	
		HepB #2			HepB #3							
Diphtheria,Tetanus, Pertussis[3,9]			DTaP	DTaP	DTaP		DTaP			DTaP	Td	
Haemophilus Influenzae Type b			Hib	Hib	Hib	Hib						
Inactivated Polio[9]			IPV	IPV		IPV				IPV		
Measles, Mumps, Rubella[4]						MMR #1				MMR #2	MMR #2	
Varicella[5]						Varicella					Varicella	
Pneumococcal[6]			PCV	PCV	PCV	PCV			PCV		PPV	
Hepatitis A[7]											HepA series	
Influenza[8]						Influenza (yearly)						

– – – – Vaccines below this line are for selected populations – – – –

1 [░░] Indicates age groups that warrant special effort to administer those vaccines not given previously.

2 **Hepatitis B vaccine (HepB).** Infants born to HBsAg-positive mothers should receive hepatitis B vaccine and 0.5 ml hepatitis B immune globulin (HBIG) within 12 hours of birth at separate sites. The 2nd dose is recommended at age 1–2 months. The last dose in the vaccination series should not be administered before age 6 months. These infants should be tested for HBsAg and anti-HBs at 9–15 months of age. Infants born to mothers whose HBsAg status is unknown should receive the 1st dose of the HepB vaccine series within 12 hours of birth. Maternal blood should be drawn as soon as possible to determine the mother's HBsAg status; if the HBsAg test is positive, the infant should receive HBIG as soon as possible (no later than age 1 week). The 2nd dose is recommended at age 1–2 months. The last dose in the vaccination series should not be administered before age 6 months.

3 **Tetanus and diphtheria toxoids (Td).** Subsequent routine Td boosters are recommended every 10 years.

4 **Measles, mumps, and rubella vaccine (MMR).** No evidence that MMR causes autism (NEJM 347:1477, 2002).

5 **Varicella vaccine.** Primary vaccine failures may occur (NEJM 347:1909, 2002). Benefit outweighs risk (JID 188:945, 2003).

6 **Pneumococcal vaccine. Pneumococcal polysaccharide vaccine (PPV)** is recommended in addition to PCV for certain high-risk groups. See MMWR 49(RR-9):1, 2000.

7 **Hepatitis A vaccine.** Hepatitis A vaccine is recommended for children and adolescents and for certain high-risk groups (MMWR 48(RR-12):1, 1999).

8 **Influenza vaccine** [see MMWR 51(RR-3):1, 2002]. Children aged ≤12 years should receive vaccine in a dosage appropriate for their age (0.25 ml 6–35 months or 0.5 ml if ≥3 years). Children aged ≤8 years who are receiving influenza vaccine for the first time should receive 2 doses separated by at least 4 weeks. A self-limited 48-hr oculorespiratory syndrome post-vaccine recognized (CID 37:1059 & 1136, 2003). Trivalent (types A & B) live, cold adapted, attenuated influenza virus vaccine (FluMist™) for intranasal application in subjects 5–49 yrs old approved by U.S. FDA 6/2003.

9 **DTaP, HepB, IPV** available in combined vaccine (Pediarix™) which is given at 2, 4, and 6 months of age (MMWR 52:203, 2003).

Additional information about vaccines, including precautions and contraindications for vaccination and vaccine shortages, is available at www.cdc.gov/nip or at the National Immunization information hotline, 800-232-2522 (English) or 800-232-0233 (Spanish). Copies of the schedule can be obtained at www.cdc.gov/nip/recs/child-schedule.htm. Approved by the **Advisory Committee on Immunization Practices** (www.cdc.gov/nip/acip), the **American Academy of Pediatrics** (www.aap.org), and the **American Academy of Family Physicians** (www.aafp.org).

Catch-Up Schedule For Children Aged 4 Months–6 Years Who Start Late Or Are >1 Month Behind

Dose 1 (minimum age)	Minimum interval between doses			
	Dose 1 to dose 2	Dose 2 to dose 3	Dose 3 to dose 4	Dose 4 to dose 5
DTaP (6 wks)	4 wks	4 wks	6 mos.	6 mos.[1]
IPV (6 wks)	4 wks	4 wks	4 wks[2]	
HepB[3] (birth)	4 wks	8 wks (& 16 wks after 1st dose)		
MMR (12 mos.)	4 wks[4]			
Varicella (12 mos.)				
Hib[5] (6 wks)	4 wks: if 1st dose given at age <12 mos. 8 wks (as final dose): if 1st dose given at age 12–24 mos. No further doses needed: if 1st dose given at age ≥15 mos.	4 wks[5]: if current age <12 mos. 8 wks (as final dose)[4]: if current age ≥12 mos. & 2nd dose given at age <15 mos. No further doses needed: if previous dose given at age ≥15 mos.	8 wks (as final dose): this dose only necessary for children aged 12 mos.–5 yrs who received 3 doses before age 12 mos.	
PCV[7] (6 wks)	4 wks: if 1st dose given at age <12 mos. & current age <24 mos. 8 wks (as final dose): if 1st dose given at age ≥12 mos. or current age 24–59 mos. No further doses needed: for healthy children if 1st dose given at age ≥24 mos.	4 wks: if current age <12 mos. 8 wks (as final dose): if current age ≥12 mos. No further doses needed: for healthy children if previous dose given at age ≥24 mos.	8 wks (as final dose): this dose only necessary for children aged 12 mos.–5 yrs who received 3 doses before age 12 mos.	

TABLE 20A (2)

[1] **Diphtheria and tetanus toxoids and acellular pertussis vaccine (DTaP):** The 5th dose is not necessary if the 4th dose was given after the 4th birthday.

[2] **Inactivated polio (IPV):** For children who received an all-IPV or all-OPV series, a 4th dose is not necessary if 3rd dose was given at age ≥4 yrs. If both OPV and IPV were given as part of a series, a total of 4 doses should be given, regardless of the child's current age.

[3] **Hepatitis B vaccine (HepB):** All children and adolescents who have not been vaccinated against hepatitis B should begin the hepatitis B vaccination series during any visit. Providers should make special efforts to immunize children who were born in, or whose parents were born in, areas of the world where hepatitis B virus infection is moderately or highly endemic.

[4] **Measles, mumps, and rubella vaccine (MMR):** The 2nd dose of MMR is recommended routinely at age 4–6 yrs, but may be given earlier if desired.

[5] **Haemophilus influenzae type b (Hib):** Vaccine is not recommended generally for children aged ≥5 years.

[6] **Hib:** If current age is <12 months and the first 2 doses were PRP-OMP [PedvaxHIB® or ComVax (Merck)®], the 3rd (and final) dose should be given at age 12–15 months and at least 8 weeks after the 2nd dose.

[7] **Pneumococcal conjugate vaccine (PCV):** Vaccine is not recommended generally for children aged ≥5 years unless post-splenectomy.

Catch-Up Schedule for Children Aged 7–18 Years Who Start Late or Are >1 Month Behind

Vaccine	Minimum interval between doses		
	Dose 1 to dose 2	Dose 2 to dose 3	Dose 3 to booster dose
Td[1]	4 wks	6 mos.	**6 mos:** if 1st dose given at age <12 mos. & current age <11 yrs **5 yrs:** if 1st dose given at age ≥12 mos. & 3rd dose given at age <7 yrs & current age ≥11 yrs **10 yrs:** if 3rd dose given at age ≥7 yrs
IPV[2]	4 wks	4 wks	
HepB	4 wks	8 wks (& 16 wks after 1st dose)	
MMR	4 wks		
Varicella[3]	4 wks		

[1] **Tetanus toxoid:** For children aged 7–10 years, the interval between the 3rd & booster dose is determined by the age when the 1st dose was given. For adolescents aged 11–18 years, the interval is determined by the age when the 3rd dose was given.

[2] **Inactivated polio (IPV):** Vaccine is not recommended generally for persons aged ≥18 years.

[3] **Varicella:** Give 2-dose series to all susceptible adolescents aged ≥13 years.

Conjugate pneumococcal vaccine (PCV): For all infants and high-risk children (e.g., HIV, asplenia, nephrotic syndrome, sickle cell anemia) between 2 and 5 years of age (Med Lett 42:25, 2000; PIDJ 19:181, 2000; PIDJ 19:371ff, 2000). Also approved for prevention of otitis media (Med Letter 45:27, 2003) and for cochlear implant recipients (MMWR 52:739, 2003). Use of vaccine associated with decline in invasive pneumococcal disease (NEJM 348:1737, 2003).

Immunization schedule: (see Schedule, page 136)

Age at first dose (0.5 ml)	Total number of doses	Timing
Infants	4	2, 4, 6, and 12–15 months
7–11 months	3	2 doses at least 4 wks apart; 3rd dose after 1 year birthday, separated from 2nd dose by at least 2 months
12–23 months	2	2 doses at least 2 months apart
≥24 months	1*	

* For children ≥24 months old who are chronically ill or immunosuppressed, ICIP recommends 2 doses of PCV admin. 2 mos. apart, followed by 1 dose of a 23-valent pneumococcal vaccine 2 or 3 mos. after 2nd PCV dose (MMWR 50:10, 2001).

TABLE 20B: ADULT IMMUNIZATION IN THE UNITED STATES (MMWR 51:904, 2002)
(Travelers: see Med Letter 38:17, 1996)

Recommended Adult Immunization Schedule—United States, 2002–2003

Vaccine	Age group (years)		
	19–49	50–64	≥65
Tetanus, diphtheria (Td)[1]	1 dose booster every 10 years		
Influenza	1 dose annually to persons with medical or occupational indications or household contacts of persons with indications	1 annual dose	
Pneumococcal (polysaccharide)	1 dose for persons with medical or other indications (1 dose revaccination for immunosuppressive conditions)[2]		1 dose for unvaccinated persons 1 dose revaccination[2]
Hepatitis B[1]	3 doses (0, 1–2, 4–6 months) for persons with medical, behavioral, occupational, or other indications[3]		
Hepatitis A	2 doses (0, 6–12 months) for persons with medical, behavioral, occupational, or other indications[4]		
Measles, mumps, rubella (MMR)[1]	1 dose if MMR vaccination history is unavailable; 2 doses for persons with occupational, geographic, or other indications[5]		
Varicella[1]	2 doses (0, 4–8 weeks) for persons who are susceptible[6]		
Meningococcal (polysaccharide)	1 dose for persons with medical or other indications[7]		

☐ For all persons in this age group	▓ For persons with medical/exposure indications	▨ Catch-up on childhood vaccinations

[1] Covered by the Vaccine Injury Compensation Program.

TABLE 20B (2)

[2] Revaccination with pneumococcal polysaccharide vaccine: 1-time revaccination after 5 years for persons with chronic renal failure or nephrotic syndrome, functional or anatomic asplenia (e.g., sickle cell disease or splenectomy), immuno-suppressive conditions (e.g., congenital immunodeficiency, HIV infection, leukemia, lymphoma, multiple myeloma, Hodgkin's disease, generalized malignancy, & organ or bone marrow transplantation), chemotherapy with alkylating agents, antimetabolites, or long-term systemic corticosteroids. For persons aged ≥65 yrs, 1-time revaccination if they were vaccinated ≥5 yrs previously & were aged <65 yrs at the time of primary vaccination *[MMWR 46(RR-8), 1997]*.

[3] Medical indications: hemodialysis pts & pts who receive clotting-factor concentrates. Occupational indications: health-care workers & public-safety workers who are exposed to blood in the workplace; persons in training in schools of medicine, dentistry, nursing, lab technology, & other allied health professions. Behavioral indications: injection-drug users, persons with more than 1 sex partner during the preceding 6 months, persons with a recently acquired STD, all clients in STD clinics, & men who have sex with men (MSM). Other indications: household contacts & sex partners of persons with chronic hepatitis B virus (HBV) infection, clients & staff of institutions for the developmentally disabled, international travelers who will be located for >6 months in countries with high or intermediate prevalence of chronic HBV infection, & inmates of correctional facilities *[MMWR 40(RR-13), 1991]*.

[4] For the combined hepatitis A-hepatitis B vaccine, use 3 doses at 0, 1, & 6 months. Medical indications: persons with clotting-factor disorders or chronic liver disease. Behavioral indications: MSM & users of injection-drug & noninjecting illegal drugs. Occupational indications: persons working with hepatitis A virus (HAV)-infected primates or with HAV in a research lab setting. Other indications: persons traveling to or working in countries that have high or intermediate endemicity of hepatitis A *[MMWR 48(RR-12), 1999]*.

[5] Measles component: Adults born before 1957 might be considered to be immune to measles. Administer 2 doses of MMR to adults with at least one of the following conditions & without vaccination history: • adults born after 1956; • persons vaccinated with killed-measles virus vaccine during 1963–1969; • students in post-secondary education institutions; • healthcare workers; • susceptible international travelers to countries in which measles is endemic. Mumps component: 1 dose of MMR should be adequate for protection. Rubella component: Administer 1 dose of MMR to women whose rubella vaccination history is unreliable & counsel women to avoid becoming pregnant for 4 weeks after vaccination. For women of childbearing age, regardless of birth year, determine rubella immunity & counsel women routinely regarding congenital rubella syndrome. Do not vaccinate pregnant women or those planning to become pregnant during the next 4 weeks. If pregnant & susceptible, vaccinate as early in postpartum period as possible *[MMWR 47(RR-8), 1998]*.

[6] Recommended for all persons without evidence of prior varicella zoster virus (VZV) infection; healthcare workers & family contacts of immunocompromised persons; those who live or work in environments in which transmission is likely (e.g., teachers of young children, day care employees, & residents & staff members in institutional settings); persons who live or work in environments in which VZV transmission can occur (e.g., college students, inmates & staff members of correctional institutions, & military personnel); adolescents & adults living in households with children; women who are not pregnant but who might become pregnant in the future; & international travelers who are not immune to infection. Do not vaccinate pregnant women or those planning to become pregnant during the next 4 weeks. If pregnant & susceptible, vaccinate as early in postpartum period as possible *[MMWR 45(RR-11), 1996; MMWR 48(RR-6), 1999]*.

[7] Meningococcal vaccine (quadrivalent polysaccharide for serogroups A, C, Y, & W-135). Medical indications: consider vaccination for adults with terminal complement-component deficiencies or with anatomic or functional asplenia. Other indications: travelers to countries in which disease is hyperendemic or epidemic [e.g., the "meningitis belt" of sub-Saharan Africa & Mecca (Saudi Arabia) during Hajj]. Revaccination at 3–5 years might be indicated for persons at high risk for infection (e.g., persons residing in areas in which disease is epidemic). Counsel college freshmen, especially those who live in dormitories, about meningococcal disease & the vaccine so that they can make an educated decision about receiving the vaccination *[MMWR 6(RR-5), 1997]*. Healthcare providers need not initiate discussion of the meningococcal quadrivalent polysaccharide vaccine as part of routine medical care.

Recommended Immunizations for Adults with Medical Conditions—United States, 2002–2003

Medical condition	Vaccine						
	Tetanus-diphtheria (Td)[1]	Influenza	Pneumo-coccal (poly-saccharide)	Hepatitis B[1]	Hepatitis A	Measles, mumps, rubella (MMR)[1]	Varicella[1]
Pregnancy		A					
Diabetes, heart disease, chronic pulmonary disease, & chronic liver disease, including chronic alcoholism		B	C		D		
Congenital immunodeficiency, leukemia, lymphoma, generalized malignancy, rx with alkylating agents, antimetabolites, radiation, or large amounts of corticosteroids			E				F
Renal failure/end-stage renal disease & recipients of hemodialysis or clotting factor concentrates			E	G			
Asplenia including elective splenectomy & terminal complement-component deficiencies			E,H,I				
HIV infection		E,J				K	

☐ For all persons in this age group   ▨ For persons with medical/exposure indications   ▢ Catch-up on childhood vaccinations   ▨ Contraindicated

[1] Covered by the Vaccine Injury Compensation Program

TABLE 20B (3)

A Vaccinate if pregnancy is at 2nd or 3rd trimester during influenza season
B Although chronic liver disease & alcoholism are not indicator conditions for influenza vaccination, administer 1 dose annually if the patient is aged ≥50.
C Asthma is an indicator condition for influenza but not for pneumococcal vaccination.
D For all persons with chronic liver disease
E Revaccinate once if ≥5 years have elapsed since initial vaccination.
F Persons with impaired humoral but not cellular immunity might be vaccinated [MMWR 48(RR-6), 1999].
G Hemodialysis patients: Use special formulation of vaccine (40 μg/ml) or two 1.0 ml 20 μg doses administered at one site. Vaccinate early in the course of renal disease. Assess antibody titers to hepatitis B surface antigen (anti-HBs) levels annually. Administer additional doses if anti-HBs levels decline to <10 mIU/ml.
H Also administer meningococcal vaccine; consider H. influenzae type b vaccine
I Elective splenectomy: Vaccinate ≥2 weeks before surgery.
J Vaccinate as close to diagnosis as possible when CD4 cell counts are highest.
K Withhold MMR or other measles-containing vaccines from HIV-infected persons with evidence of severe immuno-suppression (MMWR 45:603, 1996).

Administration schedule for vaccines: Review package insert for specific product being administered

TABLE 20C/1: ANTI-TETANUS PROPHYLAXIS, WOUND CLASSIFICATION, IMMUNIZATION

WOUND CLASSIFICATION			IMMUNIZATION SCHEDULE				
Clinical Features	Tetanus Prone	Non-Tetanus Prone	History of Tetanus Immunization	Dirty, Tetanus-Prone Wound		Clean, Non-Tetanus Prone Wound	
				Td^{1,2}	TIG	Td	TIG
Age of wound	> 6 hours	≤ 6 hours	Unknown or < 3 doses	Yes	Yes	Yes	No
Configuration	Stellate, avulsion	Linear					
Depth	> 1 cm	≤ 1 cm	3 or more doses	No^3	No	No^4	No
Mechanism of injury	Missile, crush, burn, frostbite	Sharp surface (glass, knife)					
Devitalized tissue	Present	Absent					
Contaminants (dirt, saliva, etc.)	Present	Absent					

(From ACS Bull. 69:22,23, 1984, No. 10)

1 Td = Tetanus & diphtheria toxoids adsorbed (adult)
TIG = Tetanus immune globulin (human)
2 Yes if wound >24 hours old.
For children <7 years, DPT (DT if pertussis vaccine contraindicated);
For persons ≥7 years, Td preferred to tetanus toxoid alone.
3 Yes if >5 years since last booster
4 Yes if >10 years since last booster

(From MMWR 39:37, 1990; MMWR 46(SS-2):15, 1997)

TABLE 20C/2: RABIES POST-EXPOSURE PROPHYLAXIS[1]. All wounds should be cleaned immediately and thoroughly with soap and water. This has been shown to protect 90% of experimental animals!

Post-Exposure Prophylaxis Guide, United States, 2000 (CID 30:4, 2000)

Animal Type	Evaluation and Disposition of Animal	Recommendations for Prophylaxis
Dogs, cats, ferrets	Healthy and available for 10-day observation	Don't start unless animal develops sx, then immediately begin HRIG + HDCV or RVA
	Rabid or suspected rabid	Immediate vaccination
	Unknown (escaped)	Consult public health officials
Skunks, raccoons, bats,* foxes, coyotes, most carnivores	Regard as rabid	Immediate vaccination
Livestock, rodents, rabbits; includes hares, squirrels, hamsters, guinea pigs, gerbils, chipmunks, rats, mice, woodchucks		Almost never require anti-rabies rx. Consult public health officials.

* Most recent cases of human rabies in U.S. due to contact (not bites) with silver-haired bats or rarely big brown bats (MMWR 46:770, 1997; AIM 128:922, 1998). For more detail, see CID 30:4, 2000; JAVMA 219:1687, 2001.

Post-Exposure Rabies Immunization Schedule
IF NOT PREVIOUSLY VACCINATED

Treatment	Regimen^3
Local wound cleaning	All post-exposure treatment should begin with immediate, thorough cleaning of all wounds with soap and water.
Human rabies immune globulin (HRIG)	20 IU/kg body weight given once on day 0. If anatomically feasible, the full dose should be infiltrated around the wound(s), the rest should be administered IM in the gluteal area. HRIG should **not** be administered in the **same syringe, or** into the **same anatomical site** as vaccine, or more than 7 days after the initiation of vaccine. Because HRIG may partially suppress active production of antibody, no more than the recommended dose should be given.^{3}
Vaccine	Human diploid cell vaccine (HDCV), rabies vaccine adsorbed (RVA), or purified chick embryo cell vaccine PCEC) 1.0 ml IM (**deltoid area**^{4}), one each on days 0, 3, 7, 14, & 28.

TABLE 20C (2)

IF PREVIOUSLY VACCINATED[5]

Treatment	Regimen[2]
Local wound cleaning	All post-exposure treatment should begin with immediate, thorough cleaning of all wounds with soap and water.
HRIG	HRIG should **not** be administered
Vaccine	HDCV, RVA or PCEC, 1.0 ml IM (**deltoid area[4]**), one each on days 0 and 3

CORRECT VACCINE ADMINISTRATION SITES

Age Group	Administration Site
Children and adults	**DELTOID[4]** only (**NEVER** in gluteus)
Infants and young children	Outer aspect of thigh (anterolateral thigh) may be used (**NEVER** in gluteus)

[1] From *MMWR* 48:RR-1, 1999; CID 30:4, 2000; B.T. Matyas, Mass. Dept. of Public Health

[2] These regimens are applicable for all age groups, including children.

[3] In most reported post-exposure treatment failures, only identified deficiency was failure to infiltrate wound(s) with HRIG (CID 22:228, 1996). However, several failures reported from SE Asia in patients in whom WHO protocol followed (CID 28:143, 1999).

[4] The **deltoid** area is the **only** acceptable site of vaccination for adults and older children. For infants and young children, the outer aspect of the thigh (anterolateral thigh) may be used. Vaccine should **NEVER** be administered in the gluteal area.

[5] Any person with a history of pre-exposure vaccination with HDCV, RVA, PCEC; prior post-exposure prophylaxis with HDCV, RVA, PCEC; or previous vaccination with any other type of rabies vaccine and a documented history of antibody response to the prior vaccination

TABLE 21: SELECTED DIRECTORY OF RESOURCES

ORGANIZATION	PHONE/FAX	WEBSITE(S)
ANTIPARASITIC DRUGS and PARASITOLOGY INFORMATION (CID 37:694, 2003)		
CDC	Weekdays: 404-639-3670	www.cdc.gov/ncidod/srp/drugs/drug-service.html
	Evenings, weekends, holidays:	404-639-2888
DPDx: Lab ID of parasites		www.dpd.cdc.gov/dpdx/default.htm
Gorgas Course Tropical Medicine		http://info.dom.uab.edu/gorgas
Panorama Compound. Pharm.	800-247-9767/818-787-7256	www.uniquerx.com
Parasites and Health		www.dpd.cdc.gov/dpdx/HTML/Para_Health.htm
BIOTERRORISM		
Centers for Disease Control & Prevention	770-488-7100	www.bt.cdc.gov
Infectious Diseases Society of America	703-299-0200/	www.idsociety.org
	703-299-0204	
Johns Hopkins Center Civilian Biodefense		www.jhsph.edu
Center for Biosecurity of the Univ. of Pittsburgh Med. Center		www.upmc-biosecurity.org
US Army Medical Research Institute of Inf. Dis.		www.usamriid.army.mil
HEPATITIS C (CID 35:754, 2002)		
CDC		www.cdc.gov/ncidod/diseases/hepatitis/C
Individual		http://hepatitis-central.com
Medscape		www.medscape.com
HIV		
General		
HIV InSite		http://hivinsite.ucsf.edu
Johns Hopkins AIDS Service		www.hopkins-aids.edu
Drug Interactions		
Johns Hopkins AIDS Service		www.hopkins-aids.edu
Liverpool HIV Pharm. Group		www.hiv-druginteractions.org
Other		http://AIDS.medscape.com
Prophylaxis/Treatment of Opportunistic Infections; HIV Treatment		www.aidsinfo.nih.gov
IMMUNIZATIONS (CID 36:355, 2003)		
CDC, Natl. Immunization Program	404-639-8200	www.cdc.gov/nip
FDA, Vaccine Adverse Events	800-822-7967	www.fda.gov/cber/vaers/vaers.htm
National Network Immunization Info.	877-341-6644/	www.immunizationinfo.org
Influenza vaccine, CDC	404-639-8200	www.cdc.gov/nip/flu
Institute for Vaccine Safety		www.vaccinesafety.edu
OCCUPATIONAL EXPOSURE, BLOOD-BORNE PATHOGENS (HIV, HEPATITIS B & C)		
National Clinicians' Post-Exposure Hotline	888-448-4911	www.ucsf.edu/hivcntr
Q-T_c INTERVAL PROLONGATION BY DRUGS		www.qtdrugs.org
SEXUALLY TRANSMITTED DISEASES		www.cdc.gov/std/treatment/TOC2002TG.htm
		Slides: www.hc-sc.gc.ca/pphb-dgspsp/std-mts
TRAVELERS' INFO: Immunizations, Malaria Prophylaxis, More		
Amer. Soc. Trop. Med. & Hyg.		www.astmh.org
CDC, general	877-394-8747/888-232-3299	www.cdc.gov/travel/index.htm
		www.cdc.gov/ncidod/dpd/parasites/malaria/default.htm
Prophylaxis	888-232-3228	www.cdc.gov/travel
Treatment	770-488-7788	www.who.int/health_topics/malaria
MD Travel Health		www.mdtravelhealth.com
Pan American Health Organization		www.paho.org
World Health Organization (WHO)	(41-22)-791-2122/	www.who.int/home-page
	(00-41-22)-691-0746	
VACCINE AND IMMUNIZATION RESOURCES (CID 36:355, 2003)		
American Academy of Pediatrics		www.cispimmunize.org
CDC, National Immunization Program		www.cdc.gov/nip
National Network of Immunization Information		www.immunizationinfo.org

$Q-T_c$ INTERVAL PROLONGATION BY DRUGS

TABLE 22: ANTI-INFECTIVE DRUG-DRUG INTERACTIONS

Significance/Certainty: ± = theory/anecdotal; + = of probable importance; ++ = of definite importance

ANTI-INFECTIVE AGENT (A)	OTHER DRUG (B)	EFFECT	SIGNIFICANCE/CERTAINTY
Amantadine (Symmetrel)	Alcohol	↑ CNS effects	+
	Anticholinergic and anti-Parkinson agents (ex. Artane, scopolamine)	↑ effect of B: dry mouth, ataxia, blurred vision, slurred speech, toxic psychosis	+
	Trimethoprim	↑ levels of A & B	+
	Digoxin	↑ levels of B	±
Aminoglycosides— parenteral (amikacin, gentamicin, kanamycin, netilmicin, sisomicin, streptomycin, tobramycin) NOTE: Capreomycin is an aminoglycoside, used as alternative drug to treat mycobacterial infections.	Amphotericin B	↑ nephrotoxicity	++
	Cis platinum (Platinol)	↑ nephro & ototoxicity	+
	Cyclosporine	↑ nephrotoxicity	+
	Neuromuscular blocking agents	↑ apnea or respiratory paralysis	+
	Loop diuretics (e.g., furosemide)	↑ ototoxicity	++
	NSAIDs	↑ nephrotoxicity	+
	Non-polarizing muscle relaxants	↑ apnea	+
	Radiographic contrast	↑ nephrotoxicity	+
	Vancomycin	↑ nephrotoxicity	+
Amphotericin B and ampho B lipid formulations	Antineoplastic drugs	↑ nephrotoxicity risk	+
	Digitalis	↑ toxicity of B if K⁺ ↓	+
	Nephrotoxic drugs: aminoglycosides, cidofovir, cyclosporine, foscarnet, pentamidine	↑ nephrotoxicity of A	++
Ampicillin, amoxicillin	Allopurinol	↑ frequency of rash	++
Amprenavir	Antiretrovirals—see Table 21B		
	Contraceptives, oral	↓ levels of A	++
	Methadone	↓ levels of A & B	++
	Rifabutin	↑ levels of B (↓ dose by 50%)	++
	Rifampin	↓ levels of A	++
Atovaquone	Rifampin (perhaps rifabutin)	↓ serum levels of A; ↑ levels of B	+
	Metoclopramide	↓ levels of A	+
	Tetracycline	↓ levels of A	++

Azole Antifungal Agents¹ [*Flu* = fluconazole, *Itr* = itraconazole, *Ket* = ketoconazole, *Vor* = voriconazole, + = occurs, *blank space* = either studied & no interaction OR no data found (may be in pharm. co. databases)]

Flu	Itr	Ket	Vor			
+	+	+		Amitriptyline	↑ levels of B	+
+	+	+	+	Calcium channel blockers	↑ levels of B	++
	+	+		Carbamazepine (vori contraindicated)	↓ levels of A	++
+	+	+	+	Cyclosporine	↑ levels of B, ↑ risk of nephrotoxicity	+
	+	+		Didanosine	↓ absorption of A	+
	+	+		H₂ blockers, antacids, sucralfate	↓ absorption of A	+
+	+	+	+	Hydantoins (phenytoin, Dilantin)	↑ levels of B, ↓ levels of A	++
	+	+		Isoniazid	↓ levels of A	+
			+	Lovastatin/simvastatin	Rhabdomyolysis reported; ↑ levels of B	++
+	+	+	+	Midazolam/triazolam, po	↑ levels of B	++
+	+	+	+	Oral anticoagulants	↑ effect of B	++
+	+	+	+	Oral hypoglycemics	↑ levels of B	++
	+	+	+	Pimozide	↑ levels of B	++
	+	+	?	Protease inhibitors	↑ levels of B	++
	+	+		Proton pump inhibitors	↓ absorption of A, ↑ levels of B	++
+	+	+	+	Rifampin/rifabutin (vori contraindicated)	↑ levels of B, ↓ serum levels of A	++
			+	Sirolimus (vori contraindicated)	↑ levels of B	++
+	+	+	+	Tacrolimus	↑ levels of B with toxicity	++
+		+		Theophyllines	↑ levels of B	+
+				Zidovudine	↑ levels of B	+
Caspofungin				Cyclosporine	↑ levels of A	++
				Tacrolimus	↓ levels of B	++
				Carbamazepine, dexamethasone, efavirenz, nelfinavir, nevirapine, phenytoin, rifampin	↓ levels of A; ↑ dose of caspofungin to 70 mg/d	++
Cephalosporins with methyltetrathiazole-thiol side-chain²				Oral anticoagulants (dicumarol, warfarin), heparin, thrombolytic agents, platelet aggregation inhibitors	↑ effects of B, bleeding	+
Chloramphenicol				Hydantoins	↑ toxicity of B, nystagmus, ataxia	++
				Iron salts, Vitamin B12	↓ response to B	++
				Protease inhibitors—HIV	↑ levels of A & B	++
Clindamycin (Cleocin)				Kaolin	↓ absorption of A	+
				Muscle relaxants, e.g., atracurium, baclofen, diazepam	↑ frequency/duration of respiratory paralysis	+

¹ Major interactions given; unusual or minor interactions manifest as toxicity of non-azole drug due to ↑ serum levels: Caffeine (Flu), digoxin (Itr), felodipine (Itr), fluoxetine (Itr), indinavir (Ket), lovastatin/simvastatin, quinidine (Ket), tricyclics (Flu), vincristine (Itr), and ↓ effectiveness of oral contraceptives.
² Cefotetan

TABLE 22 (2)

ANTI-INFECTIVE AGENT (A)	OTHER DRUG (B)	EFFECT	SIGNIFICANCE/ CERTAINTY
Cycloserine	Ethanol	↑ frequency of seizures	+
	INH, ethionamide	↑ frequency of drowsiness/dizziness	+
Dapsone	Didanosine	↓ absorption of A	+
	Oral contraceptives	↓ effectiveness of B	+
	Pyrimethamine	↑ in marrow toxicity	+
	Rifampin/Rifabutin	↓ serum levels of A	+
	Trimethoprim	↑ levels of A & B (methemoglobinemia)	+
	Zidovudine	May ↑ marrow toxicity	+
Delavirdine (Rescriptor) **NOTE**: Review all pt's meds before starting delavirdine. Interactions with other antiretrovirals, Table 22B, page 146	**Co-administration contraindicated:** **Anticonvulsants**: Phenytoin, phenobarbital, carbamazepine Antimycobacterials: Rifabutin, rifampin Ergot derivatives: Ergotamine HMG-CoA inhibitors: Lovastatin, simvastatin Neuroleptic: Pimozide **St. John's wort** Sedatives: Alprazolam, midazolam, triazolam		
	Dose change needed:		
	Antacids, H₂-blockers, proton pump inhibitors	↓ levels of A	++
	Amiodarone, lidocaine, quinidine	↑ levels of B—caution	++
	Calcium channel blockers	↑ levels of B	++
	Clarithromycin	↑ levels of B	++
	Cyclosporine, tacrolimus, rapamycin	↑ levels of B—measure levels	++
	Dexamethasone	↓ levels of A	++
	Methadone	↓ levels of B	++
	Sildenafil (Viagra)	↑ levels of B	++
	Warfarin	↑ levels of B	++
Didanosine (ddI) (Videx)	Cisplatin, dapsone, INH, metronidazole, nitrofurantoin, stavudine, vincristine, zalcitabine	↑ risk of peripheral neuropathy	+
	Ethanol, lamivudine, pentamidine	↑ risk of pancreatitis	+
	Fluoroquinolones	↓ absorption 2° to chelation	+
	Drugs that need low pH for absorption: dapsone, indinavir, itra/ketoconazole, pyrimethamine, rifampin, trimethoprim	↓ absorption	+
	Ribavirin	↑ levels ddI metabolite—avoid	++
	Tenofovir	↑ levels of A (reduce dose of A)	++
Doxycycline	Aluminum, bismuth, iron, Mg⁺⁺	↓ absorption of A	+
	Barbiturates, hydantoins	↓ serum t/2 of A	+
	Carbamazepine (Tegretol)	↓ serum t/2 of A	+
	Digoxin	↑ serum levels of B	+
	Warfarin	↑ activity of B	++
Efavirenz (Sustiva)	Clarithromycin	↓ levels of B	+
	Ergot derivatives	**levels of B; do not co-administer**	++
	Methadone	↓ levels of B	++
	Midazolam	**levels of B; do not co-administer**	++
	Rifampin	↓ levels of A	+
Ertapenem (Invanz)	Probenecid	↑ levels of A	++
Ethambutol (Myambutol)	Aluminum salts (includes didanosine buffer	↓ absorption of A & B	+

Fluoroquinolones *Cipro* = ciprofloxacin; *Gati* = gatifloxacin; *Gemi* = gemifloxacin; *Levo* = levofloxacin; *Lome* = lomefloxacin; *Moxi* = moxifloxacin; *Oflox* = ofloxacin.
NOTE: Blank space = either studied and no interaction OR no data found (pharm. co. may have data)

Cipro	Gati¹	Gemi¹	Levo	Lome¹	Moxi¹	Oflox			
+			+			+	Antiarrhythmics (procainamide, amiodarone)	↑ Q-T interval (torsade)	++
+	+		+	+	+	+	Insulin, oral hypoglycemics	↑ & ↓ blood sugar	++
+							Caffeine	↑ levels of B	+
+		+			+		Cimetidine	↑ levels of A	+
+			+			+	Cyclosporine	↑ levels of B	+
+	+		+	+	+	+	Didanosine	↓ absorption of A	++
+	+	+	+	+	+	+	Cations: Al⁺⁺⁺, Ca⁺⁺, Fe⁺⁺, Mg⁺⁺, Zn⁺⁺ (antacids, vitamins, dairy products, citrate/citric acid)	↓ absorption of A (some variability between drugs)	++
+							Foscarnet	↑ risk of seizures	+
+			+		+		Methadone	↑ levels of B	+
+		+			+		NSAIDs	↑ risk CNS stimulation/seizures	++
+							Phenytoin	↑ or ↓ levels of B	+
+			+			+	Probenecid	↓ renal clearance of A	+
+	+	+	+	+	+	+	Sucralfate	↓ absorption of A	++
+			+		+		Theophylline	↑ levels of B	++
+			+			+	Warfarin	↑ prothrombin time	+

[1] Neither gati, gemi, nor moxi interacts with Ca⁺⁺

TABLE 22 (3)

ANTI-INFECTIVE AGENT (A)	OTHER DRUG (B)	EFFECT	SIGNIFICANCE/CERTAINTY
Foscarnet (Foscavir)	Ciprofloxacin	↑ risk of seizures	+
	Nephrotoxic drugs; aminoglycosides, amphocin B, cis-platinum, cyclosporine	↑ risk of nephrotoxicity	+
	Pentamidine IV	↑ risk of severe hypocalcemia	++
Ganciclovir (Cytovene)	Imipenem	↑ risk of seizures reported	+
	Probenecid	↑ levels of A	+
	Zidovudine	↓ levels of A, ↑ levels of B	+
Gentamicin	See Aminoglycosides—parenteral		
Halofantrine	Mefloquine	Additive effect: prolong. Q-T interval	++ **(avoid)**
Indinavir	See protease inhibitors and Table 22B		
Isoniazid	**Alcohol, rifampin**	**↑ risk of hepatic injury**	++
	Aluminum salts	↓ absorption (take fasting)	++
	Carbamazepine, phenytoin	↑ levels of B with nausea, vomiting, nystagmus, ataxia	++
	Itraconazole, ketoconazole	↓ levels of B	+
	Oral hypoglycemics	↓ effects of B	+
Lamivudine	Zalcitabine	Mutual interference—do not combine	++
Linezolid (Zyvox)	Adrenergic agents	Risk of hypertension	++
	Aged, fermented, pickled or smoked foods — ↑ tyramine	Risk of hypertension	+
	Serotonergic drugs	Risk of serotonin syndrome	+
Lopinavir	See protease inhibitors		

Macrolides   *[**Ery** = erythromycin, **Azi** = azithromycin, **Clr** = clarithromycin; **Dir** = dirithromycin, + = occurs, **blank space** = either studied and no interaction OR no data (pharm. co. may have data)]*

Ery	Dir	Azi	Clr	OTHER DRUG (B)	EFFECT	SIGNIFICANCE/CERTAINTY
+	+		+	Carbamazepine	↑ serum levels of B, nystagmus, nausea, vomiting, ataxia	++ **(avoid with erythro)**
+			+	Cimetidine, **ritonavir**	↑ levels of B	+
+				Clozapine	↑ serum levels of B, CNS toxicity	+
+			+	Corticosteroids	↑ effects of B	+
+	+	+	+	Cyclosporine	↑ serum levels of B with toxicity	+
+	+	+	+	Digoxin, digitoxin	↑ serum levels of B (10% of cases)	+
			+	Efavirenz	↓ levels of A	++
+	+		+	Ergot alkaloids	↑ levels of B	++
+	+		+	Lovastatin/simvastatin	↑ levels of B; rhabdomyolysis	++
+			+	Midazolam, triazolam	↑ levels of B, ↑ sedative effects	+
+			+	Phenytoin	↑ levels of B	+
+	+	+	+	Pimozide	↑ Q-T interval	++
+			+	Rifampin, rifabutin	↓ levels of A	+
+			+	Tacrolimus	↑ levels of B	++
+			+	Theophyllines	↑ serum levels of B with nausea, vomiting, seizures, apnea	++
+	+		+	Triazolam	↑ levels of B	+
+	+		+	Valproic acid	↑ levels of B	+
+	+		+	Warfarin	May ↑ prothrombin time	+
			+	Zidovudine	↓ levels of B	+

ANTI-INFECTIVE AGENT (A)	OTHER DRUG (B)	EFFECT	SIGNIFICANCE/CERTAINTY
Mefloquine	ß-adrenergic blockers, calcium channel blockers, quinidine, quinine	↑ arrhythmias	+
	Divalproex, valproic acid	↓ level of B with seizures	++
	Halofantrine	Q-T prolongation	++ **(avoid)**
Methenamine mandelate or hippurate	Acetazolamide, sodium bicarbonate, thiazide diuretics	↓ antibacterial effect 2° to ↑ urine pH	++
Metronidazole	Alcohol	Disulfiram-like reaction	+
	Disulfiram (Antabuse)	Acute toxic psychosis	+
	Oral anticoagulants	↑ anticoagulant effect	++
	Phenobarbital, hydantoins	↑ metabolism of A with ↓ effectiveness	+
Nelfinavir	See protease inhibitors and Table 22B		
Nevirapine (Viramune) See Table 22B, page 146	Opiates, including methadone	↓ levels of B (withdrawal)	++
	St. John's wort	↓ levels of A	++
	Tacrolimus	**↓ levels of B**	**+++**
Nitrofurantoin	Antacids	↓ absorption of A	+
Pentamidine, IV	Amphotericin B	↑ risk of nephrotoxicity	+
	Foscarnet	↑ risk of hypocalcemia	+
	Pancreatitis-associated drugs, e.g., alcohol, valproic acid	↑ risk of pancreatitis	+
Piperacillin	Cefoxitin	Antagonism vs pseudomonas	++
Primaquine	Chloroquine, dapsone, INH, probenecid, quinine, sulfonamides, TMP/SMX, others	↑ risk of hemolysis in G6PD-deficient patients	++

TABLE 22 (4)

ANTI-INFECTIVE AGENT (A)	OTHER DRUG (B)	EFFECT	SIGNIFICANCE/ CERTAINTY

Protease Inhibitors—Anti-HIV Drugs. (**Ampren** = amprenavir & fosamprenavir, **Atazan** = atazanavir, **Indin** = indinavir, **Lopin** = lopinavir **Nelfin** = nelfinavir; **Riton** = ritonavir; **Saquin** = saquinavir). For interactions with antiretrovirals, see Table 22B, page 146

Only a partial list—check package insert
Also see NEJM 344:984, 2001; http://aidsinfo.nih.gov

Column headers (vertical): Ampren, Atazan, Indin, Lopin, Nelfin, Riton, Saquin

Ampren	Atazan	Indin	Lopin	Nelfin	Riton	Saquin	OTHER DRUG (B)	EFFECT	SIGNIF.
							Analgesics:		
					+		1. Alfentanil, fentanyl, hydrocodone, tramadol	↑ levels of B	+
		+		+			2. Codeine, hydromorphone, morphine, methadone	↓ levels of B	+
+	+	+	+	+	+	+	**Anti-arrhythmics: amiodarone, lidocaine, mexiletine, flecainide**	↑ levels of B	+
		+	+	+	+	+	**Anticonvulsants: carbamazepine, clonazepam, phenytoin, phenobarbital**	↓ levels of A, ↑ levels of B	++
	+						Antidepressants, all tricyclic	↑ levels of B	+
	+				+		Antidepressants, all other	↑ levels of B	+
						+	**Antihistamine:** Loratadine	↑ levels of B	++
		+					Atovaquone	↓ levels of B	+
+	+	+	+	+	+	+	**Benzodiazepines, e.g., diazepam**	↑ **levels of B—do not use**	++
							Beta blockers: Metoprolol, pindolol, propranolol, timolol	↑ levels of B	+
+	+	+	+	+	+	+	Calcium channel blockers (all)	↑ levels of B	++
		+					Clarithromycin, erythromycin	↑ levels of B if renal impairment	+
+		+	+	+	+	+	Contraceptives, oral	↓ levels of B	++
		+			+		Corticosteroids: prednisone, dexamethasone	↓ levels of A, ↑ levels of B	+
+	+	+	+	+	+	+	Cyclosporine	↓ levels of B, monitor levels	+
+	+	+	+	+	+	+	Ergot derivatives	↑ **levels of B—do not use**	++
		+			+		Erythromycin, clarithromycin	↑ levels of A & B	+
		+				+	Grapefruit juice (>200 ml/day)	↓ indinavir & ↑ saquinavir levels	++
+	+	+	+	+	+	+	HMG-CoA reductase inhibitors: lovastatin, simvastatin	↑ **levels of B—do not use**	++
+			+				Ketoconazole, itraconazole, ? vori	↑ levels of A	+
		+					Metronidazole	Poss. disulfiram reaction, alcohol	+
+	+	+	+	+	+	+	Pimozide	↑ **levels of B—do not use**	++
+	+	+	+	+	+	+	Proton pump inhibitors	↓ levels of A	++
+	+	+	+	+	+	+	Rifampin, rifabutin	↓ levels of A, ↑ levels of B	++ (avoid)
+	+	+	+	+	+	+	Sildenafil (Viagra)	Varies, some ↑ & some ↓ levels of B	++
+	+	+	+	+	+	+	**St. John's wort**	↓ **levels of A—do not use**	++
+	+	+	+	+	+	+	**Statins**	↑ **levels of B, esp. simvastatin & lovastatin—others OK**	++ (check)
		+		+			Theophylline	↓ levels of B	+
	+				+	+	Warfarin	↑ levels of B	+
Pyrazinamide		INH, rifampin	May ↑ risk of hepatotoxicity	±
Pyrimethamine		Lorazepam	↑ risk of hepatotoxicity	+
		Sulfonamides, TMP/SMX	↑ risk of marrow suppression	+
		Zidovudine	↑ risk of marrow suppression	+
Quinine		Digoxin	↑ digoxin levels; ↑ toxicity	++
		Mefloquine	↑ arrhythmias	+
		Oral anticoagulants	↑ prothrombin time	++
Rifamycins (rifampin, rifabutin) *See footnote for less severe or less common interactions[1]* Ref.: ArIM 162:985, 2002		Al OH, ketoconazole, PZA	↓ levels of A	+
		Atovaquone	↑ levels of A ↓ levels of B	+
		Beta adrenergic blockers (metoprolol, propranolol)	↓ effect of B	+
		Clarithromycin	↑ levels of A, ↓ levels of B	++
		Corticosteroids	↑ replacement requirement of B	++
		Cyclosporine	↓ effect of B	++
		Delavirdine	↑ **levels of A, ↓ levels of B—avoid**	++
		Digoxin	↓ levels of B	++
		Disopyramide	↓ levels of B	+
		Fluconazole	↑ levels of A[1]	+
		Amprenavir, indinavir, nelfinavir, ritonavir	↑ levels of A (↓ dose of A), ↓ levels of B	++
		INH	Converts INH to toxic hydrazine	+
		Itraconazole[2], ketoconazole	↓ levels of B, ↑ levels of A[2]	++
		Methadone	↓ serum levels (withdrawal)	+
		Nevirapine	↓ **levels of B—avoid**	++
		Oral anticoagulants	Suboptimal anticoagulation	++

[1] The following is a partial list of drugs with rifampin-induced ↑ metabolism and hence lower than anticipated serum levels: ACE inhibitors, dapsone, diazepam, digoxin, diltiazem, doxycycline, fluconazole, fluvastatin, haloperidol, nifedipine, progestins, triazolam, tricyclics, voriconazole, zidovudine

[2] Up to 4 weeks may be required after RIF discontinued to achieve detectable serum itra levels; ↑ levels associated with uveitis or polymyolysis

TABLE 22 (5)

ANTI-INFECTIVE AGENT (A)	OTHER DRUG (B)	EFFECT	SIGNIFICANCE/ CERTAINTY
Rifamycins (rifampin, rifabutin) *(continued)* See footnote 1 on page 139 for less severe or less common interactions Ref.: ArlM 162:985, 2002	Oral contraceptives	↓ effectiveness; spotting, pregnancy	+
	Phenytoin	↓ levels of B	+
	Protease inhibitors	**↑ levels of A, ↓ levels of B— CAUTION**	**++**
	Quinidine	↓ effect of B	+
	Sulfonylureas	↓ hypoglycemic effect	+
	Tacrolimus	↓ levels of B	++
	Theophylline	↓ levels of B	+
	TMP/SMX	↑ levels of A	+
	Tocainide	↓ effect of B	+
Rimantadine	*See Amantadine*		
Ritonavir	*See protease inhibitors and Table 22B*		
Saquinavir	*See protease inhibitors and Table 22B*		
Stavudine	Dapsone, INH	May ↑ risk of peripheral neuropathy	±
Sulfonamides	Cyclosporine	↓ cyclosporine levels	+
	Methotrexate	↑ antifolate activity	+
	Oral anticoagulants	↑ prothrombin time; bleeding	+
	Phenobarbital, rifampin	↓ levels of A	+
	Phenytoin	↑ levels of B; nystagmus, ataxia	+
	Sulfonylureas	↑ hypoglycemic effect	+
Telithromycin (Ketek)	Digoxin	↑ levels of B—do digoxin levels	++
	Ergot alkaloids	**levels of B—avoid**	**++**
	Itraconazole; ketoconazole	↑ levels of A; no dose change	+
	Midazolam	↑ levels of B	++
	Pimozide	**↑ levels of B; QT prolongation— AVOID**	**++**
	Rifampin	**↓ levels of A—avoid**	**++**
	Simvastatin	↑ levels of B	++
	Sotalol	↓ levels of B	++
Tenofovir	Didanosine (ddI)	**↑ levels of B (reduce dose)**	**++**
Terbinafine	Cimetidine	↑ levels of A	+
	Phenobarbital, rifampin	↓ levels of A	+
Tetracyclines	*See Doxycycline, plus:*		
	Atovaquone	↓ levels of B	+
	Digoxin	↑ toxicity of B (may persist several months—up to 10% pts)	++
	Methoxyflurane	↑ toxicity: polyuria, renal failure	+
	Sucralfate	↓ absorption of A (separate by ≥2 hrs)	+
Thiabendazole	Theophyllines	↑ serum theophylline, nausea	+
Tobramycin	*See Aminoglycosides*		
Trimethoprim	Amantadine, dapsone, digoxin, methotrexate, procainamide, zidovudine	↑ serum levels of B	++
	Potassium-sparing diuretics	↑ serum K⁺	++
	Thiazide diuretics	↓ serum Na⁺	+
Trimethoprim/Sulfa- methoxazole	Azathioprine	Reports of leucopenia	+
	Cyclosporine	↓ levels of B, ↑ serum creatinine	+
	Loperamide	↑ levels of B	+
	Methotrexate	Enhanced marrow suppression	++
	Oral contraceptives, pimozide, and 6-mercaptopurine	↓ effect of B	+
	Phenytoin	↑ levels of B	+
	Rifampin	↑ levels of B	+
	Warfarin	↑ activity of B	+
Vancomycin	Aminoglycosides	↑ frequency of nephrotoxicity	++
Zalcitabine (ddC) (HIVID)	Valproic acid, pentamidine (IV), alcohol, lamivudine	↑ pancreatitis risk	+
	Cisplatin, INH, metronidazole, vincristine, nitrofurantoin, d4T, dapsone	↑ risk of peripheral neuropathy	+
Zidovudine (ZDV) (Retrovir)	Atovaquone, fluconazole, metha- done	↑ levels of A	+
	Clarithromycin	↓ levels of A	±
	Indomethacin	↑ levels of ZDV toxic metabolite	+
	Nelfinavir	↓ levels of A	++
	Probenecid, TMP/SMX	↑ levels of A	+
	Ribavirin	**↓ levels of A—avoid**	**++**
	Rifampin/rifabutin	↓ levels of A	++

TABLE 22B: DRUG-DRUG INTERACTIONS BETWEEN PROTEASE INHIBITORS AND NON-NUCLEOSIDE REVERSE TRANSCRIPTASE INHIBITORS (RTIs) (*I = investigational)

(For interactions of nucleoside RTIs, see Table 22A)

(Abstracted from Guidelines for the Use of Antiretroviral Agents in HIV-Infected Adults & Adolescents; www.hivatis.org)

NAME (Abbreviation, Trade Name)	Amprenavir* (APV, Agenerase) Fosamprenavir (FOSA, Lexiva)	Indinavir (IDV, Crixivan)	Nelfinavir (NFV, Viracept)	Ritonavir (RTV, Norvir)	Saquinavir-soft gel (SQV, Fortovase)	Efavirenz (EFZ, Sustiva)	Delavirdine (DLV, Rescriptor)	Nevirapine (NVP, Viramune)
Amprenavir (APV, Agenerase)								
Indinavir (IDV, Crixivan)	Levels: APV AUC ↑ 33%. Dose: no change							
Nelfinavir (NFV, Viracept)	Levels of APV ↑, no data on dosage change	Levels: NFV ↑ 80%; IDV ↑ 50%. Dose: IDV 1200 mg bid + NFV 1250 mg bid (I)*						
Ritonavir (RTV, Norvir)	APV AUC ↑ 2.5x. Dose: (APV 600 mg bid + RTV 100 mg bid) OR (FOSA 700 mg + RTV 100 mg bid)	Levels: IDV ↑s RTV; RTV ↑s IDV. Dose: RTV 100 or 200 mg bid + IDV 800 bid	NFV levels ↑ 2x; no effect RTV. Dosage (RTV 400 mg bid + NFV 500-750 mg bid) ↑*					
Saquinavir—softgel (SQV, Fortovase)	APV AUC ↓ 32%. Dose: Insufficient data	Levels: SQV ↑ 4-7x; no effect IDV. Antiviral antagonism. Do not combine	SQV levels ↑ 3-5x; no effect (usual dosage). SQV: 800 mg tid or 1200 mg bid	SQV levels ↑ 20x. RTV no effect. Dosage: 100 mg SQV + 100 mg RTV bid				
Efavirenz (EFZ, Sustiva)	APV levels ↓ 30%; ↑. Dose: No change if FOSA/RTV bid + EFV	IDV levels ↓ 30%; ↑ IDV dose:1000 mg q8h; EFV standard	Usual dosage of each	Modest ↑ levels of both drugs. RTV 600 mg bid, or 1200 mg standard dose	↓ levels of SQV. Do not combine. Consider - SQV/RTV			
Delavirdine (DLV, Rescriptor)	APV levels ↑, DLV levels ↓. Do not combine	IDV levels ↑ 40%; no change DLV. Dose: IDV 600 mg q8h	DLV levels ↓ 50%. Usual dosage—watch for neutropenia	RTV levels ↑ 70%. Dosage: Consider RTV to 400 mg bid	↑ SQV levels ↑ 5x. Dose: SQV 800 mg tid + DLV standard	No data		
Nevirapine (NVP, Viramune)	APV levels ↓, no data on dosage change	IDV levels ↓ 28%; no effect. Dose or IDV: IDV 1000 mg q8h	Standard dose of both	No interaction	SQV levels ↓ 25%. Avoid combination		Do not use together	
Lopinavir/ritonavir (LP/R, Kaletra)	↓ APV to 750 mg bid + LP/R 4 pills bid	↓ IDV to 600 mg bid; IDV/R standard dose		No data	SQV 1000 mg bid + standard LP/R	Standard therapy		↑ LP/R to 533/133 mg bid + NVP standard
Atazanavir (Reyataz)				Atazan 300 mg qd + RTV 100 mg qd	SQV levels ↑; dosage adjustment unclear		No data	

* APV data apply to FOSA unless otherwise indicated

TABLE 23: LIST OF GENERIC AND COMMON TRADE NAMES

GENERIC NAME: TRADE NAMES	GENERIC NAME: TRADE NAMES	GENERIC NAME: TRADE NAMES
Abacavir: Ziagen	Diloxanide furoate: Furamide	Nafcillin: Unipen
Acyclovir: Zovirax	Dirithromycin: Dynabac	Nelfinavir: Viracept
Adefovir: Hepsera	Doxycycline: Vibramycin	Nevirapine: Viramune
Albendazole: Albenza	Drotrecogin alfa: Xigris	Nitazoxanide: Alinia
Amantadine: Symmetrel	Efavirenz: Sustiva	Nitrofurantoin: Macrobid, Macrodantin
Amikacin: Amikin	Enfuvirtide (T-20): Fuzeon	Nystatin: Mycostatin
Amoxicillin: Amoxil, Polymox	Ertapenem: Invanz	Ofloxacin: Floxin
Amox./clav.: Augmentin, Augmentin ES-600; Augmentin XR	Erythromycin(s): Ilotycin *Ethyl succinate:* Pediamycin *Glucoheptonate:* Erythrocin *Estolate:* Ilosone	Oseltamivir: Tamiflu
Amphotericin B: Fungizone		Oxacillin: Prostaphlin
Ampho B-liposomal: AmBisome		Palivizumab: Synagis
Ampho B-cholesteryl complex: Amphotec	Erythro/sulfisoxazole: Pediazole	Paromomycin: Humatin
Ampho B-lipid complex: Abelcet	Ethambutol: Myambutol	Pentamidine: NebuPent, Pentam 300
Ampicillin: Omnipen, Polycillin	Ethionamide: Trecator	Piperacillin: Pipracil
Ampicillin/sulbactam: Unasyn	Famciclovir: Famvir	Piperacillin/tazobactam: Zosyn
Amprenavir: Agenerase	Fluconazole: Diflucan	Piperazine: Antepar
Atazanavir: Reyataz	Flucytosine: Ancobon	Podophyllotoxin: Condylox
Atovaquone: Mepron	Fosamprenavir: Lexiva	Praziquantel: Biltricide
Atovaquone + proguanil: Malarone	Foscarnet: Foscavir	Primaquine: Primachine
Azithromycin: Zithromax	Fosfomycin: Monurol	Proguanil: Paludrine
Aztreonam: Azactam	Furazolidone: Furoxone	Pyrantel pamoate: Antiminth
Caspofungin: Cancidas	Ganciclovir: Cytovene	Pyrimethamine: Daraprim
Cefaclor: Ceclor, Ceclor CD	Gatifloxacin: Tequin	Pyrimethamine/sulfadoxine: Fansidar
Cefadroxil: Duricef	Gemifloxacin: Factive	Quinupristin/dalfopristin: Synercid
Cefazolin: Ancef, Kefzol	Gentamicin: Garamycin	Ribavirin: Virazole, Rebetol
Cefdinir: Omnicef	Griseofulvin: Fulvicin	Rifabutin: Mycobutin
Cefditoren pivoxil: Spectracef	Halofantrine: Halfan	Rifampin: Rifadin, Rimactane
Cefepime: Maxipime	Idoxuridine: Dendrid, Stoxil	Rifapentine: Priftin
Cefixime^{NUS}: Suprax	INH + RIF: Rifamate	Rimantadine: Flumadine
Cefoperazone: Cefobid	INH + RIF + PZA: Rifater	Ritonavir: Norvir
Cefotaxime: Claforan	Interferon alfa: Roferon-A, Intron A	Saquinavir: Invirase, Fortovase
Cefotetan: Cefotan	Interferon, pegylated: PEG-Intron, Pegasys	Spectinomycin: Trobicin
Cefoxitin: Mefoxin		Stavudine: Zerit
Cefpodoxime proxetil: Vantin	Interferon + ribavirin: Rebetron	Stibogluconate: Pentostam
Cefprozil: Cefzil	Imipenem + cilastatin: Primaxin	Silver sulfadiazine: Silvadene
Ceftazidime: Fortaz, Tazicef, Tazidime	Imiquimod: Aldara	Sulfamethoxazole: Gantanol
Ceftibuten: Cedax	Indinavir: Crixivan	Sulfasalazine: Azulfidine
Ceftizoxime: Cefizox	Iodoquinol: Yodoxin	Sulfisoxazole: Gantrisin
Ceftriaxone: Rocephin	Itraconazole: Sporanox	Telithromycin: Ketek
Cefuroxime: Zinacef, Kefurox, Ceftin	Ivermectin: Stromectol	Tenofovir: Viread
Cephalexin: Keflex	Kanamycin: Kantrex	Terbinafine: Lamisil
Cephradine: Anspor, Velosef	Ketoconazole: Nizoral	Thalidomide: Thalomid
Chloroquine: Aralen	Lamivudine: Epivir, Epivir-HBV	Thiabendazole: Mintezol
Cidofovir: Vistide	Levofloxacin: Levaquin	Ticarcillin: Ticar
Ciprofloxacin: Cipro, Cipro XR	Linezolid: Zyvox	Tipranavir: Texega
Clarithromycin: Biaxin, Biaxin XL	Lomefloxacin: Maxaquin	Tobramycin: Nebcin
Clindamycin: Cleocin	Lopinavir/ritonavir: Kaletra	Tretinoin: Retin A
Clofazimine: Lamprene	Loracarbef: Lorabid	Trifluridine: Viroptic
Clotrimazole: Lotrimin, Mycelex	Mafenide: Sulfamylon	Trimethoprim: Proloprim, Trimpex
Cloxacillin: Tegopen	Mebendazole: Vermox	Trimethoprim/sulfamethoxazole: Bactrim, Septra
Cycloserine: Seromycin	Mefloquine: Lariam	
Daptomycin: Cubicin	Meropenem: Merrem	Valacyclovir: Valtrex
Delavirdine: Rescriptor	Mesalamine: Asacol, Pentasa	Valganciclovir: Valcyte
Dicloxacillin: Dynapen	Methenamine: Hiprex, Mandelamine	Vancomycin: Vancocin
Didanosine: Videx	Metronidazole: Flagyl	Voriconazole: Vfend
Diethylcarbamazine: Hetrazan	Minocycline: Minocin	Zalcitabine: HIVID
	Moxifloxacin: Avelox	Zanamivir: Relenza
	Mupirocin: Bactroban	Zidovudine (ZDV): Retrovir
		Zidovudine + 3TC: Combivir
		Zidovudine + 3TC + abacavir: Trizivir

TABLE 23 (2)
LIST OF COMMON TRADE AND GENERIC NAMES

TRADE NAME: GENERIC NAME	TRADE NAME: GENERIC NAME	TRADE NAME: GENERIC NAME
Abelcet: Ampho B-lipid complex	Gantrisin: Sulfisoxazole	Relenza: Zanamivir
Agenerase: Amprenavir	Garamycin: Gentamicin	Rescriptor: Delavirdine
Albenza: Albendazole	Halfan: Halofantrine	Retin A: Tretinoin
Aldara: Imiquimod	Hepsera: Adefovir	Retrovir: Zidovudine (ZDV)
Alinia: Nitazoxanide	Herplex: Idoxuridine	Reyataz: Atazanavir
AmBisome: Ampho B-liposomal	Hiprex: Methenamine hippurate	Rifadin: Rifampin
Amikin: Amikacin	HIVID: Zalcitabine	Rifamate: INH + RIF
Amoxil: Amoxicillin	Humatin: Paromomycin	Rifater: INH + RIF + PZA
Amphotec: Ampho B-cholesteryl complex	Ilosone: Erythromycin estolate	Rimactane: Rifampin
	Ilotycin: Erythromycin	Rocephin: Ceftriaxone
Ancef: Cefazolin	Intron A: Interferon alfa	Roferon-A: Interferon alfa
Ancobon: Flucytosine	Invanz: Ertapenem	Septra: Trimethoprim/sulfa
Anspor: Cephradine	Invirase: Saquinavir	Seromycin: Cycloserine
Antepar: Piperazine	Kaletra: Lopinavir/ritonavir	Silvadene: Silver sulfadiazine
Antiminth: Pyrantel pamoate	Kantrex: Kanamycin	Spectracef: Cefditoren pivoxil
Aralen: Chloroquine	Keflex: Cephalexin	Sporanox: Itraconazole
Asacol: Mesalamine	Kefurox: Cefuroxime	Stoxil: Idoxuridine
Augmentin, Augmentin ES-600, Augmentin XR: Amox./clav.	Ketek: Telithromycin	Stromectol: Ivermectin
	Lamisil: Terbinafine	Sulfamylon: Mafenide
Avelox: Moxifloxacin	Lamprene: Clofazimine	Suprax: Cefixime^AUS
Azactam: Aztreonam	Lariam: Mefloquine	Sustiva: Efavirenz
Azulidine: Sulfasalazine	Levaquin: Levofloxacin	Symmetrel: Amantadine
Bactroban: Mupirocin	Lexiva: Fosamprenavir	Synagis: Palivizumab
Bactrim: Trimethoprim/ sulfamethoxazole	Lorabid: Loracarbef	Synercid: Quinupristin/dalfopristin
	Macrodantin, Macrobid: Nitrofurantoin	Tamiflu: Oseltamivir
Biaxin, Biaxin XL: Clarithromycin	Malarone: Atovaquone + proguanil	Tazicef: Ceftazidime
Biltricide: Praziquantel	Mandelamine: Methenamine mandel.	Tegopen: Cloxacillin
Cancidas: Caspofungin	Maxaquin: Lomefloxacin	Tequin: Gatifloxacin
Ceclor, Ceclor CD: Cefaclor	Maxipime: Cefepime	Texega: Tipranavir
Cedax: Ceftibuten	Mefoxin: Cefoxitin	Thalomid: Thalidomide
Cefizox: Ceftizoxime	Mepron: Atovaquone	Ticar: Ticarcillin
Cefobid: Cefoperazone	Merrem: Meropenem	Timentin: Ticarcillin-clavulanic acid
Cefotan: Cefotetan	Minocin: Minocycline	Tinactin: Tolnaftate
Ceftin: Cefuroxime axetil	Mintezol: Thiabendazole	Trecator SC: Ethionamide
Cefzil: Cefprozil	Monocid: Cefonicid	Trizivir: Abacavir + ZDV + 3TC
Cipro, Cipro XR: Ciprofloxacin & extended release	Monurol: Fosfomycin	Trobicin: Spectinomycin
	Myambutol: Ethambutol	Unasyn: Ampicillin/sulbactam
Claforan: Cefotaxime	Mycobutin: Rifabutin	Unipen: Nafcillin
Combivir: ZDV + 3TC	Mycostatin: Nystatin	Valcyte: Valganciclovir
Crixivan: Indinavir	Nafcil: Nafcillin	Valtrex: Valacyclovir
Cubicin: Daptomycin	Nebcin: Tobramycin	Vancocin: Vancomycin
Cytovene: Ganciclovir	NebuPent: Pentamidine	Vantin: Cefpodoxime proxetil
Daraprim: Pyrimethamine	Nizoral: Ketoconazole	Velosef: Cephradine
Diflucan: Fluconazole	Norvir: Ritonavir	Vermox: Mebendazole
Duricef: Cefadroxil	Omnicef: Cefdinir	Vfend: Voriconazole
Dynapen: Dicloxacillin	Omnipen: Ampicillin	Vibramycin: Doxycycline
Epivir, Epivir-HBV: Lamivudine	Pediamycin: Erythro. ethyl succinate	Videx: Didanosine
Factive: Gemifloxacin	Pediazole: Erythro. ethyl succinate + sulfisoxazole	Viracept: Nelfinavir
Famvir: Famciclovir		Viramune: Nevirapine
Fansidar: Pyrimethamine + sulfadoxine	Pegasys, PEG-Intron: Interferon, pegylated	Virazole: Ribavirin
		Viread: Tenofovir
Flagyl: Metronidazole	Pentam 300: Pentamidine	Vistide: Cidofovir
Floxin: Ofloxacin	Pentasa: Mesalamine	Xigris: Drotrecogin alfa
Flumadine: Rimantadine	Pipracil: Piperacillin	Yodoxin: Iodoquinol
Fortaz: Ceftazidime	Polycillin: Ampicillin	Zerit: Stavudine
Fortovase: Saquinavir	Polymox: Amoxicillin	Ziagen: Abacavir
Fulvicin: Griseofulvin	Priftin: Rifapentine	Zinacef: Cefuroxime
Fungizone: Amphotericin B	Primaxin: Imipenem + cilastatin	Zithromax: Azithromycin
Furadantin: Nitrofurantoin	Proloprim: Trimethoprim	Zovirax: Acyclovir
Furoxone: Furazolidone	Prostaphlin: Oxacillin	Zosyn: Piperacillin/tazobactam
Fuzeon: Enfuvirtide (T-20)	Rebetol: Ribavirin	Zyvox: Linezolid
Gantanol: Sulfamethoxazole	Rebetron: Interferon + ribavirin	

INDEX TO MAJOR ENTITIES

PAGES (page numbers bold if major focus)

Abacavir — 57, 62, **117**, **120**, 124, 135
Abbreviations — **45**
Abortion, prophylaxis/septic — 16, **126–127**
Acanthamoeba — **9**, 94
Acinetobacter — 14, 31, 34, **48**, 52–54, **56**
Acne rosacea and vulgaris — **34**, 101, 113
Actinomycosis — 9, 48, 52–54, **74**
Activated Protein C (Drotrecogin) — 13
Acyclovir — 57, 61, 108–110, **113**, 114, 128, 133
Adefovir — 57, 61, **105**, 114, 133
Adenovirus — 8, 24–25, 29, 47, 104, 111
Adverse reactions
  Antibacterials — 63–65
  Antifungals — 82–84
  Antimycobacterials — 91–92
  Antiparasitic drugs — 101–103
  Antiretroviral drugs — 120–121
  Antiviral drugs — 113–115
Aeromonas hydrophila — 11, 37, 48, 52–54
AIDS — **3**, **6**, **9**, **10**, **12**, 13, 16, 17, 24, 27, **29**, 30, 34, 38, 42, 51, 56, 75, 76, **77**, 78, **79, 80**, 81, 84, 85, 88, 89, 91, 93, 96, 97, 100, 106, 107, 109, 110–113, **116**, 121, 123, 124
Albendazole — 57, 61, 94, 98, 99, **101**
Amantadine — 57, 111, **115**, 133
Amebiasis — 11, 13, 24, **93**
Amebic meningoencephalitis — **94**
Amikacin — 48, 49, 54, 57, 59, 63, **73**, 81, 88–91, 129, 130
Aminoglycosides, single daily dose — **73**, 130
Amnionitis, septic abortion — 16
Amoxicillin — 46, 48–50, 52, 55, 56, 58, 63, 66, 74, 82, 122, 124–129, 131, 132
Amoxicillin/clavulanate — 48, 49, 50–52, 58, 63, 66, 82, 90, 122, 124, 126, 129, 132
Amphotericin B, ampho B — 57, 60, 73–**82**, 94, 101, 113, 132, 135
  lipid ampho B preps — 60, 74–76, 79, 80, **82–83**, 94, 132
Ampicillin — 48–50, 52, 54–56, 58, 63, **66**, 74, 122, 127–129, 131, 132, 135
Ampicillin/sulbactam — 48–50, 52, 55, 56, 58, 63, **66**, 125, 129, 132, 135
Amprenavir — 57, 62, 88, **118**, **120**, 135
Anaplasma (Ehrlichia) — 38, 48
Angiostrongylus — 6, **97**
Anisakiasis — 98
Anthrax — 26, **28**, **34**, 46, 48
Antifungals — 74–**84**
Antimony compounds — 94, **101**
Antiretroviral drugs & therapy/ Antiviral drugs — 104–121
Aphthous stomatitis — **30**, 40, 77, 92, 118
Appendicitis — 12, **31**, 77
Arcanobacterium haemolyticum — **32**, 48
Artesunate — **95**, 101
Arthritis, septic — 15, 20–**21**, 39–41, 51, 69, 101, 112
reactive (Reiter's) — **21**
Ascariasis — 98
Aspergillosis — 9, 10, 20, 27, 33, 42, 44, 47, **74**, 76, 82–84, 128
Aspiration pneumonia — 28
Asplenia — 35, 38, 42, 94, 124, 125, 137–139
Atabrine — **101**
Atazanavir — 62, **117**, **118**, 121, 135
Atherosclerosis & Chlamydia pneumoniae — 18
Athlete's foot — 36, **80**
Atovaquone; atovaquone + proguanil — 57, 61, 62, 94–97, **101**
Azithromycin — 46, 48–51, 54, 56, 57, 60, 65, **69**, 88, 89, 90, 93, 94, **97**, 125, 127, 129, 133
Azole antifungals — 74–81, **82–84**
AZT (zidovudine) — 57, 62, 88, 113, 116–**118**, **120**, 123, 124, 134
Aztreonam — 48, 49, 50, 52, 56, 57, 59, 63, **67**, 68, 129, 132

Babesia, babesiosis — **38**, 39, **94**, 124

PAGES (page numbers bold if major focus)

Bacillary angiomatosis — 34, **38**, 48
Bacillus anthracis (anthrax) — 26, **28**, **34**, 46, 48
Bacillus cereus, subtilis — **10**, 48
Bacitracin — 48
Bacterial endocarditis — 13, 18–**20**, 38, 51, 69, **127–128**
Bacterial peritonitis — 11, 14, 16, 24, **31**, 77, 83, 126, 77, 83, 128
Bacterial vaginosis — **17**, 49
Bacteriuria, asymptomatic — **23**, 51, 122, 126
Bacteroides species — 3, 10, **14**, 16, 17, 24, 26, 28, 29, 31, 35–37, 44, 48, 52, 54
Balanitis — **17**, 21
Balantidium coli — 93
Bartonella henselae, quintana — 20, 24, 30, 34, **38**, 40, 48
BCG — 85, **88**
Bell's palsy — **108**
Benzathine penicillin — 48, 56, 66
Benznidazole — 57, 97, **101**
Bicillin — 48, 58, 66
Biliary sepsis — **10**, 14, 42
Biological weapons — **46**
Bites — 18, 21, **35**, 37, 39, 40, 109, 112, 126, 139
Bithionol — 93, 103
BK virus, post-renal transplant — 112
Blastocystis hominis — **93**
Blastomycosis — 35, **75**, 81
Blepharitis — **8**
Boils (furunculosis) — 35–**36**
Bordetella pertussis (whooping cough) — 24, 48, 137, 139
Borrelia burgdorferi, B. garinii, B. afzelii — 21, 38, **39**, 48
Borrelia recurrentis — **39**, 48
Botulism (food-borne, infant, wound) — **43**, **46**
Brain abscess — **3**, 8, 33, 49, 81
Bronchitis, bronchiolitis — 24, 25, 26, 111
Bronchopneumonia — 24–**28**
Brucellosis — 20, 21, **40**, 48, 51, 54
Brugia malayi — 98
Buccal cellulitis — 30
Burkholderia (Pseudomonas) cepacia — **29**, 48, 52–54
Burkholderia pseudomallei (melioidosis) — **27**, 38, 48
Burns — **36**, 43, 44, 139
Bursitis, septic — **22**
Buruli ulcer — **88**

C–Section — 16, 109, 122, 124, 126–127
Calymmatobacterium granulomatis — 15
Campylobacter jejuni, fetus — 11–13, 21, 48, **56**
Canaliculitis — 9
Candida albicans, krusei, lusitaniae — 13, 17, 32, **75–77**, 84
"Candida syndrome" — 77
Candidemia, candidiasis — 9, 10, 13, 17, 18, 20, 27, 30, 32, 36, 38, 42, 44, 47, **75–77**, 82–84, 128
CAPD peritonitis — **31**, 77, **135**
Capillariasis — **35**, 42, 48
Capnocytophaga ochracea, canimorsus — 57, 86, 90, **92**
Capreomycin — 48–52, 59, 63, 67, 130
Carbapenems — 48–52, 59, 63, 67, 130
Caspofungin — 57, 61, 74–77, **80**, 83, 135
Cat bite — **35**
Catfish sting — **35**
Cat-scratch disease — 3, 24, **30**, 34, 35, 38
Cavernous sinus thrombosis — **44**
CDC Drug Service — 93, 94, 97, 101
Cefaclor, Cefaclor-ER — 53, 58, 64, **68**, 129
Cefadroxil — 53, 58, 64, **68**, 129
Cefazolin — 48, 53, 58, 64, **67**, 122, 125, 126, 129, 131, 135
Cefdinir — 53, 59, 64, **68**, 129
Cefditoren pivoxil — 53, 59, 64, **68**
Cefepime — 50, 53, 55, 59, 64, **68**, 129, 131
Cefixime — 49, 53, 59, 64, **68**, 125
Cefotaxime — 48–50, 53, 55, 59, 64, **67**, 68, 129, 131
Cefotetan — 48, 53, 58, 64, **67**, 125, 126, 131
Cefoxitin — 48, 53, 58, 64, **67**, 68, 89, 125, 126, 129, 131
Cefpirome — 64, **68**
Cefpodoxime proxetil — 49, 53, 55, 59, 64, **68**, 129

Bold numbers indicate major considerations. Recommendations in Table 1 not indexed; antibiotic selection often depends on modifying circumstances and alternative agents.

PAGES *(page numbers bold if major focus)*

Cefprozil 53, 58, 64, **68**, 129
Ceftazidime 48–50, 53, 56, 59, 64, **67**, 68, 129, 131, 135
Ceftibuten 53, 59, 64, **68**, 129
Ceftizoxime 53, 59, 64, **67**, 125, 129, 131
Ceftriaxone 48–51, 53, 55, 56, 59, 64, **68**, 74, 125, 126, 129, 135
Cefuroxime 48, 49, 53, 55, 58, 64, **67**, 68, 125, 126, 129, 131
Cefuroxime axetil 48, 53, 58, 64, **68**
Cellulitis (erysipelas) 10, 35, **36**, 43, 51
Cephalexin 48, 53, 58, 64, **68**, 127, 129
Cephalosporins, overall/generations 53, 58–59, 67–68
Cervicitis **14–16**, 51
Cestodes (tapeworms) **99–100**, 103
Chagas disease 97, 128
Chancroid **14**, 30, 49
Charcot foot 10
Chickenpox 43, 109–110, 136–138
Chlamydia pneumoniae 18, **24–26**, 48, 52
Chlamydophila pneumoniae 18, **24–26**, 48, 52
Chlamydia trachomatis 8, 14, **15–17**, 21, 22, **25**, 32, 48, 52, 125
Chloramphenicol 46, 48–51, 54, 55, 57, 60, 65, **69**, 74, 129, 133
Chloroquine 48, 57, 95, **101–103**
Cholangitis 10, 24, 125
Cholecystitis 10, **125**
Cholera 11, **12**, 50
Cholestyramine 11, **12**, 50
Chromomycosis 78
Chryseobacterium/Flavobacterium 78
Cidofovir 46, 57, 104, 107, 109, 111–**113**, 133
Ciprofloxacin 46, 48–52, 56, 57, 59, 65, **70**, 71, 86, 87, 89, 90, 92, 93, 122, 125, 126, 129, 131, 135
Citrobacter 48, 52, 53
Clarithromycin 46, 48–50, 54, 56, 57, 60, 65, **69**, 71, 88–90, 92, 94, 97, 127, 129, 131
Clindamycin 46, 48–50, 54, 57, 60, 65, **69**, 74, 79, 94–97,103, 122, 126, 127, 129, 135
Clofazimine 57, 81, 88–90, **92**
Clonorchis sinensis 99
Clostridial myonecrosis **30**, 37, 51
Clostridium difficile colitis 11, 48, 52–54, 66, 67, 68, 91
Clostridium perfringens 16, 30, 37, 48, 51
Clotrimazole 76, 77, 80, 82, **83**
Cloxacillin 52, 63, 66, 129
CMV 10, 13, 25, 47, **107**, 113, 114, 128, 134
CMV retinitis 10, 47, **107**, 113
Coccidioidomycosis 6, 28, 36, 47, **78**
Colitis, antibiotic-associated 11, 66, 69, 91
Conjunctivitis (all types) 3, **8**, 14, 21, 40, 109, 115
Contaminated traumatic wound 37
Corneal laceration 10
Coronavirus 29, **104**
Corticosteroids and meningitis **4–6**
Corynebacterium jeikeium 44, 48, 52–54
Coxiella burnetii 26, **48**
Coxsackievirus 32
"Crabs" (Phthirus pubis) 15, **100**
Creeping eruption 98
Crohn's disease **13**, 41
Cryptococcosis 6, 17, 47, 77, **78, 79**, 81, 82
Cryptococcus neoformans **6**, 17
Cryptosporidium 11–13, 79, 93
CSF 3–6, 28, 39, 46, 58–62, 69, 71, 79, 83, 84, 87, 92, 96, 97, 104, 108, 113, 126
Cycloserine 57, 86, 89, 90, **92**
Cyclospora 11–13, **93**
Cyclosporine 70, 73, 83, 132
Cystic fibrosis 2, **28**, 73, 74, 129
Cysticercosis **99**, 103
Cystitis 22, 51, 66, **77**
Cytomegalovirus 10, 13, 25, 47, **107**, 113, 114, 128, 134

D4T (stavudine) 57, 62, 116, **117**, **120**, 124, 134
Dacrocystitis 8
Dandruff (seborrheic dermatitis) 6, **36**, 123
Dapsone 57, 61, 90, **92**, 96, 96, 97, **102**

Daptomycin 50, 54, 55, 65, 71, **131**
ddC (zalcitabine) 57, 62, 90, **118**, **120**, 134
ddI (didanosine) 57, 62, 116, **117**, 118, **120**, 124, 133
Decubitus ulcer **36**
Dehydroemetine **93**, 101
Delavirdine 57, 62, **118**, **120**, 135
Dengue **104**
Dermatophytosis **79, 80**
Desensitization—penicillin & TMP/SMX **56**
Desquamative interstitial pneumonia 72
Diabetic foot 2, **10**, **36**
Dialysis 31, 77, 114, 126, **130–134**
Diarrhea **11–13**, 40, 51, 63–71, 83, 84, 89, 92–94, 101–104, 111, 113–121, 123
Dicloxacillin 52, 58, 63, **66**, 129
Didanosine (ddI) 57, 62, 116, **117**, 118, **120**, 124, 133
Dientamoeba fragilis 93
Diethylcarbamazine **93**, 98, **103**
Diiodohydroxyquin 101
Diloxanide **93**, 101
Diphtheria; C. diphtheriae **32**, 48, 51, 136–139
Dipylidium caninum 99
Dirithromycin 49, 50, 54, 60, 65, 69, 135
Dirofilariasis (heartworms) 99
Disulfiram reactions 69, 72, 83, 91, 101, 118
Diverticulitis 11, **14**, **31**
Dog bite (also see Rabies) **35**
Donovanosis **15**
'DOT' bacteroides (non-fragilis bacteroides) 48
Doxycycline 46, 48–51, 54–57, 60, 65, **70**, 74, 89, 90, 93, 95, 125, 126, 129, 135
Dracunculus (guinea worm) 98
Drotrecogin alfa (activated protein C) 43
Drug-drug interactions 26, 61–65, 69, 70, 72, 83, 84, 88, 91, 101, 114, 121, **141–146**
Duodenal ulcer (Helicobacter pylori) 13, 49, 51
Dysentery, bacillary 13, 51, 93

Ear infections **6–8**, 51
Ebola/Marburg virus 104
EBV (Epstein-Barr virus) **29**, 45, 47, **108**
Echinococcosis 99
Efavirenz (Sustiva) 57, 62, 116–**118**, **120**,124, 135
Eflornithine 57, 97, **102**
Ehrlichiosis, monocytic & granulocytic **38–39**, 48, 94
Eikenella 48
Elephantiasis (filariasis) 20, 33, 35, **48**
Empyema, lung 29
Empyema, subdural 3
Emtricitabine 105, **117**, 120
Encephalitis 3, 30, 39, 107, **108**,109
Encephalitozoon sp. 94
Endocarditis, native valve 18–20, 38, 49, 51, 69, 76
  culture-negative 20
  prophylaxis 127–128
  prosthetic valve 20, 55, 76, 127
Endomyometritis 14, 16, 31
Endophthalmitis 9–10, 44, 75, 76
Endotoxin shock (septic shock) 41–43
Enfuvirtide (T20, fusion inhibitor) 57, 62, 119, 121
Enoxacin 50, 54, 57
Entamoeba histolytica 11–13, 24, **93**
Enteric fever 11, 41
Enterobacter 7, 36, 41, 49, 52–54, 67, 68
Enterobius vermicularis **98**,103
Enterococci 4, 10, 14, 17, **18–20**, 22–24, 30, 31, 36, 37, 42, 49, 51–54, 66, 125
Enterococci, drug-resistant **19**, 49, 52–55, 67
  vancomycin-resistant 11, 41, 49, **55**, 67
Enterococcus faecalis **19**, 36, 49, **52–55**
Enterococcus faecium **19**, 49, 52, 54, **55**, 67
Enterocolitis, pseudomembranous **11–12**, 51, 52, 68, 122
  or neutropenic 3, **94**
Enterocytozoon bieneusi **12**, 94
Enterovirus 3, 31, 32, **104**
Eosinophilic meningitis 6, 97
Epididymitis **17**
Epiglottitis 32–**33**, 49
Epstein-Barr virus (infectious mono) **29**, 45, 47, **108**
Ertapenem 48–50, **52**, 55–57, 59, 63, **67**,130

PAGES (page numbers bold if major focus)

Erysipelas 10, **36**, 43
Erysipelothrix 49
Erythema multiforme **36**, 68, 120
Erythema nodosum 36, 90, 92
Erythrasma **36**, 79
Erythromycin 46, 48–50, 54–57, 60, 65, **69**, 71, 73, 74, 79, 90, 122, 126, 129, 131
Escherichia coli 3, 4, 10–**13**, 22, **23**, 31, 34, 36, 41, 49, 52–54, 93
  0157:H7 **11–12**, 44
   enterotoxigenic (traveler's diarrhea) 13
Etanercept 13, 22, 41
Ethambutol 57, 61, 86–**91**, 123
Ethionamide 57, 86, 87, 90, **92**, 133
Extended-spectrum β-lactamases (ESBL) 31, 49, 56
Eyeworm (Onchocerca volvulus) 98

Famciclovir 57, 61, 108–110, **113**, 133
Fansidar (pyrimethamine sulfadoxine) 57, 95, 102, 103
Fasciola buski, hepatica **99**
Fever blisters (cold sores) 109
Filariasis 98–**99**, 103
Flucloxacillin 66
Fluconazole 57, 61, 75–**83**, 84, 94, 122, 128, 132, 135
Flucytosine 57, 61, 76, 78, 79, 82, **83**, 94, 132
Fluke infestation (Trematodes) 99
Fluoroquinolones 46, 48–52, 55–57, 65, **70**, **71**, 87, 89, 90, 92
Folliculitis; hot tub folliculitis 36, 38
Fomivirsen 107, 113
Foot, diabetic 2, **10, 36**
Fosamprenavir 57, 62, 118, 120, 135
Foscarnet 57, 61, 71, 107–110, **113**, 134
Fosfomycin 49, 50, 54, 55, 57, 60, **71**
Fournier's gangrene **37**
Francisella tularensis 16, **29**, 30, **40**, 46, 49, 51, 54
Fumagillin 94, 102
Furazolidone 93, 101
Furunculosis **35–36**
Fusariosis 80
Fusidic acid 50, 54, 55, **71**
Fusobacterium necrophorum 9, 28, 32–35

G6PD deficiency 22, 35, 72, 92, 95, 101, 102
Ganciclovir 57, 61, 107, 109, **113**, 128, 134
Gardnerella vaginalis 17, **49**
Gas gangrene 30, 37, 51
Gastric ulcer, gastritis (H. pylori) **13**, 49, 51
Gastroenteritis **11–13**, 111
Gatifloxacin 46, 49, 50, 52, 55–57, 65, **70, 87**, 89, 90, 131
Gemifloxacin 49, 52, 55–57, 59, 65, **70**, 131
Genital herpes 3, 18, 108, 109
Gentamicin 46, 48–51, 54, 55, 57, 59, 63, **73**, 126, 128–130, 135
Giardiasis 12, 13, **93**, 101, 102
Gnathostoma 6, 99
Gonococcal arthritis; disseminated GC **15**, 21, 51
Gonococcal ophthalmia 8, 14
Gonorrhea 8, **14–15**, 16–17, 21, 49, 52–54, 125, 126
Granuloma inguinale **15**
Griseofulvin 57, 79, 80, **83**
Group B strep, including neonatal 2, 4, 11, 16, 17, 21, 25, 36, 37, 41, **43**, 50, **122**
Guillain-Barre syndrome 11, **122**

HACEK acronym; infective endocarditis **20**
Hafnia 49
Halofantrine 95, 102
Hantavirus pulmonary syndrome **29**, 104
Heartworms (dirofilariasis) 99
Helicobacter pylori **13**, 49, 51
Hemodialysis 2, 44, 69, 114, **130–134**, 138, 139
Hemolytic uremic syndrome **11**, 12, 23, 114
Hemophilus aphrophilus, H. ducreyi 8, 9, 94, 109
Hemophilus influenzae 2, 4, **5**, **6**, **7**–10, 21, 24–26, 32, 33, 41, 44, 49, 51–54, **124**, 136, 137, 139
Hemorrhagic bullae (Vibrio skin infection) 37
Hemorrhagic fevers 46, **104, 105**
Hepatic abscess **24**, 44, **93**

Hepatic disease/drug dosage adjustment **135**
Hepatitis A, B & C 21, 24, 47, 91, **105, 106**, 114, 115, 117, 120, 122, 123, 125, 128, 126–139
Hepatitis B prophylaxis **105**, 122, **136–137**
Herpes infections 3, 8–10, 12, 14, 15, 18, 22, 30, 37, 42, 107–110, 113, 128
  mucocutaneous **109**
Herpes simiae 35, **109**
Herpes simplex 3, 8–10, 13, 15, 18, 30, 32, 47, **108–109**, 128
Herpes zoster 37, 108, **110**
Heterophyes (intestinal fluke) 99
HHV-6, HHV-7, HHV-8 infections 32, **108**
Hidradenitis suppurativa **37**
Histoplasmosis 6, 28, 29, 47, **80–82**
HIV **3**, 6, 10, 12–16, 28, **29**, 30, 32, 34, 38, 61, 62, 66, 71, 75, 77–79, 81–91, 93, 94, 96,102, 104, 106–110, 112–114, **116–121**, 122–125, 130, 135, 137–139
  Prophylaxis/
    needlestick/occupational exposure **123–124**
    mother-to-infant 124
Hoignes syndrome (reaction to procaine) 66
Hookworm 98
Hordeolum (stye) 8
Hot tub folliculitis **38**
Hymenolepis 99
Hyperalimentation, sepsis 44

Imidazoles, topical **83**
Imipenem 48–50, 52, 55–57, 59, 63, **67**, 81, 82, 89, 90, 129, 130
Imiquimod 112, 115
Immune globulin, IV (IVIG) 3, 40, 43, 71, 104, 107, 112, 115
Immunizations (see Table 20, children & adults, *pp.* **136–140**) 2, 4, 30, 110, 111, 124, **136–140**
Impetigo **37**
Inclusion conjunctivitis 8
Indinavir 57, 62, 88, 116, **119**, **121**, 124, 134, 135
Infectious mononucleosis (see EBV) **32**, 66, 107, **108**
Inflammatory bowel disease 13, 36, 101
Infliximab 13, 22, 41, 80
Influenza A 29, 47, 78, **111**, 115, 122, 136, 138
INH (isoniazid) 57, 61, 85–**91**, 92, 133, 135
Interferons 48, 88, 104–106, 109, 111, 112, **114**, 115
Iodoquinol 93, 101
Isepamicin 57, **73**, 130
Isospora belli 12, 13, **93**
Isotretinoin **34**
Itraconazole 57, 61, 69, 74–82, **84**, 94, 133, 135
IV line infection & prophylaxis 10, **44**, 47, 56
Ivermectin 57, 61, 98–100, **103**

Jock itch (T. cruris) 80

Kala-azar 94, 102
Kanamycin 49, 59, 63, **73**, 86, 89, 91
Kaposi's sarcoma 29, **108**
Katayama fever 99
Kawasaki syndrome **40**, 71, 127
Keratitis 8, **9**, 94, 109
Ketoconazole 57, 69, 76, 79, 80–82, **84**, 94
Kikuchi-Fujimoto (necrotizing lymphadenitis) **29**, **30**
Klebsiella species 7, 28, 31, 41, 49, 52–54, **56**, 66

Lactobacillus sp. 11, 44, 49
Lamivudine (3TC) 57, 62, 105, 114, 116, **117**, **120**, 124, 128, 134
Larva migrans **98**
Laryngitis **33**
Lassa fever, Ebola 46, **104**
Legionnaire's disease/
    Legionella sp. **26–27**, 29, 49, 51–54
Leishmaniasis 30, 47, 82, **94**, 102
Lemierre's disease (jugular vein phlebitis) 33
Leprosy 90, 92, **98**
Leptospirosis 3, 24, **40**, 49, 70
Leuconostoc 44, 49
Leukemia, acute 42, 66, 71, 74, 85, 138

PAGES (page numbers bold if major focus)

Levofloxacin — 46, 48–50, 52, 55–57, 59, 65, **70**, 86, 87, 126, 131
Lice: body, head, pubic, & scabies — 15, 20, 38, **100**, 103
Lincomycin — 69
Lindane — 100
Line sepsis — 10, **44**, 47, 56
Linezolid — 49, 50, 54, 55, 57, 60, 63, **70**, 81, 87, 89, 90, 129, 131, 135
Listeria monocytogenes — 3, **4–6**, 9, 12, 25, 41, 47, 49, 51–54
Liver abscess — 24, **93**
Liver disease/drug dosage adjustment — **135**
Loa loa — 98
Lobomycosis — 81
Lomefloxacin — 50, 52, 57
Lopinavir/ritonavir & lopinavir — 57, 62, 116, 119, **121**, 135
Loracarbef — 53, 58, **68**, 129
Ludwig's angina — 30, 33
Lung abscess, putrid — 28, 51
Lyme disease — 6, 21, 29, 38, **39**, 51, 108, 124
Lymphadenitis — **29–30**, 34, 38
Lymphangitis, nodular — 38
Lymphedema (congenital = Milroy's disease) — 36
Lymphogranuloma venereum — 15, 30

MAC, MAI (Mycobacterium avium-intracellulare complex) — **88, 89**, 90
Macrolide antibiotics — 50, **54**, 56, 57, 60, 65, 69, 89, 90, 122, 129, 131
Madura foot — **80**, 81
Malacoplakia (pyelonephritis variant) — 23
Malaria — 62, 70, 93, **95, 96**, 101–103, 124
Malarone (atovaquone + proguanil) — 57, 95, 101
Malassezia furfur (Tinea versicolor) — 36, 44, 79, 80
Malathion — 100
Mansonella — **98**
Mastitis — **3**
Mastoiditis — 8
Measles, measles vaccine — 65, **111**, 136–139
Mebendazole — 57, 97–99, **103**
Mefloquine — 57, 61, 71, 88, 95, **102**, 103
Melbomianitis — 8
Melarsoprol — 93, 97, **102**
Meleney's gangrene — **37**
Melioidosis (Burkholderia pseudomallei) — 27, 38, **48**
Meningitis, aseptic — 3, 6, 71, 72, **104**
bacterial (acute and chronic) — **4–6**, 39, 49, 55, 56, 63, 68, 69, 87, 122, 129
Meningococci — **4–6**, 10, 21, 41, 42, 49, 51–54, 70, 122, 124, 125, 137–139
Meningococcus, meningitis — **4–6**, 10, 21, 49, 51–54, 122
prophylaxis — **6**
Meropenem — 48–50, 52, 55–57, 59, 63, **67**, 129, 130
Mesalamine — 13
Metagonimus — 99
Metapneumovirus — 29, 111
Methamine mandelate & hippurate — **71**
Methicillin — 49, 50, 52–56, 72
Methicillin-resistant Staph. aureus (MRSA) — 2–4, 19–22, 25, 27, 28, **35**–37, 41–45, 50, 52–56, 72, 125, 135
Metronidazole — 48, 49, 54, 57, 60, 63, 65, **72**, 93, 98, 101, 118, 125, 126, 129, 131, 135
Miconazole — 76, 77, 80, 81, 83, **84**, 94
Microsporidia — 12, **94**, 96
Miltefosine — 94, 102
Minocycline — 48–50, 54, 55, 60, 65, **70**, 81, 89, 90, 135
Monkey bite — **35**, 109, 111
Monkey pox — 111
Monobactams — 59, 63, **67**
Moraxella catarrhalis — 7, 10, 25–27, 33, 49, 52–54
Morganella species — 49, 52, 53
Moxifloxacin — 46, 49, 50, 52, 55–57, 59, 65, **71**, 89–90, 135
MRSA — 2–4, 19–22, 25, 27, 28, **35**–37, 41–45, 50, 52–56, 72, 125, 135
carriage — **36**
Mucormycosis — 10, 33, 44, **80**
Multidrug-resistant TB — **86, 87**
Mumps — 31, 136–138

Mupirocin — 72, 125
Mycobacteria — 6, 21, 22, 25, 28–31, 54, 70, **85–92**
Mycobacterium abscessus, M. bovis, — 18, 19, 22, 30, M. chelonae, M. genavense, M. — 70, **88–90** gordonae, M. haemophilum, M. kansasii, M. marinum, M. scrofulaceum,M. simiae, M. ulcerans, M. xenopi,M. leprae
Mycobacterium tuberculosis
directly observed therapy (DOT) — 85, **86, 87**
drug-resistant — **88**
pulmonary — 28, 29, 85, **86, 87**
Mycoplasma, pneumoniae — 24–26, 32, 49, 52, 54
genitalium — **14**
Myositis — 30, 43

Naegleria fowleri — **94**
Nafcillin — 49, 50, 52, 58, 63, 66, 129, 135
Naftifine — 80
Necrotizing enterocolitis — **11**, 122
Necrotizing fasciitis — 10, 30, 36, **37**, 43
Needlestick: HIV, Hepatitis B & C — **122–124**
Neisseria, gonorrhoeae — 8, **14–15**, 16, 17, 21, **49**, 52–54, 125
meningitidis — 5, 6, 10, 21, 49, 51–54, **122**
Nelfinavir — 57, 62, 88, 116, **119, 121**, 124, 134
Nematodes (roundworms) — **97–99**, 103
Neomycin — 59, **73**, 101,126
Neonatal sepsis — **41**, 122
Netilmicin — 54, 57, 63, **73**, 130
Neurosyphilis — **15–16**, 79
Neutropenia — 12, 27, 33, 36, 41, 42, 44, **63–65**, 66, 69, 70, 74–77, 80–82, 84, 94, 102, 113, 122
Neutropenic afebrile patients — 122
Nevirapine — 57, 62, **118, 120**, 124, 134, 135
Nifurtimox — 93, 97, **102**, 128
Nitazoxanide — 57, 61, 93, 102
Nitrofurantoin — 49, 50, 54, 55, 57, **72**, 126, 131
Nocardia brasiliensis, asteroides — 30, 49, 70, 80, **81**
Nocardiosis — 3, 30, 47, 49, 70, 80, **81**
Norovirus (Norwalk-like virus) — 111
Norwegian scabies — 100
Novobiocin — 50, 55
Nursing (breast milk) & antibiotics — **124**
Nystatin — 76, 77, **84**

Ofloxacin — 48, 49, 50, 52, 57, 59, 65, **71**, 86, 89, 90, 90, **92**,131
Onchocerciasis — 98, 103
Onychomycosis — 10, **79**, 84
Ophthalmia neonatorum — **8**
Opisthorchis (liver fluke) — 99
Orbital cellulitis — **10**
Orchitis — **17**
Organ transplantation, infection & prophylaxis — **47**, 128
Oseltamivir — 57, 61, 62, **111**, 115, 134
Osteomyelitis, hematogenous — 2, 3, 51
chronic — **3**, 51
contiguous (post-operative, post-nail puncture) — **2**
vertebral — **2**
Otitis externa—chronic, malignant, & swimmer's ear — **6**
Otitis media — 3, **7–8**, 51, 72, 124, 137
Oxacillin — 49, 50, 52, 58, 63, 66, 129

Palivizumab — 112, **115**
Pancreatitis, pancreatic abscess — **30**, 41, 68, 102, 117–121
Papillomavirus — 47, **111**, 112
Papovavirus/Polyoma virus — **112**
Paracoccidioidomycosis — 81
Paragonimus — 99
Parapharyngeal space infection — 30, 33
Parasitic infections — 93–103
Paromomycin — 73, 93, 101
Paronychia — 18, 76, 121
Parotitis — **31**
Parvovirus B19 — 21, **112**
PAS (para-aminosalicylic acid) — **92**
Pasteurella multocida — **35**, 49, 52, 53

PAGES *(page numbers bold if major focus)*

Pediatric dosages 129
Pefloxacin 50, 52, 57, 90
Pegylated interferon 105, 106, 114, 115
Peliosis hepatis 24, **38**
Pelvic inflammatory disease
(PID) 4, **16**, 34, 51, 112, 126
Pelvic suppurative phlebitis 44
Penciclovir 108, 109, 113
Penicillin allergy 2, 4, 5, 15, 16, 18, 19, 31–33, 35,
36, 39, 56, 66–68, 74, 127
Penicillin desensitization
Penicillin G 46, 48–50, 52, 55, 58, 63, **66**, 74, 122,
126, 129, 132
Penicillin V 52, 58, **66**, 74, 124, 125, 129
Penicilliosis 81
Pentamidine 57, 71, 94, 96, 97, **102**, 113, 132, 133
Peptostreptococcus 3, 28, 35, 50, **52–54**
Pericarditis **20**, 51, 87
Perinephric abscess 23
Perirectal abscess 12, 14
Peritoneal dialysis, infection 31, 77, 126, **135**
Peritonitis, bacterial/spontaneous 11, 14, 16, **31**, 77
spontaneous—prevention 31
Pertussis 24, 48, 137, 139
Phaeohyphomycosis 81
Pharmacokinetics, pharmacology 58–62
Pharyngitis 15, 20, 21, **32**, 51, 54, 129
Phlebitis, septic—various 8, **16**, 33, 36, 44
Photosensitivity 34, **57**, 63, 64, 70, 72, 83, 84, 91,
101, 103
PID 4, **16**, 34, 51, 112, 126
Pinworms **98**, 103
Piperacillin 50, 52, 56, 63, **66**, 125, 129
Piperacillin/tazobactam 48, 49, 50, 52, 56, 58, 63, **66**,
125, 129, 132
Plague 26, **39**, **46**, 50
Plesiomonas shigelloides 11, 49
PML (progressive multifocal leucoencephalopathy) 112
Pneumococci (see S. pneumoniae)
Pneumococci, drug-resistant 4, 7, 25, 26, 28, 33,
42, 50, **55**
Pneumocystis carinii 29, 47, 51, 72, **96**, 126, 129
Pneumonia, adult **25–29**, 36, 40, 47, 51, 55, 96,
104, 107, 108, 110, 112, 115
aspiration 28
chronic 28
community-acquired **26–27**
hospital-acquired **26–27**
neonatal/infants/children 25
ventilator-acquired 27
Podofilox 111
Podophyllin 111
Polio vaccine **136–137**
Polymyxin B 48, 60
Polyoma virus **112**
PPD (TST) 41, 85, 86
Praziquantel 57, 61, 99, **103**
Pregnancy, antibiotics in 5, 12–14, 16, 17, 22, 23, 27,
28, 34, 38, 39, 46, **57**, 70, 78, 83, 86, 87,
91–93, 95, 96, 98, 103, 106, 109–111,
114–116,118, 120, 122–125, 138, 139
Pregnancy, risk from anti-infectives 57
Primaquine 95, 96, **102**, 103
Proctitis 12, 15
Progressive multifocal leucoencephalopathy (PML) **112**
Prophylaxis (see Table 15, pages 122–128)
Prostatitis, prostatodynia 15, **17–18**, 23, 51
Prosthetic joint infection/prophylaxis 2, 21, 22, 126
Prosthetic valve endocarditis **19–20**, 55, 125
Protease inhibitors 77, 88–90, **118–121**
Protein binding 58–62
Pseudallescheria boydii (Scedosporium sp.) 80, **81**, 84
Pseudomembranous enterocolitis 51, 69
Pseudomonas aeruginosa 2–5, 8–10, 12, 14, 17, 20, 23,
25–29, 31, 34, 36–38, 50, 52, **56**, 58, 67, 68
Pseudotumor cerebri 70
Psittacosis **30**
Puncture wound 2, **43**, 123
Pyelonephritis **23**, 42, 51, 71
Pyomyositis 30

Pyrantel pamoate **98**, 103
Pyrazinamide 57, 61, 85–**91**, 133, 144
Pyrethrin **100**
Pyridoxine 87, 88, 90–92
Pyrimethamine 57, 61, 93, 95–97, **102**, 103, 135

Q fever **20**, 26, 48
QT, prolongation 65, 69, 77
Quinacrine HCl 93, 101, **102**
Quinidine gluconate 57, 71, 95, **96**, **102**
Quinine 38, 57, 94–96, **102**, 103, 133
Quinolones 15, 26, 65
Quinupristin/dalfopristin **19**, 49, 50, 54–56, 65, **70**

Rabies, rabies vaccine 3, **35**, 101, 112, **139–140**
Rape victim 125
Rat bite 35
Red neck syndrome & vancomycin 69
Reiter's syndrome 21
Relapsing fever 39
Renal failure, dosing **130–135**
Resistant bacteria 52–54, **55–56**
Resource directory 140
Respiratory syncytial virus
(RSV) 24, 25, 29, 47, 111, **112**, 115
Retinitis **10**, 30, 47, 96, 107
Reverse transcriptase inhibitors 116, **117**, **118**, 120,
133, 134
Rheumatic fever **20**, 21, **32**, 42, 44, 124, 127
Rheumatoid arthritis septic joint **21**, 51
Rhinosinusitis 33–34
Rhinovirus 7, 25, 33, **112**
Rhodococcus equi 50
Ribavirin 57, 61, 104, 106, 111, 112, 114, **115**, 134
Ribavirin + interferon 106, 114
Rickettsial diseases **39–40**, 41, 50, 54
Rifabutin 57, 86–90, **92**, 135
Rifampin, Rifamate, Rifater 46, 48–50, 54–57, 60, 61, 65,
80, 84–**91**, 92, 94, 122, 129, 133, 135
Rifamycins 88
Rifapentine 86, 88, 90, **92**, 135
Rimantadine 57, 61, 111, **115**, 134, 135
Ringworm 79, 80
Ritonavir 57, 62, 88, 116–**119**, 121, 134
Rocky Mountain spotted fever 39, 51
Rubella vaccine 21, 136, 137

Salmonellosis, bacteremia 2, **11–13**, 21, **40**–41, 50,
52–54
Salpingitis 16
Saquinavir 57, 62, 117, **119**, **121**, 134
SARS 29, 104
SBE 18–20, 127
SBP (spontaneous bacterial peritonitis) 31
Scabies **15**, 100, **103**
Scedosporium species (Pseudallescheria boydii) 80, **81**,
84
Schistosomiasis 99, 103
Scrofula **30**
Seborrheic dermatitis (dandruff) 6, 36, 123
"Sepsis" and "septic shock" 10, 35–37, **41–43**, 88, 125
Sepsis, abortion; amnionitis **16**, 126
Sepsis, neonatal 126
Septata intestinalis 12, 94
Serratia marcescens 50, 52–54, 68
Serum levels of selected anti-infectives 58–62
Severe acute respiratory distress
syndrome (SARS) 29, 104
Sexual contacts/assaults 8, **14**, 17, 30, 63, 123–**125**, 126
Shigellosis **11–13**, 21, 50, 52–54, 72
Shingles 37, **110**
Sickle cell disease 2, **21**, **124**, 125, 137, 138
Sinusitis 3, 24, **33–34**, 51, 74, 80, 81, 115
Smallpox **46**, 112
Snake bite, spider bite 35
Sparganosis **100**
Spectinomycin 49, 73
Spiramycin 96, 109
Splenectomy 35, 38, 42, 94, **124**, 125, 137–139
Splenic abscess 38

PAGES (page numbers bold if major focus)

Sporotrichosis 30, 81, 82
Spotted fevers 39, 40, 51
Staph. aureus 2–10, 18–23, 25–38, 41–44, 50–55,
56, 68, 72, 125
  carriers 35
  endocarditis 19, 51, 69
Staph. epidermidis 2, 4, 8, 9, 11, 20, 30, 31, 35, 36,
41, 44, 50, 52–55
Staph. hemolyticus 23, 50
Staph. scalded skin syndrome 38
Stavudine (d4T) 57, 62, 116, 117, 120, 124, 134
Stenotrophomonas maltophilia 27, 28, 50, 52–54
Stibogluconate 93, 94, 101
Stomatitis 30, 33, 40, 77, 92, 109, 118
Streptobacillus moniliformis 35, 50
Streptococcal toxic shock 36, 37, 43
Streptococci 2–4, 7, 8, 10, 16–21, 24, 25, 28–30,
32–38, 40–44, 50–55, 59, 67, 122
Streptococcus, bovis 18–19, 38
  group B, prophylaxis 122
  milleri complex 3, 28–29, 50, 52
  pneumoniae 4, 5, 7–10, 20, 25, 26, 28, 29, 32,
33, 41, 50–55, 122, 125, 136–139
  pyogenes 3, 8, 9, 21, 32, 36, 37, 43, 50
Streptomycin 46, 48–51, 55, 57, 61, 73, 85–88,
90, 91, 130, 133
Strongyloidiasis 47, 98, 103
Stye 8
Subdural empyema 3
Sulfadiazine 81, 94, 96, 97, 102, 103
Sulfadoxine + pyrimethamine 57, 95, 102, 103
Sulfasalazine 13
Sulfisoxazole 7, 25, 41, 72, 81, 96, 129
Sulfonamide desensitization 56
Sulfonamides 49, 50, 57, 60, 72, 81, 96, 103, 131
Suppurative phlebitis 16, 33, 36, 44
Suramin 97, 102, 103
Surgical procedures, prophylaxis 125–126
Swimmer's ear 6
Synercid® (quinupristin/dalfopristin) 19, 49, 50, 54–56,
65, 70
Syphilis 6, 12, 15–16, 25, 29, 30, 79, 125

Tapeworms: Taenia saginata, T. solium,
  D. latum, D. caninum 99
Teicoplanin 50, 54, 55, 69, 131
Telithromycin 48, 49, 50, 54, 57, 60, 63, 69, 131
Tenofovir 57, 62, 105, 116, 117, 120, 134
Terbinafine 57, 78–81, 84, 133
Tetanus, Clostridium tetani 35, 37, 43, 48, 136–139
Tetanus prophylaxis 35, 137, 139
Tetracycline 48–50, 55, 60, 65, 70, 93, 97, 103, 129, 132
Thalidomide 57, 90, 92
Thiabendazole 97, 98, 103
Thrombophlebitis, septic (suppurative) 36, 44
  jugular vein (Lemierre's) 33
  pelvic vein(s) 16, 44
Thrush 76, 77, 123
Ticarcillin 50, 52, 56, 58, 63, 66, 67, 129, 132
Ticarcillin/clavulanate 48–50, 52, 56, 58, 63, 67, 125, 129
Tinea capitis, corporis, cruris, pedis, versicolor 36, 79,
80, 100
Tipranavir 119, 121
Tobramycin 46, 49, 50, 54, 57, 59, 63, 66, 73,
89, 129, 130
Torsades de pointes 65, 69, 71
Toxic shock syndrome (strep. & staph.) 36, 37, 43
Toxocariasis 99
Toxoplasma gondii,
  toxoplasmosis 3, 29, 30, 47, 79, 96, 97, 128
Trachoma 8

Transplantation, infection 47, 74, 78, 105, 107, 128
  prophylaxis 107, 128
Traveler's diarrhea 13
Trematodes (flukes) 99, 103
Trench fever 20, 38, 40
Trichinosis 99
Trichomoniasis (vaginitis) 14, 17, 97
Trichostrongylus 98
Trichuris 98
Tricuspid valve endocarditis, S. aureus 19
Trifluridine 109, 113
Trimethoprim/sulfamethoxazole 46, 48–51, 54–56, 60,
65, 71, 72, 81, 82, 89, 90, 93, 94, 96, 97,
100, 102, 103, 122, 124–126, 128, 129, 135
Trypanosomiasis 47, 97, 102, 103, 128
Tuberculosis 6, 13, 22, 25, 28, 29, 41, 45, 47, 57,
79, 81, 85–87, 88–90, 92, 135
  multidrug-resistant 86, 87
  prophylaxis 85
  tuberculin skin test (TST) 85, 86
Tularemia (Francisella tularensis) 26, 29–30, 40,
46, 49, 51, 54
Tumor necrosis factor (TNF) blockade 41
Typhlitis—neutropenic enterocolitis 11–12
Typhoid fever 11, 12, 41, 51
Typhus group (louse-borne, murine, scrub) 40, 70

Ulcerative colitis 13, 93
Urethral catheter, indwelling 23, 71, 74, 127
Urethritis, non-gonococcal 14, 16, 22, 51
Urinary tract infection 22–23, 43, 47, 49, 50, 52, 54–56,
66, 72, 77, 129

Vaccinia, contact 112
Vaginitis 17, 22, 77, 83
Vaginosis, bacterial 17, 49
Valacyclovir 57, 61, 108–110, 114, 134
Valganciclovir 57, 61, 107, 113
Vancomycin 48–50, 54–57, 60, 65, 67, 69, 73, 122,
125, 126, 128, 129, 131, 135
Varicella zoster 9, 10, 43, 47, 107, 108, 109–110,
125, 136–138
Ventilator-associated pneumonia 27, 115
Vibrio cholerae, parahaemolyticus, vulnificus 12, 37, 50, 54
Vincent's angina 32
Viral infections 104–115
Visceral larval migrans 99
Voriconazole 57, 61, 74–78, 80, 81, 84, 133, 135
VRE (vancomycin-resistant enterococci) 19, 41, 49,
55, 67

Warts 16, 111, 112, 115
Wegener's granulomatosis 125
West Nile virus 3, 104
Whipple's disease 6, 13, 20
Whipworm 98
Whirlpool folliculitis (hot tub folliculitis) 36, 38
Whitlow, herpetic 18, 109
Whooping cough 24, 48, 137, 139
Wound infection, post-op, post-trauma 30, 37, 47
Wuchereria bancrofti 98

Xanthomonas (Stenotrophomonas)
  maltophilia 28, 50, 52–54

Yersinia enterocolitica & pestis 12, 21, 24, 30, 36, 39,
46, 50, 52–54

Zalcitabine (ddC) 57, 62, 90, 118, 120, 134
Zanamivir 57, 111, 115
Zidovudine (ZDV, AZT) 57, 62, 88, 113, 116–118, 120,
123, 124, 134

NEW FOR 2004

You can now order these other editions directly from us:

Sanford Guide to Antimicrobial Therapy 2004 Chinese Edition

Edited by a distinguished panel of Chinese infectious disease experts at the premier hospitals and medical schools in Beijing, Shanghai and Guanzhou, the 2004 Chinese edition translates into Mandarin (simplified characters), the entire text of the 2004 English language edition. Available in June 2004. Price: $15.00

Sanford Guide to Antimicrobial Therapy 2004 Spanish Edition

For Spanish-speaking health care professionals in the U.S. and elsewhere, we are now offering a new verbatim Spanish language translation of the 2004 English pocket-sized edition. Available in May 2004. Price: $9.50

Sanford Guide to HIV/AIDS Therapy 2003 Electronic Edition

The Sanford Guide to HIV/AIDS Therapy is now available in electronic form for handheld PDA devices (Palm OS and Windows Pocket PC). The installer is available by download or on CD. Available in May 2004. Price: $25.00

TO ORDER:

Web: www.sanfordguide.com (secure online ordering)

Phone: 802 888 2855 (9-5 U.S. Eastern Time, M-F)

Fax: 802 888 2874

Mail: Antimicrobial Therapy, Inc.
P.O. Box 70
229 Main Street
Hyde Park, VT 05655 USA

Email: info@sanfordguide.com